Cardiovascular

Computed
Tomography

Oxford Specialist Handbooks published and forthcoming

General Oxford Specialist Handbooks

A Resuscitation Room Guide
Addiction Medicine
Hypertension
Perioperative Medicine,
Second Edition
Post-Operative Complications,
Second Edition
Pulmonary Hypertension
Renal Transplantation

Oxford Specialist Handbooks in Anaesthesia

Cardiac Anaesthesia
Day Case Surgery
General Thoracic Anaesthesia
Neuroanaethesia
Obstetric Anaesthesia
Paediatric Anaesthesia
Regional Anaesthesia, Stimulation
and Ultrasound Techniques

Oxford Specialist Handbooks in Cardiology

Adult Congenital Heart Disease
Cardiac Catheterization and
Coronary Intervention
Cardiac Electrophysiology
Cardiovascular Computed
Tomography
Cardiovascular Magnetic
Resonance
Echocardiography
Fetal Cardiology
Heart Failure
Nuclear Cardiology
Pacemakers and ICDs
Valvular Heart Disease

Oxford Specialist Handbooks in Critical Care

Advanced Respiratory
Critical Care

Oxford Specialist Handbooks in End of Life Care

End of Life Care in Dementia
End of Life Care in Nephrology
End of Life in the Intensive
Care Unit

Oxford Specialist Handbooks in Neurology

Epilepsy
Parkinson's Disease and
Other Movement Disorders
Stroke Medicine

Oxford Specialist Handbooks in Paediatrics

Paediatric Dermatology
Paediatric Endocrinology
and Diabetes
Paediatric Gastroenterology,
Hepatology, and Nutrition
Paediatric Haematology and
Oncology
Paediatric Intensive Care
Paediatric Nephrology
Paediatric Neurology
Paediatric Palliative Care
Paediatric Radiology
Paediatric Respiratory Medicine

Oxford Specialist Handbooks in Psychiatry

Child and Adolescent Psychiatry
Old Age Psychiatry

Oxford Specialist Handbooks in Radiology

Interventional Radiology
Musculoskeletal Imaging
Pulmonary Imaging

Oxford Specialist Handbooks in Surgery

Cardiothoracic Surgery
Colorectal Surgery
Hand Surgery
Liver and Pancreatobiliary Surgery
Operative Surgery, Second Edition
Oral Maxillofacial Surgery
Otolaryngology and Head and
Neck Surgery
Paediatric Surgery
Plastic and Reconstructive Surgery
Surgical Oncology
Urological Surgery
Vascular Surgery

Oxford Specialist Handbooks in Cardiology
Cardiovascular Computed Tomography

Edited by

Ed Nicol

Consultant Cardiologist
Royal Brompton and Harefield NHS Foundation Trust,
and Chelsea and Westminster NHS Foundation Trust,
London, UK

James Stirrup

Clinical Research Fellow
Cardiac Imaging
Royal Brompton and Harefield NHS FoundationTrust,
London, UK

Andrew Kelion

Consultant Cardiologist
Royal Brompton and Harefield NHS Trust,
London, UK

Simon Padley

Consultant Radiologist
Royal Brompton and Harefield NHS Foundation Trust,
and Chelsea and Westminster NHS Foundation Trust,
London, UK

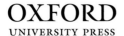

OXFORD
UNIVERSITY PRESS

OXFORD
UNIVERSITY PRESS

Great Clarendon Street, Oxford OX2 6DP

Oxford University Press is a department of the University of Oxford.
It furthers the University's objective of excellence in research, scholarship,
and education by publishing worldwide in

Oxford New York

Auckland Cape Town Dar es Salaam Hong Kong Karachi
Kuala Lumpur Madrid Melbourne Mexico City Nairobi
New Delhi Shanghai Taipei Toronto

With offices in

Argentina Austria Brazil Chile Czech Republic France Greece
Guatemala Hungary Italy Japan Poland Portugal Singapore
South Korea Switzerland Thailand Turkey Ukraine Vietnam

Oxford is a registered trade mark of Oxford University Press
in the UK and in certain other countries

Published in the United States
by Oxford University Press Inc., New York

British Library Cataloguing in Publication Data
Data available

Library of Congress Cataloging-in-Publication-Data
Data available

Typeset by Glyph International, Bangalore, India
Printed in Great Britain
on acid-free paper by
Ashford Colour Press Ltd, Gosport, Hampshire

ISBN 978–0–19–957259–5

10 9 8 7 6 5 4 3 2 1

Foreword

Over recent years, multislice computed tomography (MSCT) angiography has become increasingly implemented in the daily routine analysis of patients with cardiovascular disease. Drs Nicol, Stirrup, Kelion, and Padley have provided a comprehensive and up-to-date handbook on the use of cardiovascular CT (CCT) in practice.

The handbook starts with a variety of chapters dedicated to the technical aspects of CCT. A wide range of important topics is covered, including the different generations of scanners and particular coverage of the latest and newest CT scanners ("Beyond 64-slice CT"). Detailed chapters are also dedicated to radiation physics and protection – very important topics in the use of CCT – and the "in and outs" of iodinated intravenous contrast media. Thereafter follows a discussion of different scan protocols and an intensive and detailed explanation of image reconstructions and artefacts. Knowledge of these areas is fundamental for MSCT analysis and interpretation.

The second part of the handbook is focused on non-invasive coronary angiography. From a clinical perspective, this topic is very extensively discussed. All scenarios, ranging from calcium scoring to detection of coronary stenoses, are addressed. At present, the accuracy of MSCT is extremely high for assessment of coronary stenoses, and specifically the negative predictive value is excellent. This implies that absence of stenoses on MSCT virtually excludes the presence of significant stenoses on invasive coronary angiography. In this regard, a good summary of the available studies comparing these two techniques is provided. A point of attention remains that the presence of atherosclerosis per se does not always imply that there is myocardial ischemia. This is important in the clinical setting, specifically when considering the potential therapeutic consequences of MSCT findings. To this end, comparison of MSCT with functional cardiac imaging is dealt with in a dedicated chapter. Attention is also paid separately to assessment of coronary plaque composition, which may have potential value for identification of vulnerable plaques.

Further chapters are devoted to the prognostic performance of MSCT and the usefulness of the technique for evaluating bypass grafts/anastomoses and coronary artery stents. With regards to prognosis, recent studies have demonstrated the strong prognostic value of MSCT angiography. Normal MSCT is associated with an excellent outcome, whereas stenoses in the left main coronary artery, proximal left anterior descending coronary artery or multiple coronary arteries are all associated with a poorer outcome. This topic is covered in detail in the handbook. Coronary stent evaluation remains difficult, and stents with small luminal diameters are difficult to evaluate. The possibilities and limitations of stent imaging with MSCT receive full coverage.

In addition to evaluation of the coronary arteries, MSCT is also able to visualize the cardiac venous anatomy. This is particularly important in cardiac resynchronization therapy, where positioning of the left ventricular pacing lead depends on the presence of suitable cardiac veins.

Other cardiac structures that can be visualized include the ventricles, atria, myocardium and pericardium, heart valves and large vessels. Precise assessment of left and right ventricular function is possible with MSCT and correlates well with other imaging modalities such as magnetic resonance imaging and echocardiography. Ventricular geometry may also be assessed by MSCT, a useful feature when assessing cardiomyopathies and myocardial infiltration. Exact visualization of the heart valves and surrounding structures using MSCT is becoming increasingly important, particularly prior to percutaneous valve procedures. Novel developments in MSCT, such as the assessment of myocardial scarring and perfusion, also receive attention in the handbook.

Finally, a large part of the thorax is imaged during MSCT and non-cardiac findings, including 'incidentalomas', are often observed. Recognition of these findings is also addressed at large in the current handbook.

All in all, this superb handbook will provide all the information needed for those involved in the use of cardiovascular CT.

Jeroen J. Bax
Professor of Cardiology
Leiden University Medical Center
The Netherlands

Preface

Cardiac imaging has become a complex sub-specialty. Many techniques are now available and indications for each may overlap. Cardiovascular computed tomography (CCT) has emerged in the last decade as the primary technique for the non-invasive evaluation of the coronary arteries and the cardiovascular system in general. Some have argued that the increased use of CCT has occurred because we *can* do it rather than we *should* do it. Although there is some merit to this argument, it often reflects a lack of understanding of CCT and the information that it can provide when used appropriately. This lack of understanding may result from both the rate of change in CT technology (which often outstrips the evidence for its utility) and the lack of training opportunities in CCT. Whilst many courses exist for CCT training, it is only through hands-on experience that true clinical competence results.

Our hope is that the reader will carry this handbook with them whilst they accrue this hands-on experience. It is aimed at all students, clinicians, physicists, and radiographers involved in CCT. It is meant to be a broadly applicable résumé of CCT rather than a fully comprehensive manual for the use of every CT scanner. Indeed, the latter would be impossible given the pace of change of CT technology, coupled with the different engineering approaches used by each CT vendor. Nonetheless, details that relate to specific CT scanners are provided in the text. Four broad themes are dealt with in the handbook: the components of a (generic) CT scanner and the physics associated with them; practical aspects of cardiovascular CT, including patient set-up, contrast media and scan protocols; cardiac CT, particularly CT coronary angiography and evaluation of cardiac structure and function; and finally broader vascular imaging using CT. A recurring message in this book is that CCT is one of many imaging techniques available to assess the heart and broader cardiovascular system. We hope to reinforce this context in the final chapter with some background of the other available cardiac imaging techniques.

This book is written in the familiar, easily accessible Oxford Handbook style and draws together the experience and opinions of most UK experts in CCT. To date, we have found many textbooks on the market that cover either the engineering and physics of CCT or its clinical application. It is however rare to see a book that covers both. We hope that this handbook fills this gap.

EN
JS
AK
SP
June 2011

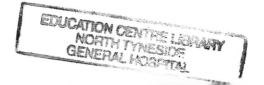

Contents

Detailed contents

Contributors

Dr Anu Balan
Consultant Radiologist
Addenbrooke's Hospital
Cambridge, UK

Dr Russell Bull
Consultant Radiologist
Bournemouth Hospital
Bournemouth, UK

Dr Roger Bury
Consultant Radiologist
Royal Victoria Hospital
Blackpool, UK

Dr Elly Castellano
Medical Physicist
Department of Medical Physics
Royal Marsden Hospital
Fulham Road
London, UK

Dr Deepa Gopalan
Consultant Radiologist
Papworth Hospital
Cambridge, UK

Dr Oliver Gosling
Cardiac MRI and CT Research
Fellow
Peninsula Clinical Research Facility
Exeter, UK

Dr Mark Hamilton
Consultant Radiologist
Bristol, UK

Dr Andrew Kelion
Consultant Cardiologist
Royal Brompton and Harefield
NHS Foundation Trust,
London, UK

Dr Paul Leeson
Consultant Cardiologist
John Radcliffe Hospital
Oxford, UK

Dr Nathan Manghat
Consultant Cardiovascular
Radiologist
Bristol Heart Institute
Bristol Royal Infirmary
Bristol, UK

Dr Paula McParland
Specialist Registrar in Radiology
Bournemouth Hospital
Bournemouth, UK

Dr Grant Mitchell
Consultant Radiologist
Derriford Hospital
Plymouth, UK

Dr Tarun Mittal
Consultant Radiologist
Harefield Hospital
Uxbridge
Middlesex, UK

Dr Gareth Morgan Hughes
Consultant Cardiologist
Derriford Hospital
Plymouth, UK

Dr Ed Nicol
Consultant Cardiologist
Royal Brompton and Harefield
NHS Foundation Trust, and
Chelsea and Westminster
NHS Foundation Trust,
London, UK

Dr Simon Padley
Consultant Cardiologist
Royal Brompton and Harefield
NHS Foundation Trust, and
Chelsea and Westminster
NHS Foundation Trust,
London, UK

Ms Trupti Patel
Superintendent Radiographer
Royal Brompton Hospital
London, UK

Dr Francesca Pugliese
Cardiac Radiologist
London Chest Hospital
London, UK

Dr Vimal Raj
Fellow Cardiothoracic Radiology
Papworth Hospital
Cambridge, UK

Dr Eliana Reyes
Nuclear Cardiology Fellow
Royal Brompton Hospital
London, UK

Dr Giles Roditi
Consultant Radiologist
Glasgow, UK

Professor Carl Roobottom
Consultant Radiologist
Derriford Hospital
Plymouth, UK

Dr Michael Rubens
Consultant Radiologist
Royal Brompton Hospital
London, UK

Dr James Rudd
Consultant Cardiologist
Addenbrooke's Hospital
Cambridge, UK

Dr Nik Sabharwal
Consultant Cardiologist
John Radcliffe Hospital
Oxford, UK

Dr James Stirrup
Clinical Research Fellow,
Cardiac Imaging
Royal Brompton and Harefield
NHS Foundation Trust,
London, UK

Dr Andrew Taylor
Consultant Radiologist
Great Ormond Street Hospital
London, UK

Symbols and abbreviations

📖	cross reference
℘	online resource/web address
↑	increase
↓	decrease
ACA	anomalous coronary arteries
ACCF	American College of Cardiology Foundation
ACHD	adult congenital heart disease
AF	atrial fibrillation
AIVG	anterior interventricular groove
ALARA	as low as reasonable achievable
AP	aortopulmonary
AR	aortic regurgitation
ARVC	arhythmogenic right ventricular cardiomyopathy
ASD	atrial septal defects
AV	atrioventricular
AVA	aortic valve area
AVNRT	atrioventricular nodal re-entrant tachycardia
AVSD	atrioventricular septal defect
BAC	broncheoalveolar cell carcinoma
BMI	body mass index
BMS	bare-metal stents
bpm	beats per minute
BSCI	British Society of Cardiovascular Imaging
CABG	coronary artery bypass grafting
CAD	coronary artery disease
CCS	coronary artery calcium score
CCT	cardiovascular CT
ccTGA	congenitally corrected transposition of the great arteries
cMPR	curved MPR
CMR	cardiovascular magnetic resonance
CT	computerized tomography
CTA	CT coronary angiography
CTDI	CT dose index
CTPA	CT pulmonary angiography
DECT	dual-energy CT
DES	drug-eluting stents

DLP	dose–length product
DRL	diagnostic reference level
DSCT	dual-source CT
EBCT	electron beam CT
ECG	electrocardiogram
EDE	effective dose equivalent
eGFR	estimated glomerular filtration rate
EP	electrophysiology
ESC	European Society of Cardiology
ESR	erythrocyte sedimentation rate
^{18}F-FDG	^{18}F-fluorodeoxyglucose
FFR	fractional flow reserve
FOV	field of view
GTN	glyceryl trinitrate
HR	heart rate
HU	Hounsfield units
ICA	invasive coronary angiography
ICD	implantable cardiac defibrillator
ICRP	International Commission on Radiological Protection
IMA	internal mammary artery
IMH	intramural haematoma
IVC	inferior vena cava
IVUS	intravascular ultrasound
LAA	left atrial appendage
LAD	left anterior descending
LAVG	left atrioventricular groove
LCx	left circumflex artery
LIMA	left internal mammary arteries
LMS	left main stem
LN	lymph nodes
LPH	lipomatous hypertrophy
LSVC	left superior vena cava
LV	left ventricular
LVEDV	left ventricular end-diastolic volume
LVEF	left ventricular ejection fraction
MACE	major adverse cardiac events
MAPCA	major aorto-pulmonary collateral artery
MFH	malignant fibrous histiocytoma
MIBG	metaiodobenzylguanidine
MIP	maximum-intensity projection

MPR	multiplanar reformatting
MPS	myocardial perfusion scintigraphy
MR	mitral regurgitation
MRI	magnetic resonance imaging
MSCT	multi-slice CT
MVA	mitral valve area
NICE	National Institute for Health and Clinical Excellence
NPV	negative predictive value
NSF	nephrogenic systemic fibrosis
PA	pulmonary artery
PAH	pulmonary artery hypertension
PCI	percutaneous coronary intervention
PDA	posterior descending coronary artery
PDA	patent ductus arteriosus
PET	positron emission tomography
PFO	patent foramen ovale
PICC	peripherally inserted central catheter
PIVG	posterior (inferior) inter-ventricular groove
PMT	photomultiplier tubes
POBA	plain old balloon angioplasty
PPV	positive predictive value
PR	pulmonary regurgitation
PTL	pre-test likelihood
PV	pulmonary vein
PVC	premature ventricular complexes
PVR	pulmonary vascular resistance
RAVG	right atrioventricular groove
RCA	right coronary artery
RF	radiofrequency
RIMA	right internal mammary arteries
RML	right middle lobe
RNV	radionuclide ventriculography
ROA	regurgitant orifice area
ROI	region of interest
RUL	right upper lobe
RV	right ventricular
RVEF	RV ejection fraction
RVEDV	right ventricular end-diastolic volume
RVESV	right ventricular end- systolic volume
RVOT	right ventricular outflow tract

SCCT	Society of Cardiovascular CT
SLE	systemic lupus erythematosis
SNR	signal-to-noise ratio
SPECT	single photon emission computed tomography
SPL	secondary pulmonary lobule
SSCT	single-slice CT
SSD	shaded-surface display
ST	sinotubular
STS-MIP	sliding thin slab MIP
SVC	superior vena cava
SVG	saphenous vein graft
TAVI	transcatheter aortic valve implantation
TGA	transposition of the great arteries
TOE	transoesophageal echocardiography
TR	tricuspid regurgitation
TTE	transthoracic echocardiography
VA	ventriculoarterial
VHD	valvular heart disease
VR	volume rendering
VSD	ventricular septal defects

Development of cardiovascular CT

Introduction

The use of X-ray computed tomography (CT) to image the heart has ↑ exponentially over the last decade. This increase is largely the result of technological improvements that have rendered cardiac images less susceptible to artefacts arising from cardiac motion. However, these artefacts have not been abolished entirely. The ability to reliably acquire high-quality cardiovascular CT (CCT) datasets is predicated in part on an understanding of the hardware and software used to generate them, which in turn may be better understood by reviewing briefly the development of the CT scanner from initial models to the current state-of-the-art equipment.

Origins of X-ray computed tomography

The invention of X-ray CT is credited to Sir Godfrey Hounsfield, an engineer working for EMI Laboratories, and Allan Cormack, a South African physicist at Tufts University, Massachusetts.

The major hurdle to the initial development of CT was mathematical. Acquiring image data through multiple projections was straightforward, but converting this into a resultant image was not. The theoretical basis for determining the nature of heterogenous tissues that attenuate a transmitted X-ray beam was laid out by Allan Cormack in the early 1960s but remained unexploited as it had uncertain practical application. Unaware of this work, Godfrey Hounsfield pursued an engineering solution to the problem, which led to the development of a CT scanner prototype in the late 1960s and, ultimately, the first clinical CT scanner, which was installed in Atkinson Morley Hospital, London in 1971. This scanner was dedicated to imaging the brain and took around 4min to acquire each axial image. A whole-body CT scanner was to follow. For their combined work, Cormack and Hounsfield shared the Nobel Prize for Physiology and Medicine in 1979.

Scanner development

To date, four broad generations of conventional CT scanners have been developed (Fig. 1.1). Each modifies the geometric arrangement of X-ray tube and detector array. Although intuition would suggest that current scanners are of the fourth generation, this is not the case. In fact, all modern CT scanners are based on third-generation technology. The technical aspects of modern CT are easier to understand with a little background knowledge of successive iterations of CT scanner geometry.

First-generation CT

The original CT scanner developed by Godfrey Hounsfield in the 1970s. A single X-ray source was collimated to produce a thin beam of X-rays, which were detected on the opposite side of the patient by two detectors lined up along the axis of rotation. The assembly was then translated across the patient to begin a new measurement. Once the entire field had been covered, the assembly was rotated by 1° and the translation procedure started afresh ('translate–rotate' motion). This was repeated over an arc of 180° to generate the data required to reconstruct an axial slice. Although by modern standards the image acquisition time was lengthy (around 6min), at the time of introduction the technique was truly revolutionary.

Second-generation CT

This generation improved on the inital CT design by using multiple narrow fan-beam X-ray sources and detectors with multiple elements. Images were still acquired using a translate–rotate mechanism, but scan times were reduced substantially due to simultaneous data acquisition from multiple detector channels. The major factor limiting the advancement of second-generation CT scanners was difficulty in engineering X-ray source detector configurations through the translate–rotate mechanism.

Third-generation CT

CT technology was improved further still by widening the X-ray fan-beam to encompass the patient. The patient lies in the centre of an imaginary circle, on the circumference of which lie the X-ray source on one side and an arc of detector elements on the other. The entire mechanism is rotated around the patient, but translation is no longer necessary. Acquisition times are substantially improved (down to 165ms on conventional 64-slice scanners).

Fourth-generation CT

This generation evolved only slightly later than third-generation CT and offers no significant advantages. A 360° array of fixed detectors is positioned around the patient, with only the X-ray source rotating

Fourth-generation scanners have a few disadvantages (scatter is a particular problem), but were dealt a mortal blow by the advent of multislice CT. Although an issue even for third-generation scanners, the costs of engineering this technology for fourth-generation scanners were impossibly prohibitive.

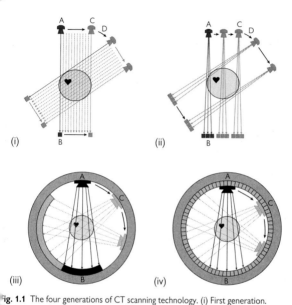

Fig. 1.1 The four generations of CT scanning technology. (i) First generation. X-rays are emitted from the source (A) to reach the detector (B). The assembly is then translated in stages across the patient (C) until complete coverage is obtained. The assembly is rotated (D) and the process is repeated. (ii) Second generation. Similar to first-generation technology, although fan-beam X-rays used and detector numbers ↑. (iii) Third generation. X-rays are emitted from the source (A), pass through the patient and reach the detectors (B). The whole assembly then rotates round the patient to a new view (C). Translation is no longer necessary. (iv) Fourth generation. Similar to third-generation CT, except that the detctor array (B) is arranged circumferentially around the patient and does not move during the acquisition.

Electron beam CT

Although third-generation conventional CT scanners were in use by the 1980s, their temporal resolution was rather poor, precluding cardiac scanning. Electron beam CT (EBCT) scanners were developed to circumvent this limitation and are occasionally referred to as fifth-generation scanners. Rather than using a rotating X-ray gantry, EBCT employs a fixed electron beam that is selectively targeted by means of electromagnetic deflection coils onto a 210° arc of tungsten anodes located beneath the patient (Fig. 1.2). The electron beam has a current in the region of 640mA; when it strikes the tungsten anodes, X-rays are emitted in a process similar to current passing through the tungsten anode of a conventional X-ray tube (see 📖 X-ray tube, p. 12). The fan-shaped X-ray beam is collimated to travel vertically; X-rays are attenuated as they pass through the patient and are detected by an array of detectors on the opposite side.

The absence of moving parts, coupled with the speed at which the electron beam can be swept over the tungsten anodes, means that the temporal resoultion (see 📖 Temporal resolution, p. 28) of EBCT is significantly faster (~33ms) than even modern multislice CT (MSCT) scanners (65–165ms). Radiation exposure is comparable to a prospectively gated calcium score acquisition using MSCT.

Three factors limit the usefulness of EBCT. Firstly, the spatial resolution (see 📖 Chapter 3 p. 26) is relatively poor (1.5mm, compared with 0.5mm for MSCT). Secondly, EBCT scanners are essentially limited to cardiac applications and are less suitable for general purpose CT radiology. Thirdly, EBCT scanners are relatively more expensive than their 64-slice MSCT equivalents.

The major clinical use of EBCT is coronary calcium scoring (see 📖 Coronary artery calcium scoring (1), p. 194), although the technology has been largely superceded by MSCT.

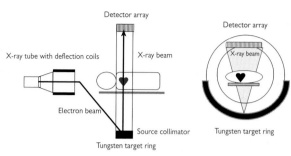

Fig. 1.2 Electron beam CT.

MSCT scanner components

Gantry

Modern CT scanners use a rotating gantry onto which the X-ray tube and detectors are mounted. Limitations in gantry technology led to the introduction of EBCT for cardiac imaging, but third-generation CT scanners eventually supplanted this technology as a result of two main advances:
- Slip ring technology
- Switch-mode power supply.

Slip-ring technology

Previously, conventional CT required power to be supplied via electric cabling, necessitating a reversal of gantry rotation after every few turns to allow unwinding of the cable. Slip-ring technology dispenses with the power cable: both power and data are transferred to and from the gantry using metal brushes fixed to the housing of the scanner, but in permanent electrical contact with the rotating gantry. This allows continuous rotation of the gantry, and paved the way for helical CT scanning (see 📖 Acquisition mode, p. 36).

Switch-mode power supply

A major problem for rotating gantry CT was the construction of a power supply that was small enough to be mounted on the gantry but powerful enough to generate the voltages required. The advent of switch-mode power supplies solved this problem, allowing higher efficiency power supplies with reduced size and weight. Most switch-mode power supplies work by converting AC to DC current via a switching circuit. The DC current is then converted back to AC but at a much higher frequency than that supplied by the mains. The ↑ efficiency allows higher tube voltages to be achieved with only limited generation of heat.

Gantry rotation time

This is the time taken for one full rotation of the X-ray tube/detector array around the axis of rotation. The speed of gantry rotation was the limiting factor in early CT, particularly before the advent of slip ring technology. For many contemporary scanners, approximately half a revolution (180°) is needed to acquire a single image (the angle of the X-ray fan beam must also be considered, so in practice a ~220° arc is required). This is known as a half-scan algorithm (see 📖 Temporal resolution, p. 28). A 64-slice CT scanner may have a gantry rotation time of 330ms and hence can acquire a single image set in ~165ms. Thus the temporal resolution of this scanner is around 165ms.

X-ray tube

Production of X-rays

In CT X-rays are produced by an X-ray tube (Fig. 2.1):

- Electrons are emitted by heating the filament with an electric current. This is called thermionic emission.
- A voltage is applied between the cathode and the anode which accelerates the electrons towards the positively charged anode. The flow of electrons is described by the tube current (see 📖 X-ray tube current, p. 22), measured in milliamperes (mA). The electrons gain energy equivalent to the applied voltage: in CT, this is typically 120kVp (see 📖 X-ray tube voltage, p. 23).
- The electron beam strikes the anode at the focal spot. Most of the electron energy is dissipated as heat; about 4% is released as X-rays.

The X-ray spectrum

X-rays are emitted with a range of energies between a few kiloelectron-volts and the applied tube voltage. The distribution of energies is described by the X-ray spectrum (Fig. 2.2).

There are two types of X-ray:

- Characteristic X-rays, which appear as peaks with discrete energies corresponding to the energy transitions between electron shells
- Bremsstrahlung X-rays, which form a continuum that falls in intensity towards the higher energies.

The average energy of the X-ray beam is referred to as the effective energy. In CT this is typically 60–70keV.

X-ray energies at the lower end of the spectrum are absorbed before reaching the detectors and thus contribute to patient dose but not to the image. Lower energy X-rays are removed from the X-ray beam by the X-ray tube housing and specialized filters that preferentially attenuate low-energy X-rays ('filtration').

The X-ray beam

The X-ray beam is defined by the tube exit port and the collimator. Most of the other X-rays are stopped by the tube housing. As the X-rays emanate from a single point, the intensity of the X-ray beam decreases with the inverse of the distance squared. For example, when the distance is doubled, the X-ray intensity is quartered.

When traversing matter, the intensity of the X-ray beam will also decrease as X-ray photons interact with the atoms in the material. The transmitted intensity, I, is given by

$$I = I_o e^{\mu x}$$

where I_o is the initial beam intensity, x is the thickness of the material and µ is the linear attenuation coefficient of the material. µ depends on photon energy and the atomic number of the material, and is generally higher at lower energies.

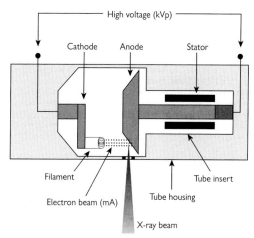

Fig. 2.1 X-ray tube.

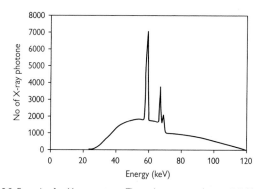

Fig. 2.2 Example of an X-ray spectrum. The peaks represent characteristic X-rays released by the transition of electrons from a higher to a lower energy shell. The smooth curve represents Bremsstrahlung X-rays generated from the deceleration of free electrons as they pass the heavy nuclei of the anode material. As the lower energy X-rays would be predominantly absorbed by the body prior to reaching the detector, they are first removed from the X-ray beam by a process known as filtration.

Collimators

Collimation describes the process of restricting the X-ray beam to a given area. It may be performed at the X-ray source (pre-patient) or at the detectors (post-patient).

Pre-patient collimators
- Determine the shape of the emitted X-ray beam.
- A fixed collimator determines the width of the maximum permitted beam.
- An adjustable collimator allows fine tuning of the beam to the desired slice width.

Post-patient collimators
- Allow only X-rays travelling along the direction of the $1°$ beam to strike the detectors.
- Reduce the effects of scatter detection.

Detectors

The most common form of detector used in modern CT scanners is the solid-state detector. Historically, these were constructed from a variety of materials, including caesium iodide and cadmium tungstate. All current CT detectors are made from rare earth ceramics. All are scintillators, releasing light photons via the photoelectric effect following absorption of an incident X-ray. The number of light photons released is dependent on the X-ray intensity (X-ray photons striking the detector per unit time). Light photons are detected by photodiodes, which convert the energy into an electrical signal for processing.

To be suitable for CT scanning, detectors must:

- Respond linearly to the energy of incident X-rays
- Respond quickly to activation by incoming X-rays—if the response time is delayed, the gantry will have rotated and the calculated ray will be back-projected incorrectly (see 📖 Image reconstruction and processing, p. 129)
- Scintillate for only a brief period after stimulation—the continuing release of light photons after the incident X-ray has been absorbed is known as 'afterglow' (brief periods of afterglow are common in all detectors, but persistence leads to blurring of images)
- Have a high absorption efficiency—detectors which let X-rays pass straight through them without detection are unsuitable
- Deliver linear responses over a wide range of X-ray intensities (dynamic range).

Signal to noise ratio

The detection of incident X-rays constitutes the 'signal' that is used to generate the CT image. Inevitably, there are statistical variations in the response of a detector element to incident X-rays. These variations lead to noise in the final image that is inversely proportional to the number of detected X-rays.

The 'quality' of a CT image may be judged according to the signal-to-noise ratio (SNR). Any modification that increases the number of X-rays (e.g. increasing X-ray tube current, see 📖 X-ray tube current, p. 22) increases the SNR. Reducing the number of detected X-rays (such as when scanning an obese patient, see 📖 Practical aspects, p. 69) has the opposite effect.

Detector terminology

Detector element size

This is the width of the detector row in the *x.y*-axis (Fig. 2.3) and is a principal determinant of in-plane (transverse) spatial resolution (see 📖 Spatial resolution, p. 26).

Detector row width

This is the width of the detector row in the *z*-axis (Fig. 2.3). This determines the minimum slice thickness and is the 1° determinant of through-plane (longitudinal) spatial resolution (see 📖 Spatial resolution, p. 26).

Detector array configuration and slice thickness

The *z*-axis configuration of the detector array varies between vendors.

Isotropic configuration

The width of each row is equal, e.g. 64 rows each of 0.625mm width (Fig. 2.4). Detector rows can be combined to give a slice-thickness that is a multiple of the detector width. For example, 64 rows each of 0.625mm width can give 64 slices of 0.625mm width, 32 slices of 1.25mm width, 16 slices of 2.5mm width, etc. This has the advantage of improving contrast resolution through a reduction in image noise. However, longitudinal spatial resolution is reduced. Although CT coronary angiography depends on maximizing spatial resolution, there are many applications that do not, including coronary calcium scoring (see 📖 Imaging atherosclerotic plaque, p. 191).

Anisotropic configuration

Also known as adaptive or hybrid configuration, the width of each detector row is variable. The most common configuration is for the central rows to be narrower than those at the periphery of the array (Fig. 2.5). To generate images at the minimum slice thickness, only the central detector rows can be used. Thicker slices can be acquired by combining the central rows and recruiting the outer rows. This kind of hybrid detector design is more common in 4- and 16-slice scanners.

Although combining data from multiple detector rows is a choice made during scanning, it is possible to reconstruct thicker slices using appropriate software after the scan has taken place. For example, images acquired on a large patient might be reconstructed using a slice thickness of 1mm rather than the standard 0.75mm in order to reduce image noise. It should be noted that the *post hoc* application of this method has no beneficial effects on radiation exposure.

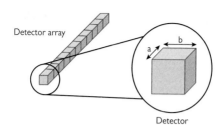

Detector array

Detector

Fig. 2.3 Single row of CT detectors. The detector element size is given by the width of the detector in the *x, y* dimension (a) and is a principal determinant of in-plane spatial resolution. The width of the detector element in the *z*-axis (b) determines the minimum slice thickness and thus the through-plane resolution.

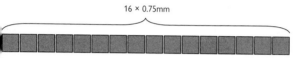

16 × 0.75mm

Fig. 2.4 16-slice isotropic detector array. Each detector row is of equal size; rows may be combined in multiples to generate thicker slices.

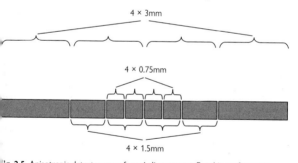

4 × 3mm

4 × 0.75mm

4 × 1.5mm

Fig. 2.5 Anisotropic detector array for a 4-slice scanner. For this configuration, acquiring the minimum slice thickness requires activation of the central detector rows only. To generate thicker slices, central detectors are combined and successive outer rows recruited. It should be noted that whilst the total number of detector rows is 8, the maximum number of slices that can be generated from this configuration is 4.

Detectors, data channels, and slices

The use of the term 'multidetector' to distinguish current generations of CT scanner can cause confusion as it suggests that previous iterations of CT technology have consisted of only a single detector. In fact, CT scanners from the second generation onwards have had multiple detectors arranged along the x, y-axis (Fig. 2.6A). They have been limited, however, in the number of detector *rows* along the z-axis. The key feature of MSCT is that there are two or more (and now usually at least 64) detector rows along the z-axis of the gantry (Fig. 2.6B).

In practice, several terms are used to describe CT scanner configurations: multidetector, multichannel, and multislice CT. Although these terms are often used interchangeably, they reflect different concepts:

- Multidetector: The physical number of detector rows mounted along the z-axis of the gantry, i.e. a 64-detector scanner consists of 64 detector rows.
- Multichannel: The number of simultaneous data channels activated in the z-axis.
- Multislice: The number of image slices acquired per gantry rotation.

The numbers of detector rows and data channels are fixed physical properties of the detector array and data acquisition system, respectively. The number of image slices acquired per gantry rotation is not necessarily equal to the number of detector rows or data channels; rather it depends on how these are coupled (Fig. 2.5).

A further complicating factor is the use of *double-sampling* (Fig. 2.7). In this case, each detector row/data channel combination is sampled twice by varying the z-axis position of the focal spot of the X-ray beam (see 📖 Scanner components, p. 9). Although this does not, in general double the number of slices, it does improve through-plane resolution (see 📖 Spatial resolution, p. 26). Scanners exist that have 64 detector rows/data channels but are termed 128-slice scanners as they use double-sampling.

Given the potential for confusion, we prefer to use the nomenclature *multislice computed tomography* (MSCT) throughout.

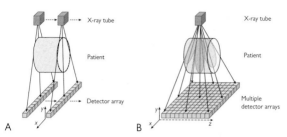

Fig. 2.6 A. Single-slice CT. Multiple detectors are arranged along the x, y-axis but there is only a single row in the z-axis. Each gantry rotation results in the acquisition of a single image slice, after which the gantry must be translated in the z-axis in order to acquire a new slice. B. Multislice CT. Multiple detector rows are arranged along the z-axis, allowing multiple slices to be acquired during each gantry rotation.

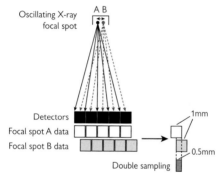

Fig. 2.7 Double sampling. The focal spot of the X-ray alternates such that each detector is sampled twice. This has the effect of improving through-plane (z-axis) resolution.

Technical principles of cardiovascular CT

X-ray tube current

This describes the number of electrons passing between the cathode and anode per second, without reference to their energy. Increasing the tube current results in more electrons striking the positively charged anode and generation of a greater number of X-rays (↑ beam intensity). The spectrum of X-ray energies is unchanged.

As radiation dose is related to the total number of X-rays that pass through the patient during the exposure, tube current is usually expressed as the product of tube current (measured in milliamperes) and exposure time (measured in seconds), to give figures with units of milliampere-seconds (mAs).

Tube current may also be expressed as *effective* mAs, which is calculated by dividing the product of tube current and exposure time by the pitch (see 📖 Scan pitch, p. 24). This value represents the mAs per slice: the total number of X-rays that contribute to a given slice. In order to keep this figure constant, any change in pitch must be matched by a similar relative change in mAs.

Scanner manufacturers may express tube current in other ways—the reader is advised to review the technical specifications of their scanner and/or consult a local CT medical physics expert for further information.

Effects of changing tube current on radiation exposure

Increasing tube current and/or exposure time increases the number of X-rays to which the patient is exposed, thus increasing radiation dose. Radiation dose increases linearly with tube current and exposure time.

Effects of changing tube current on subsequent CT image

With higher tube currents and/or exposure times, a greater number of X-rays ultimately strike the detectors. This improves the signal-to-noise ratio of the resultant image. In practice, cardiovascular CT images are often acquired at the highest current for which the X-ray tube is rated, and increases in tube current may not be possible.

X-ray tube voltage

This is the potential difference between the cathode and anode in the X-ray tube. Changes in tube voltage affect the spectrum of X-ray energies released. The greater the potential difference, the greater the energy of the electrons that are accelerated through it. This in turn increases both the number and the energy of the emitted X-rays.

Effects of changing tube voltage on radiation exposure

Increasing tube voltage (whilst leaving other parameters unchanged) increases radiation dose as a result of exposure to higher X-ray energies. Radiation dose is proportional to the square of tube voltage.

Effects of changing tube voltage on subsequent CT image

X-ray attenuation depends on both the attenuation coefficient of the tissue through which the beam is passing and the X-ray energies in the beam. For any given tissue, a beam with lower energy X-rays will be attenuated more than one with higher energies. Thus a lower energy beam will have a lower intensity on arriving at the detectors than a higher energy beam, resulting in a higher calculated attenuation coefficient. Changes in tube voltage thus lead to changes in the CT number (see 📖 CT numbers and windowing, p. 138) for a particular tissue on the resultant image.

Practical considerations

Although increasing tube voltage alone results in a higher patient dose, it also has the effect of making the X-ray beam more penetrating. Consequently, it is possible to reduce tube current to compensate for the greater X-ray flux at the detector. When concurrent adjustments are made to tube voltage and current, the net change in radiation exposure may be higher, lower, or unchanged!

Lower tube voltages result in a ↓ signal-to-noise ratio in the resultant image but may increase contrast resolution. However, in slim patients and children, the reduction in the thickness of attenuating tissue between the X-ray source and the detectors means that tube voltage may be lowered, reducing radiation dose without adversely affecting image quality. Reduced tube voltages may also have practical applications in the assessment of delayed myocardial enhancement to detect scarring (see 📖 Evaluation of myocardial scarring and perfusion, p. 259).

Scan pitch

Single-slice CT

Pitch was originally described for single-slice CT (SSCT) to relate the distance travelled by the scanning table (feed) in the z-axis per gantry rotation to slice thickness. In the era of MSCT, this value is known as 'detector pitch' and is calculated as:

$$\text{detector pitch} = \frac{\text{table feed per gantry rotation}}{\text{slice thickness}}$$

Pitch ∴ describes the degree to which X-ray beams overlap during successive gantry rotations. If the table feed during one gantry rotation is less than the slice thickness, succeeding rotations will overlap (pitch <1). Conversely, if the table feed per gantry rotation is greater than the slice thickness (pitch >1), the projection data becomes too strung out, causing problems with image reconstruction.

Multislice CT

The formula above is true for SSCT as the slice thickness is equal to the width of the X-ray beam, a factor determined by collimation (see 📖 Collimators, p. 14). In MSCT, however, slice thickness is determined by the width of the active detector elements (see 📖 Detectors, p. 15) rather than the width of the X-ray beam. A broad fan- or cone-beam is used to allow coverage of multiple detector rows, with each beam generating a number of slices. As the one-to-one relationship between X-ray beam width and slice thickness is lost, the formula above will lead to underestimation of beam overlap. For example, if the table feed per gantry rotation is equal to the slice thickness, the above formula generates a pitch factor of 1, suggesting contiguous but non-overlapping slices. In fact the broad X-ray beam fan angle leads to substantial overlap. To account for this, the following calculation is used to determine the 'beam pitch' in MSCT:

$$\text{beam pitch} = \frac{\text{table feed per gantry rotation}}{\text{number of slices} \times \text{slice thickness}}$$

For the example given, table feed per gantry rotation is equal to slice thickness, which is itself substantially less than the X-ray beam width. The beam pitch is ∴ much less than 1, indicating substantial overlap.

Effect of varying pitch

In order to acquire images of the heart in multiple phases (retrospective gating, see 📖 ECG gating (1), p. 32), 'over sampling' of data is required. In acquisition terms, this mandates significant overlap along the craniocaudal extent of the patient, requiring use of a low pitch. In cardiac CT, pitches of the order of 0.2–0.35 (which equals an over-sampling rate between approximately 5:1 and 3:1) are common.

Higher pitches equate to fewer gantry rotations per unit travelled in the z-axis and thus lower the SNR of the resultant image. In practice this is offset by increasing the tube current to maintain image quality.

Lower pitches lead to longer scan times and breath holds and, assuming that tube current is held constant, ↑ radiation doses due to the high volume of overlapping data. Many scanners adjust pitch according to heart rate and allow simultaneous adjustment of tube current by the user in order to achieve the optimum balance between image quality and radiation exposure. Newer CT scanners with higher numbers of detector rows (see 📖 Detectors, p. 15) allow greater z-axis coverage per gantry rotation and thus reduce the scan acquisition time.

Spatial resolution

This is the smallest distance at which two separate points can be distinguished as individual objects. Coronary arteries have a diameter of 2–4mm in their proximal tract and taper distally. High spatial resolution is ∴ a prerequisite for CT coronary imaging. Spatial resolution may be understood in terms of the transverse (x- and y-axes) and longitudinal (z-axis) planes.

Transverse spatial resolution
- Also known as *in-plane* spatial resolution.
- Dependent on detector element size and sampling frequency.
- The smaller the detector the better the spatial resolution.
- Typically around $0.5 \times 0.5mm^2$.
- NB: Smaller detectors → ↑random variation in photon flux (quantum mottle). Images ∴ appear noisier unless the tube current is ↑ or smoothing filters are applied.

Longitudinal spatial resolution
- Also known as *through-plane* spatial resolution.
- Determined mainly by the slice thickness.
- *Minimum* slice thickness is determined by the width of the detector row (see 📖 Detectors, p. 15), which varies between 0.5 and 0.625mm depending on the manufacturer.

Generally, the spatial resolution along the x-, y-, and z-axes is similar. Acquired voxels are ∴ virtually 'isotropic' (spatial resolution equal in all directions) and allow true three-dimensional (3D) imaging. Although invasive coronary angiography has a better bi-dimensional spatial resolution than MSCT ($0.2 \times 0.2mm^2$ vs $0.5 \times 0.5mm^2$), the ability to reconstruct multiplanar images gives CT a significant advantage.

Temporal resolution

The temporal resolution of a scanner is equal to the time required to acquire sufficient data to reconstruct a single image slice. If the object being imaged, such as the heart, moves within this time, it results in artefacts that degrade the final image and impact on the accuracy of and confidence in interpretation (Fig. 3.1A).

   Temporal resolution depends primarily on gantry rotation time (see 📖 Gantry, p. 10) and reconstruction method. To improve temporal resolution, either the speed of gantry rotation must be ↑ or methods must be sought to acquire the required data in less than a full gantry rotation.

   Faster gastry rotation results in shorter slice acquisition times and thus better temporal resolution. However, increases in gantry rotation speed are limited by the physical size of the components and the substantial centrifugal forces that result. These factors were the driving force behind the development of EBCT (see 📖 Electron beam CT, p. 6). However, several solutions exist that allow acquisition of a single image slice from less than a full rotation of projection data.

Half-scan reconstruction

Slices are reconstructed using data acquired over 180° (plus the X-ray fan-beam angle = ~220°). As acquisitions require a 220° arc rather than a full 360°, temporal resolution improves by a factor of ~40%.

Multisegment reconstruction (see 📖 Multisegment reconstruction, p. 30)

Data are acquired from successive cardiac cycles in intervals shorter than possible for a single cardiac cycle. These data are combined to produce the final image.

Dual-source CT (see 📖 Dual-source CT, p. 44)

Two X-ray sources and detector arrays are mounted at an angle of 90° on the rotating gantry. Data acquisition may be achieved in around a quarter of the gantry rotation time, improving temporal resolution twofold (Fig. 3.1B).

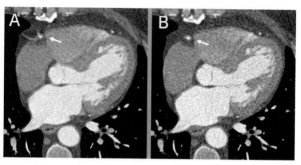

Fig. 3.1 MSCT images display the total cardiac motion over the reconstruction window, i.e. the temporal resolution, which depends primarily on the gantry rotation time. In single-source CT the reconstruction window sums image data obtained during 180° gantry rotation. In dual-source CT the reconstruction window sums image data obtained by two detectors during 90° gantry rotation. Image reconstruction using data from 180° rotation (A) may cause blurring of the coronary vessels (right coronary artery, arrow) due to insufficient temporal resolution. Image reconstruction using data from 90° rotation (B) doubles temporal resolution and reduces the artefact.

Multisegment reconstruction

For heart rates under 60bpm, the interval of minimum cardiac motion (often diastole) is usually sufficiently long for image acquisition within a single cardiac cycle. However, for faster heart rates, this interval is too short and moves beyond the temporal resolution of the scanner. This may be offset by using data from two or more cardiac cycles to generate a single image (multisegment or multiphase reconstruction, Fig. 3.2).

As data are acquired from successive cardiac cycles in intervals shorter than would be possible for single-phase reconstruction, multisegment reconstruction has the effect of improving temporal resolution. However, multisegment reconstruction relies on the heart being in an identical position during each cycle of acquisition, which is not necessarily the case even with regular heart rhythms. As the reconstructed images represent the average position of the heart in two or more cardiac cycles, image quality may be reduced. The technique is especially susceptible to motion artefact with variable heart rates.

A further limitation of multisegment reconstruction is that the area of interest must be imaged over two or more cardiac cycles rather than just one cycle for single-segment reconstruction. A much lower pitch (see 📖 Scan pitch p. 24) is ∴ required, which increases radiation dose. Finally, as scan acquisition time is ↑, a greater volume of contrast is required to ensure adequate vessel opacification.

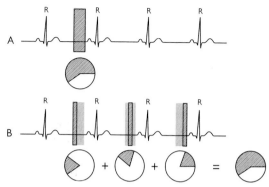

Fig. 3.2 (A) Single-segment reconstruction. A slice is acquired completely within the R–R interval of a single heartbeat. (B) Multisegment reconstruction. The slice is reconstructed by merging data acquired over several heartbeats. In the given example, three successive heartbeats are required to reconstruct a single slice, with each heartbeat providing one-third of the final data. Although this effectively improves temporal resolution threefold, the heart must be in exactly the same position during each imaging interval in order to avoid blurring of the final, 'average' cardiac image.

ECG gating (1)

The cardiac cycle may be divided into *systolic* and *diastolic* phases. In cardiac imaging, phases may also be defined according to percentage of the time between two consecutive R-waves on the ECG (R–R interval, Fig. 3.3). The number of phases that can be reconstructed within an R–R interval is typically 8–10, although this may be ↑ as required by the operator.

Typically, the heart is in end-systole and end-diastole during the 25–35% and 65–75% phases of the R–R interval, respectively. During acquisition, each unit of image data is allocated to a phase of the cardiac cycle by referencing a simultaneously recorded surface ECG. The technique of dividing the data set into time phases may also be defined according to their relative location within a given R.R internal (often expressed as a percentage, Fig. 3.3).

In a patient with a regular heart rate <65bpm, the end-diastolic phase is usually the interval of minimum cardiac motion. It is possible to acquire X-ray images exclusively during this phase of the cardiac cycle. This is known as *prospective gating*. However, it is also possible that for a given patient another phase may be optimal; this is particularly true for patients with uncontrolled heart rates. For example, the right coronary artery is only seen clearly at end-systole in ~50% of cases. In such patients, it is preferable to acquire data throughout the cardiac cycle. This is known as *retrospective gating*.

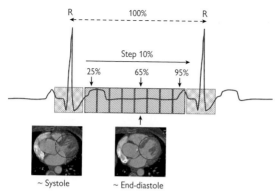

Fig. 3.3 ECG gating. The cardiac cycle is divided into percentages of the R–R interval (here shown as 10% increments from 25 to 95% of the R–R interval). End-systole and end-diastole typically occur at 25–35% and 65–75% of the R–R interval, respectively.

ECG gating (2)

Retrospective gating

- X-ray beam active for the entire cardiac cycle (Fig. 3.4).
- Retrospectively gated scans can be reconstructed using half scan reconstructions (see 📖 Temporal resolution, p. 28) or, if ↑HR, multisegment reconstructions (see 📖 Multisegment reconstruction, p. 30).
- Images may be reconstructed at any point during the cardiac cycle, allowing identification of the phase of minimum cardiac motion when not at end-diastole.
- Allows assessment of left ventricular diastolic and systolic volumes and ejection fraction, and the creation of moving cine images of cardiac structures, including valves.
- As the tube current is high throughout the scan, the radiation dose to the patient can be as high (20mSv). Modulation of tube current during the scan reduces this problem.

ECG-correlated mA pulsing

- This is a form of tube current modulation (see 📖 X-ray tube current, p. 22). Tube current is reduced during the phases of the cardiac cycle that are unlikely to be required for adequate interpretation of the dataset, but from which some diagnostic information may be obtained if necessary (Fig. 3.5).
- For CT coronary angiography, tube current is usually set to be maximal during 60–80% of the R–R interval, but is reduced in all other phases.
- Radiation dose to the patient is typically 30–50% lower than with conventional retrospective gating.
- Analysis of ventricular function is still possible, although as image quality is non-uniform throughout the cardiac cycle, accuracy may be reduced.
- ECG-correlated mA pulsing should be used routinely unless functional information is particularly required, or a high heart rate suggests that a systolic phase could be optimum.

Prospective gating

- X-ray beam only active during a pre-defined window of the cardiac cycle (Fig. 3.6).
- Significantly reduced radiation exposure (see 📖 Scan parameters and radiation dose, p. 62).
- As data are acquired only during a portion of the cardiac cycle, images can only be reconstructed for the phases examined.
- The acquisition window can be widened such that the X-ray tube is activated a short time before and deactivated a short time after the pre-defined window of the cardiac cycle (temporal padding). This allows adjustment of the reconstruction window to improve the chances of finding the interval of minimum cardiac motion.
- Prospective gating should not be used in patients with uncontrolled heart rates, arrhythmia, or in whom breath-holding may be problematic, as multiple cardiac phases are likely to be required to assess the coronary arteries adequately.

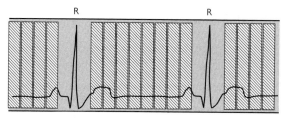

Fig. 3.4 Retrospective gating. The tube current (grey area) is at a maximum for the entire length of the scan. Phases may be reconstructed at any percentage of the R–R interval (boxes, here shown at 25–95%).

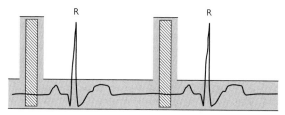

Fig. 3.5 Retrospective gating with ECG-correlated mA pulsing. The tube current (grey area) is on for the entire length of the scan, but is at a maximum for only a portion of the R–R interval (here shown at 60–80%). The current is reduced to a low level during other phases.

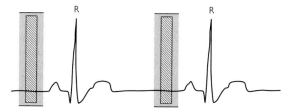

Fig. 3.6 Prospective gating. The tube current (grey area) is only on for a short percentage of the R–R interval. Although the 70% phase of the R–R interval is to be reconstructed (box), the X-ray tube is activated a short time before and deactivated a short time after the window required (temporal padding). This allows adjustment of the reconstruction window to find the optimum cardiac phase for analysis.

Acquisition mode

Axial scanning ('step-and-shoot')

- In axial scanning, data for one axial slice are acquired whilst the table is stationary.
- The table is then advanced step-wise to the next position (Fig. 3.7A).
- Sequential scans must be prospectively gated (see 📖 ECG gating (2), p. 34), usually during the diastolic phase of the cardiac cycle.
- The need for prospective gating minimizes radiation exposure but may prohibit analysis of ventricular function (see 📖 Evaluation of ventricular and atrial function, p. 229), unless the temporal padding selected includes both end systole and end-diastole.

Helical (spiral) scanning

- The table moves continuously relative to the gantry rotation (Fig. 3.7B).
- Helical scans may be prospectively or retrospectively gated (see 📖 Technical principles of cardiovascular CT, p. 21).
- Prospectively gated helical acquisitions offer the potential to reduce radiation dose whilst retaining the ability to switch to retrospective gating if tachycardia or arrhythmia develop.
- However, prospective helical acquistions require a combination of high pitch (see 📖 Scan pitch, p. 24) and slow heart rate, so are not suitable for all patients.

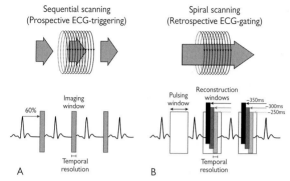

Fig. 3.7 (A) Axial scanning with prospective ECG gating. (B) Spiral scanning with retrospective ECG gating.

Beyond 64-slice CT

Limitations of 64-slice CT technology

- Long acquisition time (5–10s).
- Images obtained over multiple (typically five to eight) heartbeats, increasing susceptibility to 'banding' or misregistration artefacts (see 📖 Motion artefact, p. 156).
- 'Step' artefact occurs (particularly with prospective gating) (see 📖 Motion artefact, p. 156).
- Temporal resolution often limits use in patients with high heart rates (>65bpm), necessitating heart-rate control (see 📖 Heart-rate control, p. 78).
- Image quality may be poor in patients with atrial fibrillation or multiple ventricular ectopics due to difficulties with gating (see 📖 ECG gating (2), p. 34).
- Despite the number of detector rows, complete cardiac coverage requires several overlapping rotations in order to reconstruct slices at the periphery of the beam, leading to a small increase in radiation exposure. (NB: This is likely to be a larger issue for greater cone beam angles, i.e. >64-slice CT.)
- Radiation dose high for retrospectively gated images (10–18mSv), but lower for prospectvely gated imaging (3–5mSv).
- Temporal and spatial resolutions inferior to coronary angiography.

Some of these issues have been addressed by increasing the number of detector rows still further (see 📖 Detectors, p. 15), or by using dual-source (see 📖 Dual-source CT, p. 44) or single heartbeat acquisition (see 📖 Single heartbeat CT, p. 46) CT technology.

Cardiac CT with >64 slices

256-slice CT

Currently the only commercially available 256-slice CT scanner (Philips) has a 128-detector configuration with double sampling (see 📖 Detectors data channels, and slices, p. 18). Air bearings allow a rapid gantry rotation time of 0.27s, giving a temporal resolution of 135ms (Table 4.1). The unit is larger than a typical 64-slice scanner due to the wider detector array and the need to withstand the high g-forces generated by rapid gantry rotation.

z-axis coverage is double (8cm) that of a typical 64-slice scanner, but still short enough to require at least two gantry rotations to cover the heart completely, ∴ images may still be susceptible to step and misregistration artefacts (see 📖 Partial volume effect, p. 154). However, as fewer overlapping slices are required to cover the heart, scan acquisition time is reduced.

320-slice CT

The only commercially available 320 detector scanner (Toshiba) has an ultrawide detector width of 16cm (320 × 0.5mm), which is wide enough to cover the entire heart in a single rotation without the need to move the patient through the gantry. The 350ms gantry rotation time gives a temporal resolution of 175ms (Table 4.1) using half-scan reconstruction (see 📖 Temporal resolution, p. 28). The scanner has several technological advantages:

- *Low radiation dose*: Single-rotation cardiac acquisition allows a complete dataset to be obtained in a single prospective 'pulse'. As there is no need for overlap between successive rotations, radiation dose is reduced (typically 1–3mSv).
- *Arrhythmia management:* Single-rotation cardiac acquisition enables the scanner to 'wait' for an appropriately long R–R interval before the acquisition 'pulse'. This allows a static, isophasic dataset in all patients providing ventricular rate is well controlled (heart rate <70bpm).
- *Prospective single-beat functional analysis:* Ultrawide detector array allows acquisition of functional data from all phases of the cardiac cycle using only a single heartbeat.

However, there are also several disadvantages:
- The wide cone-beam angle (>14°) requires substantial computer processing power to produce artefact-free images, particularly to correct for scatter.
- Very wide detectors are substantially heavier than conventional detectors, resulting in higher centrifugal forces during rotation.
- As a result, temporal resolution (see 📖 Temporal resolution, p. 28) is limited to 175ms, restricting single-beat prospective scanning to patients with heart rate <65bpm.

Table 4.1 Comparison of commercially available cardiac CT scanners

Type of scanner	Temporal resolution (ms)	Spatial resolution (mm)	z-axis coverage (mm)	Minimum acquisition time for cardiac CT (s)
64-slice	165–200	0.5–0.625	32–40	5–10
64-slice dual source	83	$0.5 \times 0.5 \times 0.6$	32	4
256-slice (Philips)	135	0.625	80	2–4
320-slice (Toshiba)	175	0.5	160	1–2

Dual-source CT

Dual-source CT (DSCT) was designed to overcome the limitation in gantry rotation time by doubling the number of X-ray sources and detectors (Fig. 4.1). By mounting two X-ray sources and detector arrays at an angle of ~90° on the rotating gantry, data acquisition may be achieved in around a quarter of the gantry rotation time. This has the effect of doubling temporal resolution compared to standard MSCT. For example, a dual-source scanner with a gantry rotation time of 330ms will have a temporal resolution of 83ms. Several studies have shown the value of DSCT in producing diagnostic image quality irrespective of the heart rate.[1–] DSCT may achieve adequate image quality in patients with heart rates up to 100bpm, potentially obviating β-blockade. In practice, however, dual-source image quality is still improved if the heart rate is controlled.

Dual-source data are acquired simultaneously in the same relative phase of a patient's cardiac cycle and at the same anatomical level. The two rows of detectors in DSCT tend to vary in the area of their coverage. For example, the 1° detector array may cover the entire field of view (FOV; about 50cm), whilst the other is restricted to a smaller central FOV. The radiation burden from DSCT is roughly equivalent to a similar single-source MSCT acquisition.

Another important feature of DSCT is that the voltage and current (see 📖 X-ray tube current, p. 22) of each X-ray tube can be varied individually, allowing dual-energy CT (DECT) scans to be performed. This technique uses the phenomenon that tissues attenuate X-ray beams of different energies to differing degrees, depending on their density. Although not extensively validated, cardiac applications of DECT potentially include digital subtraction of calcium from coronary arteries (although spatial resolution is currently a limiting factor) and characterization of myocardial enhancement patterns (see 📖 Evaluation of myocardial scarring and perfusion, p. 259).

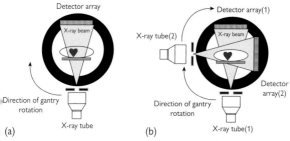

Fig. 4.1 Comparison of (a) single-source and (b) dual-source CT. Doubling the number of X-ray tube/detector array pairs reduces the arc required to obtain an image to 90°, thus improving temporal resolution two-fold.

Further reading

Achenbach S, Ropers D, Kuettner A, *et al.* (2006) Contrast-enhanced coronary artery visualization by dual-source computed tomography—initial experience. *Eur J Radiol* **57**(3), 331–335.

Johnson TR, Nikolaou K, Wintersperger BJ, *et al.* (2006) Dual-source CT cardiac imaging: initial experirence.*Eur Radiol* **16**(7), 1409–1415.

Scheffel H, Alkadhi H, Plass A, *et al.* (2006) Accuracy of dual-source CT coronary angiography: First experience in a high pre-test probability population without heart rate control. *Eur Radiol* **16**(12), 2739–2747.

Single heartbeat CT

In order to acquire CCT images within a single heartbeat, a high pitch (see 📖 Scan pitch, p. 24) is required to obtain complete cardiac coverage within the specified time window. The required pitch is generally too high for retrospectively-gated 64-slice CT as it leads to insufficient sampling along the z-axis, resulting in data gaps and problems with image reconstruction. Current 64-slice CT is ∴ limited to acquisitions taken over >1 heartbeat.

Scanners featuring wider detector arrays (128-, 256-, and 320-slice scanners) and dual-source technology allow the use of higher scan pitches (>3). Wider detector arrays may allow complete cardiac coverage in a single rotation. In the case of dual-source technology, z-axis sampling is ↑, allowing a faster spiral acquisition and thus the high pitch required to acquire images within a single heartbeat. The entire cardiac dataset may be acquired in as little as 280ms.

Such capabilities are achieved in a variety of ways depending on scanner manufacturer (e.g. Flash CT, Siemens Medical Solutions), but all allow prospectively gated acquisitions within a single heartbeat. The radiation dose associated with single-heartbeat acquistions is very low, typically 1–5mSv depending on X-ray tube settings. Exposures of <1mSv may be possible if the tube voltage is reduced to 100kV.

Single-heartbeat CT is not suitable for all patients. To ensure high-quality scans, the heart rate should be <65bpm and ideally 60bpm, so β-blockade may be required (see 📖 Heart-rate control, p. 78). Patients with irregular heart rhythms should undergo standard retrospectively gated CCT, and for others the standard weaknesses of prospectively gated acquisitions (see 📖 ECG gating (2), p. 34) apply (inability to review other cardiac phases, no functional ventricular assessment possible).

Future technology

256-slice, 320-slice, and DSCT scanners represent significant advances in cardiac CT imaging. However, motion artefact from ectopics and atrial fibrillation, blooming artefact from stents and heavily calcified vessels, and relatively high radiation doses remain clinical concerns. Future innovations addressing these three issues may include the following.

Motion artefact

- Triple-source CT will further improve temporal resolution, allowing imaging of patients with higher heart rates.

Radiation dose

- Automatic patient-centring techniques will reduce radiation exposure, particularly to the breasts.
- Organ-based automatic exposure control will reduce radiation exposure to the breasts by reducing the tube current during the anterior projection.

Blooming artefacts

- May be partly addressed by high spatial resolution algorithms or iterative reconstruction technology (although the latter involves substantial computing power).
- Dual-energy CT combined with edge-enhancing image reconstruction filters can reduce overestimation of calcium volume.

Advances in scanner technology

- Flat-panel MSCT scanners: improved spatial resolution (0.2mm compared with 0.4mm) and wider coverage, although current gantry rotation times are very slow (2s) and contrast resolution is limited (5–10 Hounsfield units (HU)).
- Although it does not yet match MSCT, there is the potential for further advances in electron-beam CT, especially given its superior temporal resolution.

The ability to acquire isophasic data for the entire heart and coronary arteries during a single heartbeat offers new possibilities for dynamic imaging, such as the assessment of true myocardial perfusion (acquiring blocks of data at multiple time points during contrast injection at rest and during adenosine stress). This might allow high-resolution anatomical imaging of the coronary arteries combined with functional evaluation of stenoses at acceptable levels of radiation exposure (<15mSv). Combined anatomical and functional assessment is already possible using image fusion software to combined cardiac CT and single-photon emission CT (SPECT) or or positron emission tomography (PET) perfusion datasets.

Radiation physics, biology, and protection

Interactions of X-rays with matter

X-rays are a type of ionizing radiation, which means that they have sufficient energy to eject an orbital electron from an atom. The ionization of an atom results in an ion pair: a positive ion (the atom) and a negative 'ion' (the electron). X-rays interact with atoms in three ways: photoelectric effect, Compton (or incoherent) scatter and Rayleigh (or coherent) scatter.

Photoelectric effect
- The X-ray photon transfers all of its energy to an inner shell electron.
- The X-ray photon is absorbed.
- The electron is ejected from the atom and carries away the surplus energy.
- The atom is ionized.
- Electrons in higher shells descend energy levels to fill the vacant inner shell; characteristic X-rays or Auger electrons may be emitted in the process.

Compton (or incoherent) scatter
- The X-ray photon transfers some of its energy to an outer shell electron.
- The X-ray photon loses energy and changes direction.
- The electron is ejected from the atom and carries away the energy transferred from the X-ray photon.
- The atom is ionized.
- The collision between a moving and a stationary billiard ball provides a good analogy.

Rayleigh (or coherent) scatter
- The X-ray photon resonates with the atom's electron cloud.
- The X-ray photon changes direction but does not lose energy.
- The atom is not ionized.

Dominant interactions
- The number of photoelectric interactions decreases with X-ray energy and increases with the cube of the atomic number of the material.
- The number of scatters decreases with X-ray energy and is independent of atomic number (as scatter involves only outer-shell electrons).
- At the X-ray energies used for CT imaging, scatter dominates in soft tissues and the photoelectric effect dominates in bone, in the detector array, and in lead.

Biological effects of ionizing radiation

Ionizing radiation can damage biological tissue by ionizing DNA directly or by ionizing water molecules to form free radicals, which in turn react with DNA. DNA repair mechanisms exist that are generally extremely effective. However, they can be overwhelmed by exposures to high doses and to high dose rates. Errors in DNA repair lead to mutations, which may be carcinogenic.

Two types of biological effect are observed in tissue.

Deterministic effects (tissue reactions)

- Acute onset.
- Observed when the radiation dose exceeds a given threshold. As the dose increases above the threshold, the probability of occurrence increases rapidly to 100%.
- The severity of the reaction increases with radiation dose.
- Examples of tissue reactions are given in Table 5.1.
- Tissue reactions have been documented in interventional radiology, cardiac X-ray imaging, and CT.

Stochastic effects (carcinogenic and heritable effects)

- Observed some time after the exposure: 2 years for leukaemias and one or two decades for solid cancers.
- The risk of cancer induction increases with radiation dose (Fig. 5.1). For radiation protection purposes the linear no-threshold model is used, which assumes that cancer risk is proportional to radiation dose. This is the basis for ensuring that radiation exposure is 'as low as reasonably achievable' (ALARA).
- However, current evidence suggests that:
  - Above 100mSv the risk of cancer induction increases following a linear or a linear-quadratic relationship.
  - Below 100mSv the risk of cancer induction cannot be demonstrated unequivocally because the additional cancer incidence attributable to radiation is of the order of the uncertainty in the data.
- Radiobiological studies suggest that a threshold exists around 100mSv, below which no cancer risk exists because of the effectiveness of repair mechanisms.
- The risk of cancer induction depends on the age of the individual: it is about three times higher for babies than for adults. A risk coefficient

Table 5.1 Estimated dose thresholds for 1% incidence of radiation-induced tissue reactions[1]

Tissue injury	Dose threshold (Gy)
Skin erythema	3–6
Cataract	1.5
Hair loss	4
Skin burns	5–10

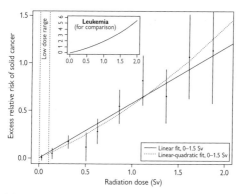

Fig. 5.1 Relationship between additional cancer risk and radiation dose. Reprinted with permission from the National Academic Press, Copyright 2006, National Academy of Sciences.

Table 5.2 Effective doses and risk estimates for imaging exams relevant to cardiology

Cardiac exam	Effective dose (mSv)	Radiological risk
Chest X-ray	0.02	1 in 1,000,000
Cardiac catheterisation[2]	7	1 in 2,800
Tc-99m myocardial imaging[3]	4–10	1 in 2,000–5,000
Tl-201 myocardial imaging[3]	14–21	1 in 950–1,400
Cardiac CT[4]	9–19	1 in 1,000–2,000

The ranges provided depend on the exact protocol used.

of 5×10^{-5} per mSv is often used as a rule of thumb for the general population.
● The risk of heritable effects has not yet been demonstrated.
Table 5.2 provides risk estimates for typical exams relevant to cardiology. Note that the effective doses are less than 100mSv.

Further reading

1 International Commission on Radiological Protection (2007) The 2007 Recommendations of the International Commission on Radiological Protection. ICRP Publication 103. *Ann ICRP* **37**(2–4), 1–332.
2 Hart D and Wall BF (2002) Radiation exposure of the UK population from medical and dental x-ray examinations. Report NRPB-W4. National Radiological Protection Board, Chilton.
3 Administration of Radioactive Substances Advisory Committee (2006) Notes for guidance on the clinical administration of radiopharmaceuticals and use of sealed radioactive sources. Health Protection Agency, Chilton.
4 Hausleiter J, Meyer T, Hermann F et al. (2009) Estimated radiation dose associated with cardiac CT angiography. *JAMA* **301**(5), 500–507.

Radiation dosimetry (1)

Absorbed dose

Absorbed dose, D, is the energy absorbed per unit mass. The SI unit is the gray (Gy).

Equivalent dose

Equivalent dose, H_T, is a measure of the biological damage caused to tissue by a given absorbed dose. The SI unit is the sievert (Sv). Equivalent dose takes into account both the harmfulness of the radiation and the radiosensitivity of the tissue. It is given by

$$H_T = w_R w_T D$$

where w_R is the radiation weighting factor and w_T is the tissue weighting factor. These weighting factors were set by the International Commission on Radiological Protection (ICRP) in 1990 and reviewed in 2007. w_R is 1.0 for X-rays and electrons. w_T ranges between 0.01 and 0.2.

Effective dose

Effective dose is the sum of 5×the equivalent doses for all irradiated organs. The SI unit is the sievert. The effective dose can be thought of as the whole-body radiation dose that would carry the same radiological risk as that from the exam, ∴ effective dose is useful for comparing different types of exposures, e.g. coronary CT coronary angiography and thallium scans, in a single patient cohort. Effective dose can, however, be misleading when comparing different patient cohorts, e.g. if they are characterized by different age and sex distributions. Effective dose will be numerically different depending on whether the ICRP 1990 or 2007 tissue weighting factors are used.

CT dose index

The CT dose index (CTDI) is given by

$$CTDI = 1/(nT) \int D_z dz$$

where D_z is the dose profile along the axis of rotation, integrated over ±50mm, and nT is the nominal X-ray beam collimation (Fig. 5.2).
   ⚠ CTDI works well for beam collimations up to about 40mm, but underestimates radiation dose for beam collimations greater than 40mm. A revised definition of or substitute for CTDI is currently being sought by the medical physics community. CTDI can be measured free in air or in standard head and body CT dose phantoms (Fig, 5.3), which are 16 and 32cm in diameter, respectively, and made of Perspex.

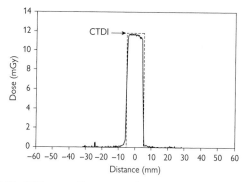

Fig. 5.2 The CTDI concept. The curve is a radiation dose profile that represents the dose received as a function of distance along the z-axis of the patient. The CTDI is given by the area under this curve.

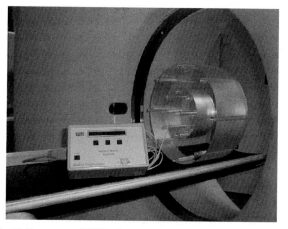

Fig. 5.3 Measurement of CTDI in the standard body phantom. The head phantom doubles up as the central section.

Radiation dosimetry (2)

Weighted CTDI

The weighted CTDI ($CTDI_w$) is given by:

$$CTDI_w = 1/3\,CTDI_c + 2/3\,CTDI_p$$

where $CTDI_c$ and $CTDI_p$ are the CTDI values measured at the centre and periphery of the CT dose phantom, respectively. $CTDI_w$ is an indicator of the average absorbed dose in the irradiated volume per gantry rotation.

Volumetric CTDI

The volumetric CTDI ($CTDI_{vol}$) is given by

$$CTDI_{vol} = CTDI_w \times p$$

where p is the pitch in spiral scanning (see 📖 Technical principles of cardiovascular CT, p. 21) or the table feed/X-ray beam collimation in axial scanning. $CTDI_{vol}$ is an indicator of the average absorbed dose in the irradiated volume per scan.

Dose–length product

The dose–length product (DLP) is given by

$$DLP = CTDI_{vol} \times R$$

where R is the irradiated length of the patient. DLP can be empirically related to effective dose E (ICRP 1990 definition) using the following expression:

$$E = c_k \times DLP$$

where c_k is a conversion coefficient, tabulated in Table 5.3 for a standard 70kg subject.

Table 5.3 Conversion coefficients for a standard 70 kg subject

Region of body	Effective dose per DLP (mSv/(mGy cm))
Head and neck	0.0031
Head	0.0021
Neck	0.0059
Chest	0.014
Abdomen and pelvis	0.015
Trunk	0.015

These conversion factors must not be used to calculate radiation dose in individual patients as they do not account for variations in size and anatomy.

Principles of radiation protection

The objective of radiation protection is to provide a level of protection for people and the environment without unnecessarily constraining the benefits of the practices requiring exposure to radiation.

International radiation protection advice

The ICRP has formulated three principles of radiation protection to ensure good practice.

Justification (see 📖 *Justification and authorization, p. 70*)

- A decision that changes the existing radiation exposure situation should do more good than harm.
- Both patient and staff exposures need to be justified.
- A patient exposure can be justified when the benefit to the patient from the clinical information gleaned exceeds the radiation risk. In reaching the decision to proceed, all applicable imaging options must be considered.

Optimization

- Radiation exposures must be ALARA, taking societal and economic factors into account.
- Both patient and staff exposures need to be optimized.
- Patient exposures are optimized by managing the radiation dose so that it is appropriate to the diagnostic task.
  - Diagnostic reference levels provide a benchmark for deciding if patient doses are consistent with good clinical practice. They can ∴ be used to prioritize reviews of scan protocols.
- Staff radiation exposures are reduced by managing patient doses effectively and considering:
  - Time—minimizing the length of the exposure
  - Distance—maximizing the distance from the X-ray tube and the patient
  - Shielding—shielding X-ray rooms and using personal protective equipment such as lead aprons when required.

Limitation

- ICRP specifies dose limits for staff and members of the public.
- The dose limits recommended by ICRP should not be exceeded in planned situations.

Radiation legislation in the UK

Two pieces of radiation legislation apply to cardiac CT. They are identified and summarized below.

Ionizing Radiations Regulations 1999

- Address the protection of workers and the public.
- Enforced by the Health and Safety Executive.
- Identify the control hierarchy required to ensure the radiological safety of individuals.
- The employer and the employee are the duty holders.
- A radiation protection adviser and a radiation protection supervisor are required to assist the employer in the discharge of their duties.

Ionizing Radiation (Medical Exposures) Regulations 2000
- Address the protection of patients and individuals undergoing medical exposures for diagnosis, treatment, screening, and research.
- Enforced by the Department of Health.
- Identify the procedures and staff training required to ensure the radiological safety of patients and individuals undergoing medical exposures.
- The employer, the referrer, the practitioner, and the operator are the duty holders.
- A medical physics expert is required to provide advice on optimization.

Patient dose and scanner design

Patient radiation dose is intrinsically linked to the design and performance of the CT scanner. Some scanner features have a greater effect on patient dose than others.

Temporal resolution

- Temporal resolution is determined by the number of X-ray sources in the scanner, the rotation time, and the reconstruction mode (single- or multi-phase) (see 📖 Technical principles of cardiovascular CT, p. 21).
- Dual-source scanners have intrinsically better temporal resolution than single-source ones, without implications for patient dose.
- Shorter rotation times improve temporal resolution without affecting the radiation dose if tube current and exposure time are unchanged.
- Multiphase reconstructions incur a dose penalty over single-phase ones because they require projection data to be acquired using retrospective ECG gating.

Tube current modulation

The tube current can be adjusted in a variety of ways (see 📖 X-ray tube current, p. 22):

- According to patient size
- Along the z-axis of the patient, i.e. higher current when covering a region of particular interest (e.g. heart) but lower current elsewhere
- As a function of angular position of the X-ray tube
- As a function of cardiac phase (ECG-correlated mA pulsing (see 📖 X-ray tube current, p. 22)).

The way in which these features are implemented depends on the CT manufacturer. In cardiac CT, it is usual for the tube current to be adjusted only according to the size of the patient and the cardiac phase. The target image quality is specified on the scanner console using a variety of image quality indicators (Table 5.4). In order for tube current modulation to work properly, the patient must be centred in the scan plane.

Detector coverage

- Detector coverage has a modest influence on patient dose. Effects are more noticeable on prospective than on retrospective ECG-gated CT.
- With narrow detector coverage, e.g. 40mm:
  - The scan range can be tailored to the subject's heart
  - The table feed may be less than the X-ray beam width, so images at the X-ray beam edges can be reconstructed and stitched together
  - A small dose penalty is incurred.
- With intermediate detector coverage, e.g. 80mm:
  - The scan range cannot be easily tailored to the subject's heart
  - The table feed will be less than the X-ray beam width
  - A modest dose penalty is incurred.
- With wide detector coverage, e.g. 160mm:
  - The heart is covered in one rotation with no table feed, but over-ranging is required to reconstruct the peripheral portions of the scan (see below)

- No adjustment of scan range to heart size can be made
- A modest dose penalty is incurred.

X-ray beam collimation

The X-ray beam is wider than the active detector length to ensure uniform irradiation of all the detector elements. This is called over-beaming. The excess radiation dose associated with it can be minimized by selecting the widest possible X-ray beam collimation compatible with the required slice thickness.

Adaptive collimation

In helical scanning, more of the patient is irradiated than is imaged along the z-axis. This is called over-ranging and is necessary to reconstruct the first and last slices. Adaptive collimators cut off the trailing edge of the X-ray beam at the start of the helical scan and the leading edge at the end of the scan, as these parts of the beam are not needed for reconstruction. Small dose savings are achievable.

Table 5.4 Image quality indicators used with tube current modulation

Manufacturer	Tube current prescription	Image quality indicator
GE	mAs	Noise index
Philips	mAs per slice	mAs per slice
Siemens	mAs (axial), effective mAs (helical)	Quality reference mAs
Toshiba	mAs	Noise in virtual image

Scan parameters and radiation dose

The scan technique and protocol selected are the principal determinants of the radiation dose delivered to the patient.

Effect of scan technique on patient dose

Prospective ECG-gated CT with step-and-shoot acquisition

- Dose-efficient because most of the projection data acquired contribute to the images.
- The patient dose is mainly determined by the mAs chosen and the degree of temporal padding (see 📖 ECG gating (2), p. 34) prescribed.

Prospective ECG-gated CT with fast helical acquisition

- Dose-efficient because most of the projection data acquired contribute to the images.
- The patient dose is mainly determined by the mAs prescribed.

Retrospective ECG-gated CT

- Dose-inefficient because considerable redundancy in the projection data is necessary for multi-phase reconstruction; doses are typically three to five times greater than for prospective ECG-gated CT.
- The patient dose is mainly determined by the mAs chosen, the degree of ECG-correlated mA pulsing (see 📖 ECG gating (2), p. 34), and possibly the helical pitch.

Scan settings that affect patient dose

Exposure parameters

- Tube voltage (see 📖 X-ray tube voltage, p. 23): Patient dose increases approximately in proportion to the square of the tube voltage (e.g. –120kV → 100kV results in ~40%↓ dose).
- Tube current, rotation time, mAs, effective mAs, or mAs per slice (see 📖 X-ray tube current, p. 22): Patient dose increases linearly with these parameters.

Helical pitch

- For scanners that specify mAs, patient dose varies inversely with pitch if the mAs is constant.
- For scanners that specify effective mAs or mAs per slice, patient dose is independent of pitch if the mAs indicator is constant.
- Note that for retrospectively gated scans the prescribed pitch increases with heart rate, and ∴ patient dose might be affected (it might decrease).

Field of view

In prospectively gated CT, larger FOVs may require a smaller table feed between rotations, resulting in an increase in patient dose.

Slice thickness

A four-fold increase in mAs is required for the noise in a 0.6mm slice to match that in a 1.2mm slice because image noise is inversely proportional to the square root of the slice thickness (see 📖 Detector terminology, p. 16). However, a more modest increase in mAs is often sufficient because the superior spatial resolution of thin slices compensates for the increase in image noise.

ECG-correlated mA pulsing

- In prospectively ECG-gated CT with step-and-shoot acquisition, patient dose is ↑ in proportion to the additional mAs delivered during temporal padding (see 📖 ECG gating (2), p. 34).
- In retrospective ECG-gated CT, reductions in patient dose of about 37% can be achieved with ECG-correlated mA pulsing.[1]

Further reading

1 Shrimpton PC, Hillier MC, Lewis MA, Dunn M (2005) Doses from computed tomography (CT) examinations in the UK. 2003 review, Report NRPB-W67. National Radiological Protection Board, Chilton.

Radiation dose management

Radiation dose management is underpinned by patient dose audit. Once typical doses for a standard 70-kg patient are available, local practice can be compared against national guidelines and/or the scientific literature. The outcome of the review will determine whether or not optimization is required.

Patient dose audit
- A sample of about 60 examinations is desirable.
- The following information for each exam is required:
  - Patient demographics (sex, height, weight)
  - $CTDI_{vol}$ and DLP (see 📖 Radiation dosimetry, p. 56) for each scan series
  - Total DLP.
- Data for patients with weight in the range 60–80kg or body mass index (BMI) 20–30 are selected.
- The median $CTDI_{vol}$ and DLP for each series (i.e. the components of the examination—control scan, test bolus, main acquisition, etc (see 📖 Scan protocols, p. 100)) and the median examination DLP are calculated.
- The median $CTDI_{vol}$ for the complete examination is obtained by summing the median $CTDI_{vol}$ values for each scan series.

Diagnostic reference levels
- The median examination $CTDI_{vol}$ and DLP can be compared with the scientific literature, taking care to match the scan technique; they can also be compared with national diagnostic reference levels (DRLs) as they become available.
- The median examination $CTDI_{vol}$ and DLP values can be set as the departmental DRLs for cardiac CT as a benchmark for future audits.
- To estimate the effective dose (E) to a representative 70-kg subject, the following formula may be used:

$$E \text{ (mSv)} = 0.0014 \times DLP \text{ (mGycm)}$$

☞ The conversion coefficient of 0.0014[1] applies to thoracic CT, not cardiac CT, and changes from time to time. Nevertheless it is liberally adopted in the scientific literature. It must not be used for individual patient calculations as body size and weight are rarely comparable to the 'representative' 70-kg subject for whom the co-efficient is valid.

When doses are too high or too low
Causes can be identified by considering the following:
- Similarity of patient cohort to that in the reference data
- Similarity of scan technique
- Number and types of series in the scan sequence
- Type and use of tube current modulation (see 📖 ECG gating (2), p. 34), particularly ECG-correlated mA pulsing
- Local expertise: patient doses tend to be lower at specialist centres.

Variation of dose descriptors with patient size

- The variation of $CTDI_{vol}$ with patient size provides an insight into how the tube current modulation is behaving.
- Figs 5.4 and 5.5 show plots of $CTDI_{vol}$ against patient cross-section for scan protocols where the tube current modulation with patient size is disabled and enabled, respectively.

⚠ In adult scan protocols, the scanner console displays $CTDI_{vol}$ and DLP values as calculated for the CT body phantom, not for the patient being scanned. True values depend on the difference between the patient and the phantom: smaller patients receive a higher radiation dose than that displayed, whilst for larger patients the dose will be lower.

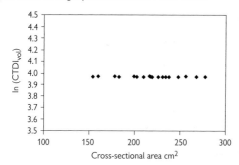

Fig. 5.4 Relationship between $CTDI_{vol}$ and patient size when tube current modulation is disabled. Exposure is the same regardless of the size of the patient.

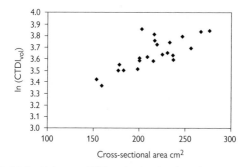

Fig. 5.5 Relationship between $CTDI_{vol}$ and patient size when tube current modulation is enabled. Tube current increases automatically for patients with larger cross-sectional areas, improving image quality.

Further reading

Shrimpton PC, Hillier MC, Lewis MA, Dunn M (2005) Doses from computed tomography (CT) examinations in the UK. 2003 review, Report NRPB-W67. National Radiological Protection Board, Chilton.

Radiation dose optimization techniques

When a patient dose audit indicates that patient doses are significantly higher (or lower) than accepted clinical practice, a review of the scan protocols, scanning techniques, and staff training is indicated.

Review of local practices

- Tailor the ECG-gating technique and the use of ECG-correlated mA pulsing to each patient by considering the clinical information required, the heart rate, and the presence of arrhythmias.
- Tailor the scan range and FOV to each patient; note that in retrospectively ECG-gated CT the irradiated length may be up to 6cm longer than the imaged length due to helical over-ranging.
- Review how the contrast bolus is administered; tube output may have been altered with the intention of improving image quality when the 1° problem was instead related to sub-optimal contrast timing.
- Scan protocols must be size-specific; this is achievable by activating tube current modulation with patient size or setting mAs according to patient weight or BMI.
- If the dose indicators are acceptable but the images are noisy, review the reconstruction algorithms (see 🕮 Convolution filters and kernels, p. 134) selected.
- Reduce the tube voltage to 100kVp for small and medium-sized patients: iodine contrast agent is more conspicuous at lower tube voltages; increase the mAs modestly to compensate for the increase in image noise (the prescribed CTDI$_{vol}$ should still be lower at 100kVp than at 120kVp). ⚠ For large patients low X-ray transmission will result in image artifacts at 100kVp.
- The CTDI$_{vol}$ and DLP predicted for the scan should be used to determine the effect of dose reduction measures *before* the scan takes place.

Education and training

- During equipment procurement, a thorough knowledge of the operation of the CT scanner must be gained as some aspects of patient dose optimization are intrinsically linked to scanner design; the local medical physics expert can provide impartial advice on technical performance and its impact on patient doses if he or she is involved in the evaluation process.
- Application training provides vital information for protocol optimization.
- The local medical physics expert will be able to provide further advice based on commissioning data.

Transferring protocols between scanners

⚠ When setting up scan protocols on a new scanner in the department, or implementing peer-reviewed scan protocols, protocol details must not be copied directly from the reference scanner. This is possible only between scanners of the same model. The following approach can be safely adopted instead:

- In collaboration with the medical physics expert, set up a scan protocol with tube voltage, rotation time, slice thickness, X-ray collimation, FOV, and ECG-correlated mA pulsing comparable to the reference scanner.
- Adjust the mAs until the predicted $CTDI_{vol}$ is comparable to that of the reference scanner; a phantom might be needed at this stage.
- Reconstruct the image data using a variety of different kernels (see 📖 Convolution filters and kernels, p. 134). Select the one that best matches the image quality achievable by the reference scanner.
- Conduct a patient dose audit—compare the $CTDI_{vol}$, DLP, and the behaviour of $CTDI_{vol}$ with patient size with values for the reference scanner.

Practical aspects of cardiovascular CT

Justification and authorization

In order for a cardiovascular CT scan to be performed, a referral must be sent to the appropriate practitioner. This practitioner remains ultimately responsible for the conduct and reporting of the test and must ∴ evaluate each referral for appropriateness. This evaluation is referred to as justification and authorization.

Justification occurs in two steps:
- Generic justification is provided by professional bodies in the form of evidence-based guidelines for referral to cardiovascular CT (see 📖 Guidelines, accreditation, and certification, p. 455).
- Individual justification is provided by the Ionising Radiation (Medical Exposure) Regulations (IRMER) practitioner based on the information supplied by the referring clinician.

Individual justification requires the following to be considered.

Is a cardiovascular CT scan needed?

The answer to this question will have the largest impact on the radiation dose to the patient.

What information is already available?

A high coronary calcium score might be a contraindication to cardiac CT (see 📖 Quantifying luminal stenosis, p. 200).

Are there alternative imaging techniques?

Techniques that provide the required clinical information at a lower radiation dose to the patient must be considered as part of the justification process:
- Echocardiography (see 📖 Echocardiography, p. 482)—does not use ionizing radiation
- Magnetic resonance imaging (see 📖 Cardiovascular magnetic resonance imaging, p. 488)—does not use ionizing radiation
- Nuclear cardiology (see 📖 Myocardial perfusion single photon emission CT (1), p. 472).

Which cardiovascular CT protocol?

The radiation dose varies between scan techniques, as shown in Table 6.1, and is particularly influenced by the decision to use prospective or retrospective ECG gating (see 📖 ECG gating (1), p. 32). In general

Table 6.1 Typical effective doses for cardiac CT scans in 2010[1,2]

Cardiovascular CT scan	Effective dose mSv*	Clinical information provided
Coronary calcium score	1	Coronary calcium score
Prospective ECG-gated CTA (step-and-shoot and fast helical acquisitions)	1–3	Coronary arteries
Retrospective ECG-gated CTA with ECG-correlated mA pulsing	7–12	Coronary arteries
Retrospective ECG-gated CTA without ECG-correlated mA pulsing	12–30	Coronary arteries, wall motion, ejection fraction, valve motility

*The scan projection radiograph (topogram, see Scan protocols, p. 99) adds about 0.2mSv to the effective doses quoted.

The more clinical information yielded by the CT scan, the greater the radiation dose associated with it.

What is the total radiation burden?

The patient's clinical work-up should be efficacious not only in terms of the clinical information gained but the radiation burden accrued. For example, there is no point in performing a cardiac CTA if a cardiac catheterization is required.

If the scan is felt to be justified clinically, the referral is authorized and the patient sent an appointment.

Further reading

Alkadhi H (2009) Radiation dose of cardiac CT—what is the evidence? *Eur Radiol* **19**, 1311–1315.
Hausleiter J, Meyer T, Hermann F, et al. (2009) Estimated radiation dose associated with cardiac CT angiography. *JAMA* **301**(5), 500–507.

Patient selection

When justified and authorized, the technical suitability of a patient for CT coronary angiography is determined by a number of factors.

Patient size
- Very heavy patients may require X-ray beam energies that exceed the rating of the X-ray tube in order to achieve adequate signal-to-noise ratio (see 📖 Large patients, p. 120). Dose limitations may apply and image quality will be poor.

Heart rate
- Ideal with regular heart rates <65bpm (see 📖 Heart-rate control, p. 78).
- Relatively contraindicated if significant dysrhythmia.

Cardiovascular status
- The presence of heart block or history of cardiac transplant are contraindications to β-blockade (see 📖 Heart-rate control, p. 78).

Respiratory status
- Depending on z-axis coverage (see 📖 Detectors, p. 15), breath-holding of up to 20s may be required for CT coronary angiography.
- Moderate to severe obstructive airways disease is a contraindication to β-blockade, and other rate-controlling agents may be used (see 📖 Heart-rate control, p. 78).

Suitability for iodinated contrast
- Absolute contraindications include previous severe contrast reaction. Recognition and management of adverse contrast reactions are described elsewhere (see 📖 Adverse contrast reactions, p. 92).
- Scanning relatively contraindicated in chronic renal failure, although low-osmolar contrast agents (e.g. Visipaque™) may be used (see 📖 Iodinated contrast media, p. 84).
- Note that metformin no longer needs to be stopped if the patient has normal renal function (see 📖 Intravenous contrast media, p. 83).

Ensure that the patient receives appropriate information for CT coronary angiography (such as a patient information leaflet) prior to the examination date. In most circumstances, this allows identification of potential contraindications to CT prior to arrival in the department. Even if no contraindications exist, the patient will have a better understanding of the procedure and be more likely to adhere to protocol.

Preparing the patient

Prior to arrival

The following information should be discussed with the patient during booking and be provided in the patient information leaflet:

- Caffeine should be avoided for 12h prior to the appointment (risk of tachycardia).
- Oral hydration should be encouraged; patients 'at risk' of contrast nephropathy should follow local protocols for avoidance of contrast nephropathy.
- Medications should be taken as usual.

Length of appointment

The time slot for the CT scan should include adequate patient preparation time prior to the CTA. The following pre-scan procedures should be undertaken: the *patient safety check, discussion of the procedure, cannulation* and *heart-rate control* (see 🕮 Heart-rate control, p. 78) if required. A 30-min appointment is usually sufficient, although departments that use oral agents to control heart rate may ask patients to arrive up to an hour in advance.

Patient safety check

- Patient safety checks and observations should take place in a dedicated room separate from the main waiting area to ensure privacy.
- Checks should include a brief, focused patient history, including family history, current medication, and possibility of pregnancy, where appropriate.
- Suitability for the following agents should also be assessed:
  - Intravenous contrast (NB: Seek specifically risk factors for adverse contrast reactions (see 🕮 Iodinated contrast media, p. 84))
  - Heart-rate controlling agents (see 🕮 Heart-rate control, p. 78) and glyceryl trinitrate (see 🕮 Glyceryl trinitrate, p. 80).
- Baseline observations of heart rate, blood pressure, and oxygen saturations should be recorded to determine suitability for the test and the need for heart-rate control.

The information above is best recorded on a standardized questionnaire/ observation chart (see 🕮 Sample patient observation chart, p. 77). This may then be audited as necessary. After completion of the questionnaire, the patient should be given the opportunity to ask questions about the procedure.

Discussion of procedure

A thorough explanation of the procedure from start to finish will ultimately lead to better quality images. A patient who knows what to expect is more likely to comply with instructions during the procedure and images are more likely to be diagnostic. Mandatory topics to cover include the side-effects of intravenous contrast, the need to adhere to breathing instructions, and the requirement to remain still during scanning.

Intravenous contrast

The rationale, action, and side-effects of intravenous contrast should be explained. The following side-effects are common but transient:

- Body-wide flushing sensation—the patient should be warned that they may feel very hot during injection
- Metallic taste in the mouth
- A feeling of bladder fullness and the need to micturate.

Injection of contrast should be painless; warn the patient to alert the radiographer if pain occurs at the site of injection during contrast administration as this may indicate contrast extravasation (see 📖 Treatment of adverse contrast reactions, p. 97).

Stages of the procedure

A brief explanation should be given of the placements of ECG electrodes and how the ECG triggering is used to produce good-quality images. The necessity for a slow, steady heart rate and the possibility of the use of β-blockade to lower the heart rate should also be discussed.

An explanation of how the scanning table will move and the noise from gantry rotation during acquisition will prepare the patient for the chain of events. If a test bolus is used, this also should be mentioned and a brief explanation of how this information is used to set the main scan may further reduce anxiety.

Compliance with breath-holding is often improved by practising the sequence of instructions used during the scanning. Shallow inspiration and absolute breath-hold is the aim.

Cannulation

Cannulate the patient in the preparation room if possible.

An 18G peripheral intravenous cannula is preferable for intravenous contrast administration, although 20G may be used with caution.

A right antecubital vein is preferred as it offers a more direct route to the heart and avoids streak artefact across the aortic arch, great vessels, and internal mammary artery origins from retained contrast in the left brachiocephalic vein.

Use of central lines should generally be avoided as these may split or rupture with the standard contrast flow rates used in CTA.

Final steps

Before the final acquisition, the following points should be discussed by the radiographer and the supervising physician/radiologist:

Patient observations and risk factors for adverse contrast reactions (see 📖 Adverse contrast reactions, p. 92)

The need for and method of administration of heart-rate control (see 📖 Heart-rate control, p. 78) and glyceryl trinitrate (see 📖 Glyceryl trinitrate, p. 80)

Appropriate CT protocol for scanning the patient.

Sample patient safety questionnaire

Patient safety questionnaire

Name: Height:
Hospital no: Weight:
Date of birth:

As part of your CT scan, you are required to undergo an injection of X-ray contrast dye. Please answer the following questions by circling or ticking the correct response.

YES	NO	Do you have any allergies (drugs, food, latex, or other)? If yes, please specify.
YES	NO	Have you had a previous injection of contrast medium (X-ray dye) for any purpose? If yes, did you have a reaction?
YES	NO	Have you had any previous surgery to your heart?
YES	NO	If you have had an invasive coronary angiogram before, did you have stenting to open up any coronary arteries?
YES	NO	Do you suffer from high blood pressure? If yes, what treatment (drugs) do you take?
YES	NO	Do you have kidney disease?
YES	NO	Are you diabetic? If yes, are you taking metformin?
YES	NO	Do you have asthma? If yes, do you use an inhaler?
YES	NO	Do you have any family history of heart disease?
YES	NO	Do you smoke? How many packs per year?
YES	NO	Have you ever smoked? If yes, how many a day for how many years?
YES	NO	Have you taken Viagra (Sildenafil) or a similar drug within the last 24h?
YES	NO N/A	Is there any possibility you might be pregnant? Please provide the date of your last menstrual period.
YES	NO	Do you consent to the use of your anonymised CT images for research, audit, or teaching?

Patient signature: Date:
Referring Physician:

Sample patient observation chart

Observation chart for adult patients receiving β-blockade ± sublingual GTN for CT coronary angiography

Name: Height:
Hospital no: Weight:
Date of birth:

	Time	HR	BP	SpO$_2$	Supp O$_2$ (L/min)
Baseline Observations					

β-blockade   Contraindications and cautions checked?   ☐

Contraindication: hypotension (blood pressure <90/60mmHg), asthma (bronchospasm), severe peripheral vascular disease, uncontrolled heart failure, sick sinus syndrome, second/third degree heart block

Metoprolol 50mg po	☐	Metoprolol 1mg/mL iv injection		☐
Dose (mg)				
Dose (mg)				

GTN   Contraindications and cautions checked?   ☐

Contraindication: hypersensitivity to nitrates, hypotension (blood pressure <90/60mmHg), use of Viagra (sildenafil), cialis (tadalafil) or Levitra (vardenifil) within last 24h, hypertrophic cardiomyopathy, aortic stenosis, cardiac tamponade, constrictive pericarditis, mitral stenosis, known severe anaemia

800 micrograms (2 puffs) sublingually just prior to CT angio scan		☐
Discharge Observations		

Prescribed by: Given by:
Signature: Signature:

Reversibility of β-blockade

Bradycardia: heart rate <40bpm or <50bpm and symptomatic
- Atropine 600mcg iv every 2–3min up to a maximum of 2400mcg

Persistent bradycardia:
- If metoprolol given: administer im glucagon 2–10mg (1 vial mixed with 5% dextrose)
- And bleep on-call cardiology specialist registrar/resident via switchboard

Heart-rate control

Introduction

Heart-rate control is a crucial step in the acquisition of high-quality CTA. The temporal resolution (see 📖 Temporal resolution, p. 28) of different CT scanners, and thus the extent to which heart rate must be lowered, varies. However, image quality is improved at heart rates between 60 and 65bpm regardless of scanner technology.

In some cases, borderline heart rates (and small fluctuations) may be controlled with arrested inspiration. With this approach it may be possible to lower the heart rate to below 65bpm without the need for pharmacological intervention.

Heart-rhythm control is also obligatory. Prevention of premature ventricular complexes (PVC) is far preferable to trying to edit the ECG (see 📖 ECG interpretation errors, p. 160) in the post-processing phase.

⚠ Cardiac monitoring during administration of rate control therapy is recommended. The administration of rate control therapy should be undertaken by appropriately trained personnel with a full understanding of the patient's underlying diagnoses, past history and current therapy.

β-blockers

Except for the contraindications listed below, β-blockade should be the first-line approach for heart-rate control in CTA. Some operators advocate β-blockers in all patients, while others tailor treatment based on resting heart rate. We suggest that the latter is mandatory but the former optional.

Suggested protocols
- Metoprolol 100mg po 1h prior to CTA
- Metoprolol 50mg po 12h and 1h prior to CTA
- Metoprolol 5mg iv whilst in scanner (titrate in 5mg increments every 2–3min up to 25mg according to heart-rate response)
- Esmolol 500mcg/kg iv whilst in scanner (titrate after 5min).

Depending on expertise, a combination of oral and intravenous beta-blockers can also be used.

⚠ Beta blockers should be used with caution in the following groups:
- Sino-atrial or conducting system disease
- Syncope
- Reversible airways disease
- Heart failure/ventricular dysfunction
- Concomitant rate-slowing medications, especially verapamil
- Known intolerance to β-blockers.

Calcium channel blockers

Short-acting rate-slowing calcium channel blockers (verapamil and diltiazem) have been suggested as an alternative to β-blockers, especially in patients unable to tolerate β-blockers. There is no efficacy data available for these drugs in the setting of CTA. Both agents act on the atrio-ventricular node and are unlikely to have any effect on PVCs.

Suggested protocols
- Verapamil 80–240mg po 1h prior to CTA.
- Diltiazem 60–240mg po 1h prior to CTA.
- Verapamil 2.5–5mg iv whilst in scanner (titrate as necessary every 5min; maximum 15mg).

Ivabradine

Ivabradine is a novel sinus node blocker that works exclusively on the I_f channel. It has been shown to reduce the heart rate in patients with angina. There is interest in its use prior to cardiac CTA and a well-controlled clinical trial is needed.

Suggested protocol
- 5mg orally twice daily for 3 days prior to CTA.
- There is currently no intravenous preparation available.

Lidocaine

Lidocaine is an intravenous sodium channel blocker that is routinely used to suppress PVCs.

Suggested protocol
- Lidocaine 50mg iv bolus; titrate upwards every 3–5min to maximum 200mg or 3mg/kg (whichever is lower).

Treatment of side-effects

All physicians and radiographers undertaking cardiac CTA should be aware of local policies for treating symptomatic bradycardia associated with heart-rate control medications. The following is a guide for the emergency treatment of drug-induced bradycardias:
- Atropine 0.6mg iv bolus; maximum dose 3mg.
- Dobutamine infusion 2.5–20mcg/kg/min.
- Temporary transvenous pacing.

Specific reversal agents
- Glucagon 2–5mg iv bolus; to reverse β-blocker.
- Calcium chloride 10% 10mL over 5min; to reverse Ca^{++} blocker.
- Salbutamol 2.5–5mg nebulized; for bronchospasm.

⚠ Urgent cardiology/medical advice should be obtained, especially if unfamiliar with the management of symptomatic bradycardia.

Glyceryl trinitrate

Mechanism of action
- Metabolized to nitric oxide, a potent vasodilator, by nitric oxide synthase lining the endothelium of blood vessels.

Use in cardiovascular CT
- Vasodilator effect increases coronary artery contrast opacification, improving visualization of distal coronary arteries.
- Most useful in those with small-caliber coronary vessels—smokers, patients with diabetes mellitus, and women.

The use of glyceryl trinitrate (GTN) is not routine in every centre. The main concerns are the potential for reflex tachycardia and hypotension, the latter being of particular concern with co-administration of β-blockade. Such problems are relatively rare but blood pressure monitoring prior to discharge is recommended in all patients receiving GTN.

Contraindications
GTN should be avoided in patients who have taken phosphodiesterase inhibitors (sildenafil, tadalafil, vardenafil, etc.) within the previous 24h as there is the potential for profound hypotension after co-administration. The patient questionnaire should ask specifically about the use of these drugs (see 📖 Sample patient safety questionnaire, p. 76).
　　Further relative contraindications include:
- Hypersensitivity to nitrates
- Hypotension
- Left ventricular outflow tract obstruction (aortic stenosis, hypetrophic cardiomyopathy)
- Cardiac tamponade
- Constrictive pericarditis
- Mitral stenosis
- Known severe anaemia.

Suggested protocol
- 1–2 puffs GTN (400–800mcg) sublingually 1–2min prior to scanning.

Preparing to scan

Setting up the CT equipment

- Load the dual-headed power injector (see 📖 Adminstration of intravenous contrast, p. 88) with contrast and saline as required by the contrast protocol (see 📖 Scan protocols, p. 100).
- Set up the ECG monitoring connections.
- Lay out saline flush and injection tray if required.
- Select appropriate contrast programme on the injector console (see 📖 Adminstration of intravenous contrast, p. 88).

Setting up the patient

- Where possible, the member of staff administering the observation/ check form should accompany the patient into the scanning room. This will ensure continuity in patient contact.
- The radiographer should continue to reassure the patient and recap on the procedure whilst positioning him or her on the scanning table.
- Position the patient feet first or head first on the scanning table, depending on the scanner model and site protocol: in our experience, most patients prefer to see where they are going!
- ECG electrodes should be applied so as to achieve a clear ECG signal. A three-lead ECG is sufficient, with electrodes placed most commonly in the right and left mid-clavicular lines just below each clavicle and at the sixth intercostal space in the mid-clavicular line.
- Points to consider when positioning the ECG electrodes include:
  - Shave the chest if there is excess body hair.
  - Clean and abrade the area if ECG contact with skin is poor.
  - Electrodes and wires should be placed outside the region of interest.
  - If the standard lead positions result in a poor-quality ECG signal, reposition the electrodes wherever necessary to correct this. All that is required is an obvious R-wave to trigger ECG gating (see 📖 ECG gating, p. 32).
- Once a good ECG signal is obtained, ask the patient to raise their arms above their head to avoid scanning through the upper limbs. Try to avoid excessive flexion of the arm with the intravenous cannula to prevent kinking it.
- Move the CT table so that the topogram/scout (see 📖 Scan protocols, p. 100) starts above the lung apices.
- Connect the contrast injector line to the patient, securing the line if necessary.
- Recap the breathing instructions, the expected effects of contrast injection, and the breathing technique practised earlier.
- Having left the scanning room, maintain communication with the patient: this provides reassurance that someone is still there!

Performing the acquisition

- Where possible, maintain direct communication with the patient at all stages of the acquisition.
- Use the images acquired during calcium scoring (see 📖 Coronary artery calcium scoring, p. 106) to determine the start and end positions for the main acquisition. If calcium scoring was not undertaken, a control scan must be performed (see 📖 Scan protocols, p. 99).
- Allowing for variation in the position of the heart during subsequent shallow inspiratory breath-holding, the start position is typically two slices above the origins of the coronary arteries and two slices below the bottom of the heart.
- Set the scan delay for the acquisition using the information gathered from the test bolus/bolus tracking method (see 📖 Optimizing scan timing, p. 102).
- Warn the patient that contrast injection is about to begin, arm the injector, and start the scan simultaneously.
- During acquisition, monitor the ECG, contrast enhancement, and heart rate.
- ⚠ Be prepared to abort the scan and contrast administration if:
  - No contrast is visible on initial real-time images—check connections and enquire about pain at injection site (contrast extravasation; see 📖 Treatment of adverse contrast reactions, p. 96) or
  - Patient demonstrates signs or symptoms of an adverse contrast reaction (see 📖 Adverse contrast reactions, p. 92).

After acquisition is complete

- Check the reconstructed image acquisition before taking the patient off the CT scanning table to establish that coverage and quality are adequate. Consult the supervising radiologist and rescan if necessary.
- Help the patient off the scanner and perform post-scan observations if necessary.
- If large doses of β-blocker have been administered, only discharge the patient if the observations are normal and the patient feels well.
- Remind the patient of the side-effects of β-blockade and the symptoms of delayed contrast reactions (see 📖 Adverse contrast reactions, p. 92). The patient should be instructed to contact the department during working hours or attend either their general practitioner or accident and emergency should they feel unwell out of working hours.

Intravenous contrast media

Iodinated contrast media (1)

Introduction

X-rays are attenuated in proportion to the density of the tissues through which they pass (see 📖 Technical principles of cardiovascular CT, p. 21). Adjacent tissues of considerably different density may be easily distinguished as a result of their natural contrast. However, adjacent soft tissues, such as a coronary artery and the blood within its lumen, have similar densities and are difficult to distinguish by natural contrast alone. In order to assess these tissue components individually, artificial contrast must be created between them. In X-ray CT, this is achieved using iodinated contrast agents.

Chemistry

Virtually all modern iodinated intravenous contrast agents are based on the tri-iodinated benzene ring. Benzene is a toxic lipophilic compound that can be made water soluble through acidification into benzoic acid. As a benzene ring contains six carbon atoms, the introduction of an acid branch onto one carbon atom leaves five others onto which other moieties may be substituted. In contrast agents, iodine is usually added to three, whilst side branches are attached to the other two, subtly altering the toxicity and water solubility. Iodine is ideal for use in contrast agents because it has high contrast density, low toxicity, and binds firmly to the benzene ring.

Properties of contrast agents

Iodinated contrast media have three important properties which balance clinical utility with toxicity: *osmolality*, *viscosity*, and *ionicity*.

Osmolality

This describes the number of contrast molecules per kilogram of water and is closely related to the ionicity (see below). High osmolality contrast media have osmolalities up to seven or eight times that of blood plasma, whilst those of low osmolality are approximately two to three times higher (Table 7.1; see 📖 Iodinated contrast media, p. 84). The likelihood of symptoms during contrast injection (see 📖 Adminstration of intravenous contrast, p. 88), particularly flushing, increases with osmolality. Adverse contrast reactions (see 📖 Adverse contrast reactions, p. 92), such as renal impairment, are also five to ten times more likely to occur with high-osmalality contrast agents. This association has led to the manufacture of *iso-osmolar* contrast agents, which have the same osmolality as plasma.

Viscosity

This describes the 'thickness' of the contrast medium. In practical terms, it determines the maximum rate at which contrast may be injected, which, for CT coronary angiography, is usually of the order of 5–6mL/s. Media that are more viscous are more difficult to inject and more likely to result in adverse contrast reactions.

Ionicity

Contrast media may be either *ionic* or *non-ionic*. A single molecule of ionic contrast medium will dissociate into two equally but oppositely charged particles when in solution. Non-ionic contrast agents do not share this property, remaining as a single electrically neutral molecule in solution. As osmolality is determined by the number of particles, ionic or otherwise, per kilogram of water, ionic contrast agents have at least double the osmolality of similarly structured but non-ionic equivalents.

Contrast agents are usually defined by the number of iodine atoms delivered per contrast molecule in solution. Clinically attractive contrast agents have low osmolality relative to the number of iodine atoms delivered. An ionic contrast agent consisting of a single benzene ring with three iodine atoms would dissociate into two ions and deliver three iodine atoms, resulting in a 2:3 ratio of osmolar components to iodine. A better ratio may be achieved in two ways:
• Use non-ionic contrast agents
• Use dimeric rather than monomeric contrast agents.

Dimeric contrast agents consist of molecules made up of two covalently bonded benzene rings containing six iodine atoms in total. Thus an ionic dimeric agent yields a ratio of 1:3 and a non-ionic dimeric agent a ratio of 1:6. Such agents ∴ represent the optimal balance of osmolality and iodine delivery.

Further reading

Katayama H, Yamaguchi K, Kozuka T, Takashima T, Seez P, Matsuura K (1990) Adverse reactions to ionic and nonionic contrast media. A report from the Japanese Committee on the Safety of Contrast Media. *Radiology* **175**(3), 621–628.

Singh J, Daftary A (2008) Iodinated contrast media and their adverse reactions. *J Nucl Med Technol* **36**(2), 69–74.

Iodinated contrast media (2)

Iodinated contrast media are usually marketed with a brand name followed by a number, e.g. Ultravist 370® (Bayer HealthCare Pharmaceuticals Inc). The number describes the concentration of iodine per millilitre of solution and is usually referred to as the *strength* of the contrast agent. Ultravist 370 ∴ contains 370 milligrams of iodine per millilitre of solution (mgI/mL).

Stronger contrast agents provide better opacification at the expense of higher viscosity and osmolality. This increases the likelihood of side-effects and adverse contrast reactions (see 📖 Adverse contrast reactions, p. 92). Selection of appropriate contrast strength depends on the organ to be imaged. In cardiovascular CT, strengths of 300–370mg/mL are typically used.

Common iodinated contrast agents used in cardiac CT are listed in Table 7.1.

Table 7.1 Common intravenous iodinated contrast agents used in cardiac CT

Type		Composition	Trade Name	Manufacturer	Iodine Concentration (mgI/mL)	Viscosity (cP)[†]	Osmolality (mOsmol/kg water)	Contrast Plasma Osmolality Ratio[‡]
Ionic	Monomer	Diatrizoate	Hypaque	GE Healthcare	370	9	2016	7.1
	Dimer	Ioxaglate	Hexabrix	Guerbet	320	7.5	600	2.1
Non-ionic	Monomer	Iohexol	Ominpaque	GE Healthcare	300	6.1	640	2.2
					350	10.6	780	2.7
		Ioversol	Optiray	Mallinckrodt	350	9	780	2.7
		Iopromide	Ultravist	Bayer Healthcare	300	4.9	607	2.1
					370	10	774	2.7
		Iomperol	Iomeron	Bracco	300	4.3	520	1.8
					350	7	620	2.2
					400	13.6	726	2.5
	Dimer	Iodixanol	Visipaque	GE Healthcare	320	11.8	290	1

[†]At 37°C

[‡]Plasma osmolality 285mOsmol/kg water

Administration of intravenous contrast

Power injectors

Before the introduction of power injectors to routine use, contrast was administered by intravenous infusion or, if a bolus was required, hand injection. Hand injection is problematic for several reasons, the most important being:

- Variable flow rate, depending in particular on the size of the intravenous cannula used
- The need for the injecting member of staff to remain in the scanning room, increasing their risk of radiation exposure
  Power injectors circumvented these issues by providing:
- Consistent flow rates and volumes, which allow better opacification
- Delivery of a tight bolus, maximizing enhancement in the area of interest
- Precise timing of contrast delivery.

Power injectors used in cardiovascular CT consist of a head unit containing two syringes ('double-headed', Fig. 7.1) filled with contrast medium and saline, respectively. The unit is connected to the patient via an administration set and controlled by a console in the control room (Fig. 7.1), allowing specification of contrast and saline flow rates and timing.

Saline flushing

Benefits include:

- Advancement of contrast bolus from the venous to the arterial circulation, improving arterial enhancement and avoiding redundant contrast load
- Reduction of venous enhancement, which decreases the likelihood of streak artefacts from brachiocephalic and superior caval veins; in cardiac CT, dense right ventricular enhancement can cause streak artefacts through the right coronary artery, potentially eroding diagnostic accuracy.

Vascular access

Power injectors are pressure-limited sytems, such that the delivery of contrast at pre-specified flow rates may be impossible if the cannula size is too small. At flow rates typical for cardiovascular CT (5mL/s or greater in adults), a 20G intravenous cannula is the minimum requirement, preferably in an antecubital vein. Injection through smaller cannulae runs the risk of rupture and contrast extravasation (see 📖 Intravenous contrast media, p. 83). Modern power injectors are designed to suspend contrast infusion if pressure in the delivery system rises above a certain threshold.

Routine use of central venous catheters, peripherally inserted central catheters (PICCs) and tunnelled central venous catheters is not recommended unless specifically CT compatible. Manufacturer specifications suggest that the flow rates required for CT coronary angiography cannot be safely achieved through central venous catheters, and published safety data is inconsistent. Patients requiring cardiovascular CT who have central access but in whom peripheral access is impossible should be considered on an individual basis.

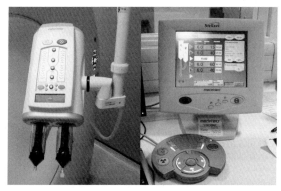

Fig. 7.1 Dual-headed power injector (left) and contrast administration console (right).

Practical aspects

General issues

According to the Medical Devices Regulations 2002 (and its amendment in 2003), a 'medicine' includes, amongst many other definitions, any substance or combination of substances that may be used in or administered to human beings with a view to making a medical diagnosis. This includes iodinated intravenous contrast media.

Responsibility for contrast administration lies with the supervising physician, although local policies, such as a patient group directive, are likely to defer the act of administration to a registered radiographer. There are several general aspects to consider when administering intravenous contrast:[1]

- An appropriately trained doctor must be available immediately in the department to deal with any severe contrast reaction.
- An individual trained in recognizing and treating severe contrast reactions, including anaphylaxis, should be available immediately within the department. This may be any appropriately trained healthcare professional (nurse, radiographer, etc.).
- After conducting the patient safety check, any risk factors for adverse contrast reactions should be discussed with the duty radiologist, who must then decide whether or not to proceed with imaging.
- In view of the potential for contrast nephrotoxicity, dehydration of patients prior to scanning is to be avoided.
- Appropriate resuscitation drugs, equipment, and facilities must be readily available.
- The patient must give informed consent (which may be verbal) prior to the administration of contrast. Information should be provided in written form within the department and discussed with the patient prior to scanning.
- No patient should be left unsupervised within the first 5min of contrast administration.
- All patients who receive contrast should be monitored for at least 15min before discharge; 30min is more appropriate if risk factors for adverse contrast reactions are present.
- All reactions should be detailed in the scan report, patient record, and radiology information system.

1 Reprinted with permission from the Royal College of Radiologists. Royal College of Radiologists. Standards for Iodinated Intravascular Contrast Agent Administration to Adult Patients, 2nd edition. London: The Royal College of Radiologists, 2010.

Adverse contrast reactions (1)

Prior to administration of contrast, certain information should be obtained in the patient history. Ideally, this information should be known when the examination is requested, but it should also be confirmed on patient arrival. Guidelines for the treatment of adverse contrast reactions in Europe and the USA are similar; the following are based on the recommendations of the Royal College of Radiologists, UK for adult patients.[2]

Previous contrast reaction

- The exact nature of the previous reaction and the responsible contrast agent should be determined.
- If the reaction was moderate (e.g. bronchospasm or urticaria requiring treatment) or severe (e.g. laryngeal oedema, severe bronchospam), assess the risk:benefit ratio of the procedure, bearing in mind that a non-diagnostic procedure may be as detrimental as the perceived risk of contrast exposure.
- If the procedure is deemed necessary:
  - Use a different (and non-ionic, low osmolar) agent to that which caused the reaction
  - Maintain close medical supervision
  - Have the resuscitation trolley close by
  - Maintain intravenous access and observe for at least 30min after administration.

Renal impairment

- In the presence of renal impairment, all contrast agents are nephrotoxic.
- Risk of contrast nephrotoxicity is related to extent of renal impairement, volume of contrast to be administered, and hydration status.
- Congestive heart failure, age >70 years, and concurrent use of nephrotoxic drugs are also risk factors.
- Estimated glomerular filtration rate (eGFR) should be used to identify patients at risk, in preference to serum creatinine. An eGFR <60mL/min/1.73m^2 indicates renal dysfunction, although local laboratory measurements may differ.
- Measurement of eGFR is mandatory in all patients with renal disease and diabetes mellitus, as well as those undergoing angiographic procedures.

2 Reprinted with permission from the Royal College of Radiologists. Royal College of Radiologists. Standards for Iodinated Intravascular Contrast Agent Administration to Adult Patients, 2nd edition. London: The Royal College of Radiologists, 2010.

- Contrast nephropathy is poorly defined; one definition is a ≥50% rise in creatinine from baseline over 24–72h after contrast administration.
- In the presence of renal impairment, assess the risk:benefit ratio of the procedure, and in particular whether an unenhanced scan (or alternative imaging modality) may provide the required information.
- If the procedure is deemed necessary, the following may reduce the risk:
  - Use the smallest possible dose of low osmolar non-ionic monomeric or iso-osmolar non-ionic dimeric contrast.
  - Ensure the patient is adequately hydrated prior to administration of contrast. Oral hydration is adequate in the outpatient setting, although intravenous hydration is preferable if high doses of contrast are to be given (suggested protocol: 100mL fluid po or iv for 12h before and after scanning).
  - There is no conclusive evidence of benefit for the prophylactic use of N-acetylcysteine in patients at high risk of contrast nephrotoxicity.[3]

---

3 If considered, the most common protocol is NAC 600mg po bd the day before and the day of scanning.

Adverse contrast reactions (2)

Asthma

- Asthmatics are six times more likely to have an adverse contrast reaction with low osmolar contrast agents (10-fold higher with high osmolar agents).
- Determine whether the patient has true asthma or chronic obstructive pulmonary disease, and whether or not symptoms are well controlled.
- For routine scans the examination should be deferred in the presence of active wheeze or uncontrolled symptoms.
- If asthma is well controlled, assess the risk:benefit ratio of the procedure, particularly whether an unenhanced scan (or alternative imaging modality) may provide the required information.
- If the procedure is deemed necessary:
  - Use a non-ionic, low osmolar contrast agent
  - Maintain close medical supervision
  - Have the resuscitation trolley close by
  - Maintain intravenous access and observe for at least 30min after administration.

Multiple allergies or documented severe allergy requiring therapy

- These patients are at ↑ risk of adverse contrast reactions.
- Assess the risk:benefit ratio of the procedure, particularly whether an unenhanced scan (or alternative imaging modality) may provide the required information.
- If the procedure is deemed necessary:
  - Use a non-ionic, low osmolar contrast agent
  - Maintain close medical supervision
  - Have the resuscitation trolley close by
  - Maintain intravenous access and observe for at least 30min after administration
- There is no conclusive evidence of benefit for the prophylactic use of steroids in the prevention of severe contrast reactions.

Diabetes mellitus

- Those with diabetes should be considered at risk of contrast nephrotoxicity, and the guidelines above should be followed.
- There is no conclusive evidence that lactic acidosis represents a real problem when administering contrast agents to those taking metformin. It is likely that more problems ensue from its discontinuation.
- If renal function is normal, metformin may be continued.
- If renal function is abnormal, the discontinuation of metformin for 48h should be discussed with the referring clinician.

Treatment of adverse contrast reactions

A local policy should be in place in all radiology departments for the treatment of adverse reactions to iodinated contrast media. Standard guidelines for resuscitation apply (ABCDE approach etc.). The following specific measures are based on those of the Royal College of Radiologists, UK.[1]

Nausea/vomiting
- Transient—supportive treatment only.
- Severe, protracted—consider standard antiemetics.

Urticaria
- Scattered, transient—supportive treatment, including observation.
- Scattered, protracted—appropriate H_1-antihistamine im, iv, or po.
- Profound—consider 0.1–0.3mL adrenaline 1:1000 im; repeat as necessary.

Bronchospasm
- 6–10L/min oxygen by facemask.
- Inhaled β_2-agonist, preferably nebulized.
- Adrenaline:
  - If blood pressure normal, give 0.1–0.3mL adrenaline 1:1000 im (lower dose if coexisting coronary artery disease or elderly)
  - If blood pressure low, give 0.5mL adrenaline 1:1000 im.

Laryngeal oedema
- 6–10L/min oxygen by facemask.
- 0.5mL adrenaline 1:1000 im; repeat as necessary.

Hypotension
- Isolated hypotension:
  - Elevate legs
  - 6–10L/min oxygen by facemask
  - Normal saline intravenous infusion (rapid)
  - If unresponsive—0.5mL adrenaline 1:1000 im; repeat as necessary.
- Vagal reaction (hypotension plus bradycardia):
  - Elevate legs
  - 6–10L/min oxygen by facemask
  - Atropine 0.6mg iv every 3–5min to a total dose of 3mg
  - Normal saline intravenous infusion (rapid).

1 Reprinted with permission from the Royal College of Radiologists. Royal College of Radiologists. Standards for Iodinated Intravascular Contrast Agent Administration to Adult Patients, 2nd edition. London: The Royal College of Radiologists, 2010.

Generalized anaphylactoid reaction

- Call for resuscitation team.
- ABCDE; airway protection is a priority—involve anaesthetist early.
- Elevate legs.
- 6–10L/min oxygen by facemask.
- 0.5mL adrenaline 1:1000 im; repeat as necessary.
- H_1-antihistamine, e.g. diphenhydramine 25–50mg iv.

Contrast medium extravasation

- Record details of the event with management advice in the patient's notes and scan report.
- Elevate affected limb.
- Apply ice packs to the affected area.
- If symptoms do not resolve quickly, admit and monitor.
- Skin blistering, paraesthesia, altered tissue perfusion, and increasing or persistent pain beyond 4h suggest severe injury; surgical (plastics) referral for advice is recommended.

Delayed skin reaction

- Skin reactions have been reported up to a week after contrast administration.
- Symptomatic treatment is generally all that is required.
- The reaction should be recorded in the patient's notes, although the significance of these reactions for future contrast administration is uncertain.

Scan protocols

Introduction

CT coronary angiography consists of a variable number of discrete image acquisitions, several of which are for set-up purposes only (to define scan range, level of the carina, contrast timing, etc.). A routine scan protocol may proceed step-wise as follows.

Topogram
- Start at the lung apices, end at the base of the heart (Fig. 8.1).
- Used to define the scan range in subsequent acquisitions.

Calcium score
- Unenhanced, prospectively gated, 3mm/3mm sequential scans acquired between 60 and 75% of the R–R interval.
- Acquired from carina to inferior border of heart.
- Data used to determine the calcium score, most commonly using the Agatston scoring system (see 📖 Coronary artery calcium scoring, p. 194).

Control scan
- Performed to locate the level of the carina.
- This step may be avoided if a calcium score is performed, as the level of the carina can be identified on this dataset.

Test bolus
- Calculates timing of optimum contrast enhancement in the ascending aorta, enabling calculation of scan delay after main contrast injection.
- This step may be avoided if bolus tracking is used (see 📖 Optimizing scan timing, p. 102).

CT coronary angiogram
- Prospectively or retrospectively gated acquisition (see 📖 ECG gating, p 34) of the heart.
- Either the control scan or the calcium score acquisition should be used to plan the acquisition.
- FOV should be collimated in both planes to include the heart.

Protocols for specific cardiac CT applications may vary from those described above. The following pages describe examples of scan protocols as performed on a Siemens Sensation 64 CT scanner. Readers are advised to review the technical specifications of their scanner and consult a local CT medical physics expert when setting up new scan protocols.

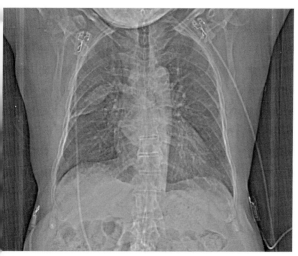

Fig. 8.1 Topogram. The ECG electrodes can be seen but are outside the required FOV for cardiac CT. The scan range for subsequent acquisitions can be determined from this view (see 🕮 Coronary artery calcium scoring, p. 106).

Optimizing scan timing

CT coronary angiography involves injection of contrast into a peripheral vein. This is potentially problematic because the contrast bolus spends an unpredictable amount of time in the venous and pulmonary circulation before reaching the coronary arteries via the ascending aorta. If image acquisition is performed when the contrast bolus is still in the right side of the circulation (too early) or after it has passed through the proximal aorta (too late), coronary artery enhancement will be inadequate and the scan non-diagnostic. Optimizing the delay between contrast injection and triggering of the acquisition is ∴ of great importance.

Currently, two equally valid methods may be used to decide the scan delay: the *test bolus* and *bolus tracking*.

Test bolus method

- A scan level is selected 1cm below the carina.
- A test bolus of contrast is injected. Typically 10–25mL of contrast is injected at 5mL/s, followed by a 40–50mL saline flush at 4mL/s.
- A series of 10-mm thick slices (usually 20–30) are acquired through the scan level defined above, with each scan separated by an interval of 1s.
- Observation of the ascending aorta demonstrates enhancement as contrast passes into the arterial circulation, followed by a reduction in enhancement during washout. Scanning is continued until it is clear that washout is occurring (Fig. 8.2a and b).
- Using contrast enhancement evaluation software on the CT workstation, a region of interest is placed in the ascending aorta and the time to peak enhancement is measured (Fig. 8.2c).
- This is used to estimate the time to peak coronary artery enhancement—as the distal coronary arteries take slightly longer to fill, the scan delay is calculated as the time to peak aortic enhancement plus 2–3s (this may vary in different centres).
- During the main scan acquisition, the calculated scan delay is entered into the scan protocol and the acquisition is triggered once this interval has elapsed after the main contrast injection.

Bolus tracking

- As for the test bolus method, a scan level 1cm below the carina is selected.
- A region of interest (ROI) is drawn in the ascending aorta.
- The scan and contrast injection are activated simultaneously.

- Bolus tracking software triggers the main acquisition once enhancement in the ROI passes a certain threshold (typically 100–150HU).
- A predefined delay after reaching the threshold (usually 5–8s) is inserted to allow for breathing instructions and table movement.
- Note that positioning the ROI close to the superior vena cava or any calcified structure may result in premature triggering of the scan.

Determinants of scan delay

Scan delay depends greatly on the patient's cardiac output and the size and position of the intravenous cannula. When using the test bolus method in a patient with known cardiac dysfunction, the number of test slices should be ↑ to allow for late filling of the ascending aorta. If this is not done, the test bolus sequence will end before aortic enhancement has occurred, necessitating repeat exposure of the patient.

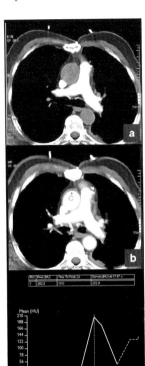

Fig. 8.2 Test bolus technique. An ROI is set in the ascending aorta (circle) and monitored after injection of 10–25mL of contrast (a, b). Images are acquired every second, the enhancement within the ROI is plotted against time, and the time to peak enhancement is derived (c).

Coronary artery calcium scoring

Indication

The clinical indications for this scan protocol are discussed elsewhere (see
📖 Coronary artery calcium scoring, p. 194). In brief, this is a low-dose
unenhanced scan used to evaluate the extent and distribution of coronary artery calcification, a surrogate marker of atherosclerosis. Although
originally described using EBCT, equivalent results may be achieved using
MSCT.

Scan components

- Calcium score acquisition

Scan parameters for coronary calcium scoring

ECG/scanning mode	Prospective/sequential at 60–75% R–R interval
Scan range	Carina to inferior border of heart (Fig. 8.3)
kVp	120
Effective mAs	30

Reconstructions

Reconstruction thickness/increment	3mm/3mm
Kernel (see 📖 Convolution filters and kernels, p. 134)	Medium-smooth
Window setting	Mediastinum

Radiation exposure

Effective dose	~1mSv

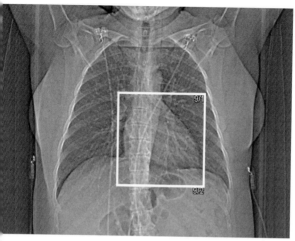

Fig. 8.3 Reconstruction FOVs for coronary calcium scoring. The upper and lower borders should be defined by the carina and inferior border of heart, respectively. The outer borders should be defined by the margins of the heart.

CT coronary angiography

Indication
See 📖 Guidelines, accreditation, and certification, p. 455.

Scan components
- Topogram.
- Calcium score/control scan.
- Test bolus (not required if bolus tracking used).
- CT coronary angiogram.

Contrast protocol
Test bolus
- 15mL iv contrast at 5mL/s followed by
- 40mL 0.9% saline at 5mL/s.

Main acquisition
- 60mL iv contrast at 5mL/s followed by
- 40mL 50:50 mix of iv contrast and 0.9% saline at 5mL/s.

Scan parameters for 64-slice CT coronary angiography

ECG/scanning mode	Prospective/sequential or helical retrospective/helical
Scan range	Carina to inferior border of heart (Fig. 8.4)*
kVp	120 (standard sized adult)
	100 (slim patient)
Effective mAs	770
Pitch	0.2

*If the patient has had previous internal mammary artery (IMA) coronary artery bypass surgery, start the scan above the expected IMA origin (just below the lung apices) and continue to the inferior border of the heart.

Reconstructions

	Lungs	Heart
Reconstruction thickness/increment	3mm/3mm	0.75mm/0.5mm
Kernel (see 📖 Convolution filters and kernels, p. 134)	Sharp	Medium-smooth (standard) Medium-sharp (stents)
Window setting	Lungs	Mediastinum

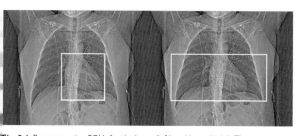

Fig. 8.4 Reconstruction FOVs for the heart (left) and lungs (right). The upper and lower borders of each should be defined by the carina and inferior border of heart, respectively. The outer borders should be defined by the margins of the heart (heart FOV) and the skin edges (lung FOV). For a patient with bypass grafts, the reconstruction FOV should be as shown for gated CT pulmonary angiography (CTPA) (Fig. 8.3 see 📖 Gated CT pulmonary angiogram, p. 110).

Radiation exposure

Effective dose	1–15mSv (depending on gating protocol, see 📖 ECG gating, p. 32)

Gated CT pulmonary angiogram

Indication

The clinical indications for this scan protocol are discussed elsewhere (see 📖 Evaluation of ventricular and atrial function, p. 229). In brief, patients undergo gated CT pulmonary angiography as part of the assessment of pulmonary hypertension and congenital heart disease.

Scan components

- Gated CT pulmonary angiogram with same scan and reconstruction parameters as CT coronary angiography (see 📖 CT coronary angiography, p. 108), except with modified scan range.

Contrast protocol

A triple-phase injection is commonly used:
- 70mL iv contrast at 5mL/s followed by
- 60mL 70:30 mix of intravenous contrast and 0.9% saline at 5mL/s followed by
- 40mL 50:50 mix of intravenous contrast and 0.9% saline at 5mL/s.

Scan range

- Lung apices to inferior border of heart (Fig. 8.5).

Specific issues

The timing of the scan delay is complex as contrast transit times are delayed in patients with 1° pulmonary arterial hypertension and variable in those with congenital heart disease. Either test bolus or bolus tracking methods (see 📖 Optimizing scan timing, p. 102) may be used, although the latter is possibly more straightforward in these patients. Two possible approaches are:
- Set the bolus-tracking ROI in the centre of the main pulmonary artery with a threshold of 100HU.
- Locate the ROI outside the patient and start the contrast injection. Start the acquisition manually once a visual enhancement threshold is reached.

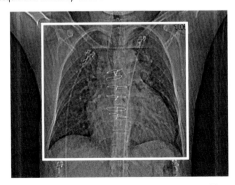

Fig. 8.5 Reconstruction FOV for gated CT pulmonary angiography. The upper and lower borders should be defined by the lung apices and inferior border of heart, respectively. The outer borders should be defined by the skin edges. This FOV should also be used for bypass graft studies.

Gated CT pulmonary venography

Indication

The clinical indications for this scan protocol are discussed elsewhere (see 📖 Left atrium and pulmonary veins, p. 276). In brief, patients undergo gated CT pulmonary venography prior to electrophysiological testing to assess left atrial and pulmonary venous anatomy.

Scan components

- Test bolus
- Gated CT pulmonary venography with same scan and reconstruction parameters as CT coronary angiography (see 📖 CT coronary angiography, p. 108).

Contrast protocol

Test bolus

- 20mL iv contrast at 5mL/s followed by
- 10mL 0.9% saline at 5mL/s

Main acquisition

A triple-phase injection is commonly used:

- 70mL iv contrast at 5mL/s followed by
- 60mL 70:30 mix of intravenous contrast and 0.9% saline at 5mL/s followed by
- 40mL 0.9% saline at 5mL/s

Specific issues

The timing of scan delay is identical to that used in CT coronary angiography except that 3s is not added to the time to peak aortic enhancement.

Prior to percutaneous aortic valve replacement

Indication

The clinical indications for this scan protocol are discussed elsewhere (see 📖 Thoracic aortic imaging, p. 395). In brief, patients undergo cardiovascular CT in order to assist in planning the procedure and to assess vascular access prior to percutaneous aortic valve implantation.

Scan components

- Topogram.
- Test bolus.
- CT coronary angiography (see 📖 CT coronary angiography, p. 108).
- Whole-body angiography: scan and reconstruction protocols (on facing page).

Contrast protocol

Test bolus

- 15mL iv contrast at 5mL/s followed by
- 10mL 0.9% saline at 5mL/s

Main acquisition

- 120mL iv contrast at 5mL/s followed by
- 50mL iv contrast at 4mL/s followed by
- 40mL 0.9% saline at 4mL/s

Specific issues

The timing of scan delay is complex as both coronary and whole-body angiography must be performed using the same bolus injection of contrast. The exact calculation depends on the CT manufacturer, but an example protocol using the test bolus technique on the Sensation 64 (Siemens Medical Solutions, Germany) is given below.

- Calculate the time to peak aortic enhancement (peak time, see 📖 Optimizing scan timing, p. 102).
- Calculate the time required to acquire the scan length of the whole-body angiogram (circle of Willis to the lesser trochanter), the whole-body scan time.
- Apply the following formula to calculate the body angiogram delay:
  - (peak time + 40s)—(whole-body scan time)
- Calculate the time required to acquire the scan length of the coronary angiogram (carina to the inferior border of the heart), the coronary scan time.
- Apply the following formula to calculate the coronary angiogram delay:
  - (peak time + 3s) + (coronary scan time)
- Apply the following formula to calculate the overall scan delay:
  - (body angiogram delay)—(coronary angiogram delay)

Scan parameters for 64-slice whole body angiography

ECG/scanning mode	Ungated/helical
Scan range	Circle of Willis to the lesser trochanter (Fig. 8.6)
kVp	120
Effective mAs	100
Pitch	1.2

Reconstructions

	Peripheral angiography		Heart
Reconstruction thickness/increment	5mm/5mm	1mm/1mm	0.75mm/0.5mm
Kernel (see ⬚ Convolution filters and kernels, p. 134)	Medium-smooth	Medium-smooth	Medium-smooth
Window setting	Abdomen	Abdomen	Mediastinum

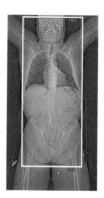

Fig. 8.6 Reconstruction FOV for whole-body angiography prior to percutaneous aortic valve replacement. The upper and lower borders should be defined by the circle of Willis and the lesser trochanters, respectively. The outer borders should be defined by the skin edges.

Radiation exposure

Effective dose	10–30mSv depending on cardiac gating protocol

Difficult scenarios

Dysrhythmia (1)

Introduction

The acquisition of high-quality images in coronary CTA requires a regular heart rate. Optimal image quality is achieved with contemporary MSCT scanners at heart rates under 65bpm. Prospectively gated acquisitions (see 📖 ECG gating, p. 34) are particularly dependent on a regular heart rate, and artefact and misregistration of data will inevitably occur in the presence of cardiac dysrhythmias. Retrospective gating (see 📖 ECG gating, p. 34) allows greater flexibility because data are acquired continuously throughout the cardiac cycle and images may be viewed at any point within the R–R interval.

General strategy

If possible, imaging should be deferred until the dysrhythmia is treated. When imaging is essential, retrospective data acquisition should be strongly considered to avoid non-diagnostic radiation exposure. Dysrhythmias can be problematic when evaluating the coronary arteries as the relative position of the coronaries can change in successive cardiac cycles, leading to misregistration artefact (see 📖 Motion artefact, p. 156).

Scan pitch (see 📖 Scan pitch, p. 24) should be lowered in patients with dysrhythmias. Although this increases radiation exposure, the likelihood of a diagnostic acquisition is improved.

Extrasystoles

Extrasystoles are a serious problem for gating in coronary CTA. The ventricular contraction pattern is altered as a result of premature atrial or ventricular contraction, leading to misregistration of data from successive cardiac cycles due to changes in the location of the heart compared with normal sinus beats (Figs 9.1 and 9.2). Extrasystoles can be unpredictable and may be worsened by the administration of contrast medium.

ECG dataset editing (if manufacturer's software allows)
- Data from the premature ventricular extrasystole is removed, although this may lead to banding artefacts in the final reconstructed images.
- Premature atrial extrasystoles are more difficult to negotiate as the pause after the extra beat is variable. In general, the slower the rate of the underlying sinus rhythm, the higher the likelihood of successful ECG editing.

First-degree atrio-ventricular block

This dysrhythmia places the P-wave in that portion of diastole where scan data are normally obtained. Atrial contraction after the P-wave displaces the right coronary and circumflex arteries, and shifts the period of least cardiac motion.

Depending on the location of the P-wave, the best phase (late diastolic or early systolic) can be anticipated for multiplanar image reconstruction. Successful prospective scanning requires recognition of first-degree AV block prior to acquisition to allow adjustment of scan triggering.

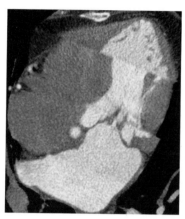

Fig. 9.1 Misregistration artefact through the mid ventricle as a result of ventricular ectopy during CTA.

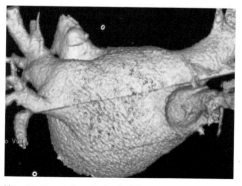

Fig. 9.2 Misregistration artefact affecting the left atrium and pulmonary veins as a result of ventricular ectopy during CTA.

Dysrhythmia (2)

Atrial tachycardia

Despite altering the ventricular filling pattern, this dysrhythmia maintains an activation pattern similar to sinus rhythm. The systolic phases may offer the best opportunity to obtain diagnostic images.

Ventricular tachycardia

There is a markedly abnormal activation pattern of the heart, and compensation through ECG editing is almost impossible. DSCT technology and/or ≥256-slice scanners may offer hope in the future, but validation is required.

Sinus tachycardia

Normal motion of the coronary arteries during the cardiac cycle is exacerbated in tachycardia, leading to motion artefact (see 📖 Motion artefact, p. 156). Various post-processing techniques can be used, involving multiple reconstructions or multisegmented reconstructions (see 📖 Multisegment reconstruction, p. 30), with variable degrees of success. If the tachycardia is regular, it may be possible to override the ECG-gating for the patient's inherent rhythm and select a gating rate at a factor of the actual heart rate (e.g. with a sinus tachycardia of 100bpm, ECG-gating at 50bpm would sample alternate complexes).

Atrial fibrillation

AF is a common dysrhythmia with a prevalence of >5% in patients older than 69 years. The variability in R–R interval limits the accuracy of ECG gating. DSCT may be of benefit in obtaining diagnostic quality images for coronary CTA in this setting. It is possible to achieve diagnostic quality images using 64-slice technology providing the ventricular rate is aggressively controlled and multiphase data are acquired. If the CT is being performed prior to electrophysiological testing and/or ablation, only left atrial and pulmonary venous anatomy may be required (see 📖 Left atrium and pulmonary veins, p. 278); accurate evaluation of the coronary arteries would ∴ be unnecessary.

Marked bradycardia

If the R–R duration exceeds the image acquisition time, image data may be lost as the acquisition stops before completion of each cardiac cycle. This leads to banding artefact. ECG-gating override can be employed, which allows scanning at a predetermined rate and still produces a gated data set. This will not conform to the true phases of the cardiac cycle but will be diagnostic (e.g. 75% reconstruction phase will not be equivalent to end diastole).

Conclusion

Careful planning, optimal heart-rate control, and judicious post processing (which may involve ECG editing) are needed to perform coronary CTA in selected patients with dysrhythmias.

Depending on the clinical question to be answered, CT requests for patients with uncontrollable dysrhythmias should in most cases be rejected and returned to the referrer along with an explanation. Such education will improve the appropriateness of future referrals.

256/320-slice CT technology may prove to be the solution for most kinds of dysrhythmia, with the prospect of whole volume cardiac imaging in a single gantry rotation.

Further reading

Pena AJ, Moselewski F, Teague SD, et al. (2005) Heart rate variation during coronary multi-detector computed tomography: implication for imaging protocol optimization. Paper presented at the 6th International Conference on Cardiac CT, July 22. Boston, MA.

Lesser JR, Flygenring BJ, Knickelbine T, et al. (2009) Practical approaches to overcoming artifacts in coronary CT angiography. *J Cardiovasc Comput Tomogr* **3**(1), 4–15.

Wolak A, Gutstein A, Cheng VY, et al. (2008) Dual-source coronary computed tomography angiography in patients with atrial fibrillation: initial experience. *J Cardiovasc Comput Tomogr* **2**(3), 172–180.

Large patients

Introduction

Sixty-five per cent of the adult population is now considered overweight (BMI ≥25). Obese patients are at ↑ risk of developing cardiovascular problems independently of other risk factors. Those who are morbidly obese (BMI >40) have a higher rate of mortality directly as a result of coronary artery disease.

Cardiac imaging has always been a challenge in obese patients with reduced diagnostic accuracy:

- SPECT imaging—↑ soft-tissue attenuation
- Stress echocardiography—difficult acoustic windows
- Invasive catheter angiography—↑ risk of procedure-related complications, reduced image quality due to impaired fluoroscopic penetration.

Coronary CTA also suffers from ↓ diagnostic accuracy in obese patients, primarily because of ↑ X-ray scatter and a resultant decrease in SNR. Excessive image noise results in especially poor delineation of smaller vessels, as well as non-calcified atherosclerotic lesions.

There are clearly opportunities for dose reduction with almost any type of CT scan.[1,2] For cardiac CT specifically, the use of bodyweight-adapted protocols has been shown to reduce the effective dose by about 12% in males and 25% in females.

Scan acquisition in obese patients

Particular adjustments need to be made in obese or morbidly obese patients to acquire diagnostic images. The trade-off between X-ray exposure and image quality when obtaining images in cardiac CT becomes more important in obese patients.

Image noise may be reduced by a number of adjustments:

- ↑ tube voltage and current (see 🕮 X-ray tube voltage, p. 22)—↑tube voltage = ↑X-ray photon energy = ↑beam penetration; ↑tube current = ↑beam intensity. Both these changes increase signal at detectors (Fig. 9.3). NB: Radiation dose is calculated for a 'standard' 70-kg adult; increasing X-ray energies in a larger patient may not increase radiation dose when compared to this standard, as
  Δdose = Δenergy/Δmass.
- ECG-gated dose modulation (see 🕮 ECG gating, p. 34)—Tube current is ↑ in specified portions of the R–R interval. This method significantly reduces overall radiation dose when gating retrospectively and should be employed in overweight patients to compensate for increasing tube current/voltage.

- Attention to heart-rate control (see 🕮 Heart-rate control, p. 78)—
  This may allow a further compensatory dose reduction. Ensuring a
  heart rate of <65bpm reduces the incidence of motion artefact.
- Use of higher strength contrast agent (370 or 400mg/mL) or higher
  flow rate (7mL/s).

Further reading

1 ICRP (2000) Managing Patient Dose in Computed Tomography. ICRP Publication 87. *Ann ICRP* **30**(4), 1–80.
2 ICRP (2007) Managing Patient Dose in Multi-Detector Computed Tomography (MDCT). ICRP Publication 102. *Ann ICRP* **37**(1), 7–9.

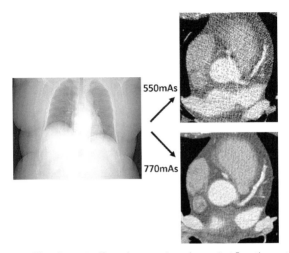

Fig. 9.3 Effect of increasing X-ray tube current in an obese patient. From the scout image (left) it is clear that the patient is significantly overweight. CTA performed using an X-ray tube current of 500mAs (top right) has more image noise than the scan obtained using 770mAs (bottom right). Although quality is improved, CTA using a higher tube current results in an ↑ radiation dose to this patient.

- Use of DSCT—In a morbidly obese patient DSCT images may be of better quality than those acquired using single-source CT.
- Special reconstruction algorithms—Those proposed for DSCT include the use of smooth convolution kernels (see 📖 Convolution filters and kernels, p. 134) and 0.75-mm slice thickness, using the best systolic and diastolic phases reconstructed from temporal resolutions of 83, 105, 125, and 165ms (eight image datasets in total). The dataset with the least amount of noise can be chosen for multiphase reconstruction.

Conclusion

Coronary imaging is possible with cardiac CT in obese or even morbidly obese patients. An increase in exposure parameters is likely to be required, which may increase radiation dose, although this may be mitigated using various technical adjustments. These may include modification of tube current or voltage, scan length, or the use of tube current modulation. The use of prospective gating may also be useful. Nevertheless, there is a trade-off between radiation dose and image quality, which must be clear to the referring physician, patient, radiographer, and responsible radiologist. If doubt exists, advice should be sought from the local medical physics expert.

Further reading

Yoshimura N, Sabir A, Kubo T, Lin PJ, Clouse ME, Hatabu H (2006) Correlation between image noise and body weight in coronary CTA with 16-row MDCT. *Acad Radiol* **13**(3), 324–328.
Chinnaiyan KM, McCullough PA, Flohr TG, Wegner JH, Raff GL (2009) Improved non-invasive coronary angiography in morbidly obese patients with dual-source computed tomography. *J Cardiovasc Comput Tomogr* **3**(1), 35–42.

Children (1)

Advances in CT, in particular dual-source technology, now allow ECG-gated cardiovascular studies to be performed in young children, even with high heart rates, without the need for β-blockade. With improved temporal and spatial resolution, it is now possible to acquire isotropic volume data providing detailed intracardiac and vascular anatomy that can be displayed in all three imaging planes.

Patient selection

Ideally, patients should be referred via a multidisciplinary meeting attended by imagers, cardiologists, cardiothoracic surgeons, and cardiac anaesthetists, with individual consideration of:
- The clinical question to be answered by imaging
- The underlying cardiac condition
- The need for airway and lung parenchyma assessment
- The age of the patient (ability to co-operate—stay still, breath-hold) and hence need for 'feed and wrap', sedation, or anaesthesia
- The likely need for invasive intervention
- On-site expertise
- The imaging modality availability.

Using this information, the patient may undergo magnetic resonance imaging (MRI), CT, echocardiography, or conventional angiography.

Indication for cardiovascular CT in children

For all patients older than 8 years, MRI can be considered the first-line investigation. MRI is also performed in those under 8 years of age under general anaesthetic when it is essential to acquire good intracardiac anatomy and/or good cardiac function (ventricular function) and good vascular flow (particularly to quantify valvular regurgitation). Cardiovascular CT is used as the 1° investigation in neonates and young infants in whom echocardiography has been able to clearly identify the intracardiac anatomy, but not the vascular anatomy (Fig. 9.4).

There are some exceptions to the above guideline, in which CT can be considered as the first-line assessment:
- Vascular rings—CT imaging of airways and lungs (Fig. 9.5)
- Imaging of stents—Routine CT 3 months following coarctation stent insertion to assess for stent fracture (Fig. 9.6) and stent-related pseudo-aneurysm
- Assessment of coronary artery stenoses (β-blockade required)
- Pulmonary hypertension—assessment of the heart and lungs
- Pulmonary venous anatomy (MRI can be problematic)
- Pulmonary atresia with major aorto-pulmonary collateral arteries (MAPCAs)—CT performed prior to cardiac catheterization identifies the number of large aorto-pulmonary collaterals and the presence of any central pulmonary arteries
- Metallic implants
- Contraindication to MRI (e.g. permanent pacemaker).

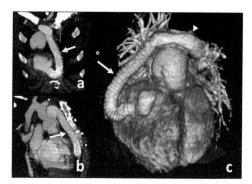

Fig. 9.4 Non-gated, contrast-enhanced cardiovascular CT of 3-year-old with complex congenital heart disease and right ventricle to pulmonary artery conduit (arrow). Images show (a) coronal and (b) sagittal reformats (note proximity of conduit to posterior sternum) of right ventricle to pulmonary artery conduit, and (c) volume-rendered 3D reconstruction viewed from the left anterior oblique plane. The left pulmonary artery is indicated (arrowhead).

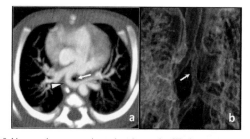

Fig. 9.5 Non-gated, contrast-enhanced cardiovascular CT of 3-month-old with left pulmonary artery sling (arrowhead). (a) Axial reformat at the level of the left pulmonary artery sling, which arises from the right pulmonary artery and passes posterior to the trachea (arrow) and anterior to the oesophagus (naso-gastric tube *in situ*). (b) Volume-rendered reconstruction of the airways, viewed from anterior aspect, showing a narrowed 'stove-pipe' trachea (arrow). Note high take-off of right upper lobe airway.

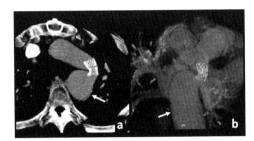

Fig. 9.6 ECG-gated, contrast-enhanced cardiovascular CT of 14-year-old with aortic coarctation stent fracture. (a) Oblique axial reformat at the level of stent. Note dilated proximal descending aorta (arrow). (b) Volume-rendered reconstruction of the aorta, viewed from behind.

Children (2)

Patient preparation

- It is important that all children are properly prepared, either through play therapy for younger children or detailed explanation of the procedure for older patients, ensuring full co-operation throughout the study.
- Children under 2–3 months of age are scanned without any intervention. They are given a feed and allowed to fall into a natural sleep—'feed and wrap'. Ideally appointments should be scheduled to coincide with their natural sleep pattern.
- For children who do not sleep after 'feed and wrap', and who are <15kg, sedation has been proposed in the past; however, because of underlying cyanotic congenital heart disease and the need for a controlled environment in these patients, general anaesthesia is increasingly used.
- Oral sedation—chloral hydrate (50mg/kg). If ineffective, supplementary sedation can be given (i.e. 0.2–0.3mg/kg Diazemuls iv in increments of 0.1mg/kg to a maximum dose of 0.3mg/kg or 10mg), but only by a doctor skilled in paediatric resuscitation.
- For older children, imaging can be performed awake. It is important to practice breath-holds with the patient to gauge ability to comply with instructions. If unable to comply, the scan should be undertaken during gentle respiration.
- Parents are encouraged to stay with their child to provide the necessary reassurance and also help hold their child in position.

Radiation dose

ECG-gating of CT studies increases radiation burden. Protocols must be adapted to reflect the age and weight of the child. Radiation dose can be minimized as follows:

- On-line dose modulation (angular and long-axis modulation) reduces tube current according to patient size.
- ECG-triggered dose modulation (see 🕮 ECG gating, p. 34) reduces tube current to 40% in the systolic phase of the cardiac cycle. Further reduction to 4% is not possible when using paediatric protocols as the mA used is at the lower limit of the generator's output.
- The phases of the cardiac cycle during which tube current is maximum is dependent on heart rate (varies between 30–70% R-R interval).
- In DSCT, scan pitch (see 🕮 Scan pitch, p. 24) is adjusted automatically between 0.2 and 0.5 depending on heart rate to ensure that image data from an entire cardiac cycle is recorded. A fast heart rate raises the pitch to 0.5, reducing scan time and thus radiation dose.

Contrast medium administration

- Iohexol (Omnipaque, GE Healthcare) 300mg/L at 2mL/kg delivered via pressure injector at a flow rate of 1.5–3.5mL/s. Slower flow rates improve enhancement in patients with heart rate >120bpm.
- Hand injection via a neonatal venous cannula is often necessary due to difficulty with venous access.
- Visual bolus tracking is preferred due to patient movement and difficulty in identification of mediastinal anatomy due to lack of fatty tissue. A region of interest is placed outside the scan field and the scan is started when contrast is seen in the target area by the operator.
- Patients with Glenn or Fontan circulations may require a dual-contrast injection via the foot and the arm to ensure enhancement of both pulmonary arteries simultaneously. Alternatively, a delayed phase scan may be acquired after equilibration of contrast within the blood pool. Care must be taken not to over-diagnose pulmonary embolus in this patient group due to poor contrast mixing.

Scanning technique

- The wide variation in weight from neonate to adolescent mandates the adoption of specific weight-based scanning parameters in order to avoid overexposure in younger children.
- 80kVp should be used in younger children to reduce radiation dose and improve contrast resolution.
- The entire thorax should be imaged, including the lung parenchyma, to highlight interstitial lung abnormalities.

Post processing and data presentation

Reporting should be done on the native 3D data in the axial, coronal, and sagittal planes. The ability to create oblique multiplanar reformats is essential. 3D and 4D reconstructions can be useful for data interpretation, but conclusions gleaned from these post-processing algorithms should always be confirmed on the native images. 3D and 4D images are extremely valuable in presentations to other clinical colleagues, and these data should be available at the time of surgery or interventional cardiac catheterisation.

Further reading

Taylor AM (2008) Cardiac imaging: MR or CT? Which to use when. *Paediatr Radiol* **38**(Suppl 3), S433–S438.

Tann OR, Muthurangu V, Young C, Owens CM *et al.* (2009) Cardiovascular CT imaging in congenital heart disease. *Prog Pediatr Cardiol* **28**(1–2), 21–27.

Image reconstruction and processing

Preparing to reconstruct

ECG timing

Regardless of ECG gating protocol, it is necessary first to define the starting point for reconstruction on the ECG prior to image reconstruction. This may be achieved in two ways.

Relative timing

The starting point of the reconstruction interval is determined as a percentage of the R–R interval. This method relies on a constant duration of both systole and diastole. Any change in the heart rate preferentially alters the duration of diastole, thus affecting the R–R allocation of successive reconstruction intervals.

Absolute timing

Reconstruction is started at a defined time in milliseconds after the R-wave. This approach depends on the duration of systole, which is not as strongly influenced by alterations in the heart rate as diastole. Thus, the R–R allocation of the reconstruction interval is less influenced by heart-rate changes.

Other considerations

There are several other factors that must be considered prior to reconstructing the CT raw data.

ECG editing

Significant variability in heart rhythm during scanning may necessitate editing of the ECG prior to reconstruction in order to improve the quality of the final images (see 📖 ECG interpretation errors, p. 160).

Reconstruction thickness and increment

The desired thickness of reconstructed slices and the reconstruction increment (the interval between reconstructed slices) should be defined according to the necessary protocol.

Convoultion filtering

This is applied to the raw data prior to reconstruction. The appropriate filter should be selected according to the clinical situation (see 📖 Convolution filters and kernels, p. 134).

Reconstruction of the CT image (1)

The mathematics involved in CT reconstruction techniques is beyond the scope of this handbook; concepts are presented here in brief.

Generation of raw data

X-rays are emitted through the patient in the transverse plane (Fig. 10.1A). At each angle on the gantry, each detector element records the X-ray beam intensity, which is proportional to the average attenuation coefficient of tissue through which the beam has passed (Fig. 10.1A). The gantry is rotated such that the X-rays are projected through the same tissue but at a different angle. Measurements are repeated (Figs 10.1B and C). Slice acquisition is complete after rotation through 180° plus the fan beam width, an arc that provides sufficient data to allow reconstruction of an axial image. All collected measurements are pre-processed (to correct for errors) to form the 'raw' data.

Image reconstruction

Raw data are processed to form the final image data using a reconstruction algorithm known as back projection.

Simple back-projection

At any given angle, the line between the beam focus and a given element in the detector array defines a 'ray path'. The number of ray paths in the X-ray beam is determined by the number of elements in the detector array. Ray paths are used to trace back the mean attenuation coefficients through which the X-ray beam has passed. By superimposing rays from data acquired at each angle of the gantry, a picture may be formed of the tissue originally imaged (Fig. 10.1D).

Filtered back-projection

Figure 10.1 illustrates the main problem arising from simple back-projection. Star artefacts result from the smearing effect of tracing back the mean attenuation coefficients along the ray paths. This artefact may be eliminated through the use of processing filters, called convolution kernels. These filters are mathematically required to eliminate star artefacts and are applied to the raw data prior to back-projection. The process is ∴ termed *filtered* back-projection. Kernels algorithms have additional effects on the image that are discussed elsewhere (see 📖 Convolution filters and kernels, p. 134).

Image resolution

The resolution of the resultant image depends in part on the number of projections during a single gantry rotation. The greater the number of projections the better the spatial resolution of the final image. For current generation CT scanners around 1000–2000 projections are acquired per gantry rotation.

The major benefit of this method over planar X-ray imaging is its superior *contrast resolution*. This parameter refers to the ability to distinguish between differences in signal intensity in an image. In CT, tissues that differ in density by only a small amount may be distinguished (low-contrast resolution). Contrast resolution is improved further through the use of intravenous contrast media (see 📖 Iodinated contrast media, p. 84).

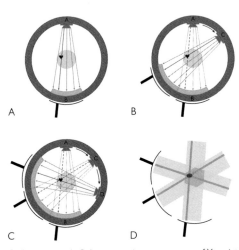

Fig. 10.1 Back-projection. A–C show successive measurements of X-ray intensity at different projections. These profiles are then projected backwards to form the image (D). The star artefact arising from back-projection seen in (D) can be eliminated by applying convolution filters to the raw data prior to back-projection (filtered back-projection).

Convolution filters and kernels

As part of image reconstruction, data are subjected to an algorithm designed to smooth or sharpen the image variably according to user preference. This process is known as *convolution filtering*.

A *convolution filter* uses a mathematical function that selectively enhances the spatial frequency content in the data, resulting in enhancement or smoothing of object boundaries as required. The mathematical function itself is known as a *kernel*. Kernels are named according to the extent to which they smooth or sharpen an image (smooth, medium-smooth, medium-sharp, sharp), although exact terminology varies with scanner manufacturer (e.g. Siemens: *b30f* (medium-smooth), *b46f* (medium-sharp), etc.).

Kernels have effects on two image properties: *spatial resolution* and *image noise*. For any kernel, one is traded off against the other. For example, a smooth kernel has the effect of smoothing object boundaries and reducing image noise, but as a result it reduces spatial resolution. In contrast, a sharp kernel will improve spatial resolution by enhancing object boundaries but at the cost of ↑ image noise.

In cardiovascular CT, the choice of kernel should be determined by the characteristics of the structure to be assessed. For instance, the choice of kernel can affect the assessment of coronary plaques. In the absence of heavy coronary calcification, smoother filters reduce image noise and allow easier assessment of the coronary lumen. In contrast, when highly attenuating structures, such as calcium and stents, are present, sharper kernels improve edge detection and decrease the blooming effect, again allowing improved luminal assessment. In a mixed plaque, this has the effect of increasing the mean attenuation of the calcified component whilst reducing the mean attenuation of the non-calcified component, allowing better assessment of plaque composition and stenosis severity.

Generally, a medium-smooth filter is a good compromise for most cardiovascular CT applications. In the presence of heavy calcification or when stent assessment is required, a sharper, edge-enhancing kernel should be applied. A medium-sharp kernel is probably the best choice in this circumstance as it provides the best trade-off between spatial resolution and image noise.

Kernels	
Smooth	Provides the lowest image noise at the expense of ↓ spatial resolution
Medium-smooth	Kernel of choice for the majority of cardiovascular CT
Medium-sharp	Kernel of choice for imaging high contrast structures such as stents or heavily calcified vessels
Sharp	Best spatial resolution but high image noise; of limited clinical use in cardiovascular CT but useful in high-resolution chest CT

Reconstruction of the CT image (2)

The digital image is made up of a pixel matrix of defined size (usually 512 × 512) into which raw data may be processed.

Pixels and voxels

A contraction of the term 'picture element', a pixel represents the smallest measurable part of an image that may be displayed in the x, y-plane. The addition of z-axis information confers a volumetric quantity to a pixel, which is thus termed a 'volume picture element' or voxel (Fig. 10.2). Pixel size is determined by the size of the FOV and the image matrix (Fig. 10.3).

Field of view

The FOV describes the ROI on the CT scan that is to be reconstructed. This is defined prior to scan acquisition (see 'Scan protocols'), typically by selecting an ROI tightly bordering the tissue to be evaluated.

Image matrix

This describes the pixel matrix (usually 512 × 512 pixels) over which the CT data is reconstructed.

Example

A FOV of 40 × 40cm results in a pixel size of ~0.6mm when using a 512 × 512 image matrix. A typical cardiac reconstruction FOV might be 20 × 20cm, resulting in a pixel size of ~0.3mm when using the same matrix.

⚠ Although 0.3mm might be the minimum dimension that *could* be displayed in the image, other properties of the system (sampling frequency and detector width, see ▫ Detectors, p. 15) determine the limiting spatial resolution of the images. There is ∴ little point in combining image matrix size and reconstruction FOV in such a way as to result in a pixel size beyond the spatial resolution of the scanner. Furthermore, image noise is inversely related to pixel size such that reducing pixel size below ~0.5mm leads to an increase in image noise without significantly improving spatial resolution.

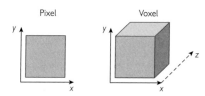

Fig. 10.2 Pixels represent the smallest measurable part of an image. The CT dataset is 3D, with longitudinal (z-axis) resolution determined by the slice thickness. Thus the CT dataset is made up of volume picture elements known as voxels.

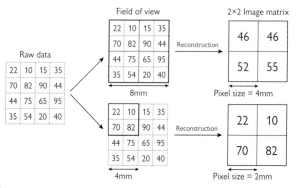

Fig. 10.3 Relationship between FOV and pixel size. Reconstructing the 8mm FOV over a 2 × 2 image matrix (top) results in a pixel size of 4mm, each of which represent an average of the attenuation values measured within that area. Reducing the FOV to 4mm spreads the data in this area over the same 2 × 2 image matrix, resulting in a smaller pixel size (2mm). Reconstructing the 8mm FOV over an 4 × 4 image matrix would have the same effect.

CT numbers and windowing

CT numbers

After filtered back-projection, each voxel is assigned a linear attenuation value corresponding to the mean attenuation of the tissue within
its volume. However, these values are difficult to interpret because of
their dependence on X-ray energy. To overcome this difficulty, each value
is normalized to the attenuation coefficient of water according to the
equation:

$$\frac{\mu_{tissue} - \mu_{water}}{\mu_{water}} \times 1000 = CT\,number$$

where μ is the linear attenuation coefficient of the material. This process
of normalization results in CT numbers, measured in *Hounsfield units*
(HU), which reflect the relative attenuation of tissue compared to water
(Fig. 10.4).

By definition ∴ water has a value of 0HU. Voxels that have average linear
attenuation values higher than water will have positive CT numbers, whilst
those that are lower will be negative. Air has a CT number of –1000HU,
whilst the upper limit detectable by current CT scanners with extended
scales may be as high as +30,000HU. From a practical perspective, bone
has a CT number of typically +400 to +1000HU. Foreign bodies, such as
metal clips or pacemaker electrodes, will be higher still.

Windowing

CT numbers in an image are mapped onto an 8-bit grey scale. As the
dynamic range of the CT number scale exceeds that of the gray scale,
the way in which CT numbers are mapped needs to be adjusted by using
windowing. The display window represents the CT number interval of
interest and is defined by two parameters: *window level* and *window width*.

Window level

This is the CT number on which the window is centred.

Window width

This is the magnitude of the range of CT numbers covered by the
window, defined as the difference between the upper and lower limits of
the window. Voxels with CT numbers above the upper limit appear white
whilst those below the lower limit appear black. The window width thus
determines the contrast in the displayed image: a narrow window spreads
a large range of grey-scale values over a small range of CT numbers
allowing detection of very small differences in tissue densities.

Typical window settings in CT imaging are given in Table 10.1.

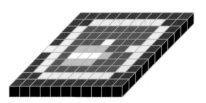

Fig. 10.4 Reconstructed image slices are made up of volume picture elements (voxels), each of which is assigned a CT number representing the average attenuation within that volume relative to water.

Table 10.1 Typical window settings in X-ray computed tomography

	Window width (HU)	Window level (HU)
Mediastinum	350	25
Lungs	1500	−500
Abdomen	400	60
Brain	80	40
Bone	1500	300

Image formats

Raw imaging data is reconstructed into a series of transaxial slices, which may be transferred to an off-line dedicated workstation. The transaxial slices should be reviewed initially to determine the quality of the study and to assess the interval of minimum cardiac motion (usually in diastole, ~65% R–R interval). The images can then be further post-processed and reviewed as multiplanar reformatted (MPR) images (see 📖 Multiplanar reformatting, p. 142), curved MPR (cMPR, see 📖 Curved multiplanar reformatting, p. 144) images, maximum-intensity projection (MIP) images (see 📖 Maximum intensity projection, p. 146), and/or 3D volume-rendered images (see 📖 3D image formats, p. 148) such as shaded-surface display (SSD) and volume rendering (VR).

Except in the most straightforward cases, a combination of these techniques is usually required to reach a firm diagnosis. High diagnostic accuracy requires interactive manipulation of all the images and review of the whole vessel volume rather than just a cursory inspection of the static reformatted images.

Dedicated workstations use a wide range of software programs and processing tools. It is essential for the reader to become familiar with the software available at his/her institution, as each vendor provides software with similar capabilities but different interfaces.

Regardless of software, the transaxial slices remain the data source for all 2D and 3D post-processing methods. The following is a brief enumeration of the various post-processing techniques and their advantages and disadvantages.

Multiplanar reformatting

Transaxial slices may be combined to create a volume data set. As the spatial resolution of the CT dataset is virtually equal in all planes (near-isotropic), this volume may be cut and viewed in any arbitrary plane without artefact or loss of information (Fig. 10.5). Once the viewing plane has been selected, only voxels that exist within this plane are displayed, with spatial resolution similar to the source images.

MPR images usually have a default thickness equivalent to the slice thickness (see 📖 Detector terminology, p. 16). However, several slices in the desired plane may be summed to give a 'thick MPR' (Fig. 10.7). This is equivalent to increasing the slice thickness during acquisition (see 📖 Detector terminology, p. 16). Resultant images represent the average attenuation values of the included slices. Although there is a consequent decrease in spatial resolution, image noise is also averaged across the slices, improving the SNR of the resulting images.

Advantages of MPR

1. Quick and easy to create.
2. Images contain all available information.
3. No editing is required.

Disadvantages of MPR

1. Only one vessel can be displayed at a time.
2. Only 2D views can be generated.
3. Can produce artefactual stenoses or underestimate real stenoses as it depends on manual orientation of the planes.

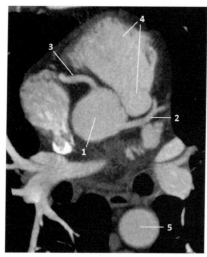

Fig. 10.5 Multiplanar reformatting. The image has been orientated such that the aortic root (1) and proximal left and right coronary arteries (2, 3) are seen in the same plane. The right ventricular outflow tract is also seen (4), as is the descending aorta (5).

Curved multiplanar reformatting

The coronary arteries course in and out of conventional flat planes used in imaging. For example, the right coronary artery typically traverses the x, y-planes in its proximal and distal course ('in-plane' see 📖 Spatial resolution, p. 26) but passes in the z-axis plane in its mid section ('through-plane' see 📖 Spatial resolution, p. 26).

cMPR is a variant of MPR, in which a 2D image is created by sampling CT volume data along a predefined *curved* plane. It is obtained by semi-automatic selection of a curved centreline based on the luminal attenuation of the coronary artery of interest. A curved plane is then assigned along this curved centreline, which is flattened and analysed as a 2D image (Fig. 10.6).

Although particularly useful for displaying tortuous vessels, cMPR should be a routine part of the analysis of the coronary arteries. cMPR images may be rotated around the coronary artery centreline to give a full 360° view of the coronary artery. Additionally, short axis cuts of the coronary artery may be obtained orthogonal to the centreline, allowing assessment of stenoses in terms of both diameter and area at any level of the coronary artery.

It is important to remember that cMPR images are only as good as the coronary artery centreline from which they are derived (see 📖 Centreline tracking errors, p. 164). An improperly generated centreline may lead to the creation of apparent stenoses (if eccentric to the true centreline) or replication of data (if the centreline loops within the coronary artery). The centreline must ∴ always be checked prior to analysis of cMPR images.

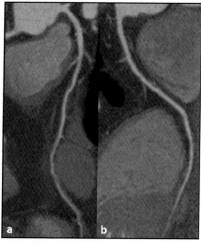

Fig. 10.6 Curved MPR of (a) left anterior descending (LAD) and (b) right coronary arteries.

Maximum intensity projection

An MIP image is formed from a stack of slices in an arbitrary plane, as described for thick MPR (see 📖 Multiplanar reformatting, p. 142). However, whereas a thick MPR image represents the average of each of the contributing slices, an MIP image displays the brightest voxel in each stack across the slices (Figs 10.7, 10.8 and 10.9).

High attenuation structures such as bone or calcification within the contributing slices may dominate an MIP image at the expense of other structures such as the coronary arteries, ∴ MIPs are unhelpful in the presence of coronary calcification. Furthermore, as the brightest voxels within a stack of slices are rarely within the same slice, MIPs may give the impression of overlapping structures in the plane of the image when they are in fact separated by a considerable through-plane distance. The extent to which this occurs depends on the MIP thickness selected, being less of an issue for smaller thicknesses.

Volume editing, using an interactive process called sliding thin-slab MIP (STS-MIP), can overcome some of these problems. This is performed by selecting a thin MPR, moving the slab through the volume, and creating an MIP at each step. Thin-slab MIP can provide a 'road map' of a vessel, charting its course for further evaluation with MPR, and is particularly suited for analysing bypass grafts.

Advantages of MIP
- Quick and easy to configure.
- Good differentiation between vessels and background (Fig. 10.9).
- Less variability in MIP reconstruction than in volume rendering because fewer parameters are involved in its creation.

Disadvantages of MIP
- Misrepresents anatomical spatial relationships.
- Requires substantial editing.
- Can overestimate stenosis severity.
- Particularly unsuitable for evaluation of stenosis severity in the presence of dense calcification or stents.
- No 3D depth information is available.

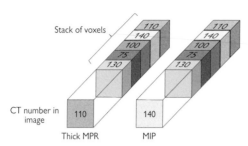

Fig. 10.7 Thick MPR versus MIP. Thick MPR displays the *average* CT number of the contributing voxels along the stack. In contrast, MIP displays the *maximum* CT number. In the example above, the same voxels result in different CT numbers in the final image.

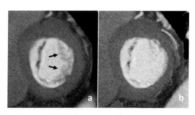

Fig. 10.8 (a) Thick MPR and (b) MIP short-axis images of the mitral valve in diastole. Both are 5mm cuts in the same plane. Note that the posterior mitral valve leaflet (arrows) is seen easily on thick MPR but is less well seen on the MIP as voxels from the contrast-opacified left ventricle are projected forward.

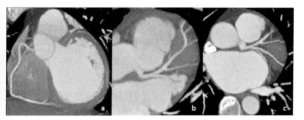

Fig. 10.9 MIP of the (a) right and (b, c) left coronary arteries. High CT numbers in the contrast-enhanced coronary arteries cause them to be projected forward in the final MIP image.

3D image formats

Shaded surface display

SSD was one of the first 3D imaging techniques available, and has largely been superseded by 3D VR techniques. It is less computationally intensive than 3D VR as it uses only approximately 10% of the acquired image data.

The user sets a clinically relevant threshold for the surface of the object that is to be rendered (e.g. soft-tissue windows to view the surface of the heart). The SSD algorithm then searches the volume dataset for voxels beneath this threshold and identifies boundaries where the threshold is exceeded. Surfaces are rendered at these boundaries and shaded according to a gray scale. A 'virtual' light source is used to determine the shading of the surface, simulating surface reflections and shadowing to enhance depth perception.

SSD has the advantages of being fast and flexible, but is not well suited to objects that have poorly differentiated boundaries. Furthermore, the binary method for selecting the surface means that all voxels above the pre-defined threshold are represented in the same way, so much imaging information is lost.

3D volume rendering

3D VR techniques now represent the main method of 3D image generation. These are derived from the entire volume dataset and are thus computationally intensive, requiring dedicated workstations with high-end graphics hardware.

A 3D image is created by considering the contribution of each voxel along a line from the viewer's eye through the volume dataset, and presenting the calculated value in the final image. Each tissue type is assigned a colour, transparency, and shading, allowing distinction from other neighbouring structures. Each voxel is classified on a continuum (rather than the binary system used for SSD), allowing better distinction of tissues of similar attenuation profiles. The presentation of the 3D image data can be modified by the user through alteration of window settings.

From a clinical point of view, VR provides excellent representation of spatial relationships (Fig. 10.10). This makes it particularly suitable for the assessment of complex anatomy, such as anomalous coronary arteries, bypass grafts, and congenital heart disease, especially when demonstrating these relationships to those unfamiliar with cardiac CT interpretation. However, images often require extensive manual editing and are of extremely limited value in assessing coronary artery stenoses.

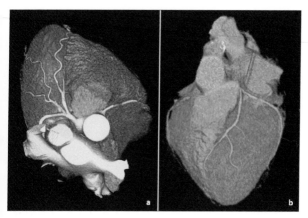

Fig. 10.10 VR images viewed in (a) craniocaudal and (b) left anterior oblique projections.

Sources of artefact

Beam hardening

As an X-ray beam passes through any given tissue, the lower energy X-rays are preferentially removed through attenuation. Thus the higher energy X-rays constitute a larger proportion of the remaining beam. This may cause two kinds of artefact: *cupping* and *streak artefact*.

Cupping

The centre of an image has inappropriately low calculated attenuation values compared to the periphery. This is because the X-ray beam has a higher mean energy in the centre of the object than around the periphery when averaged over a whole gantry rotation.

Cupping is usually avoided through beam filtration (see 📖 Collimators, p. 14) and correction factors determined by calibration using phantoms. However, the phenomenon may be encountered when imaging stents or coronary arteries with circumferential calcification, where the coronary lumen appears hypodense and may be mistaken for non-calcified plaque or even occlusion (see 📖 The blooming effect, p. 212).

Streak artefact

Streak artefact has several causes but, in the context of beam hardening, occurs predominantly behind high-contrast structures such as a contrast-filled superior vena cava, areas of dense calcification, stents, metal clips, and pacemaker wires. The high-contrast material filters out lower energy X-rays, and CT values are ∴ derived from a higher energy X-ray beam, which produces artefactually low attenuation values (Fig. 11.1). In its most severe form, virtually no photons reach the detectors, resulting in incomplete projection data (*photon starvation*).

Tricks and tips

Streak artefact from a densely enhanced superior vena cava may be minimized by flushing the contrast bolus with saline (see 📖 CT coronary angiography, p. 108). A highly enhanced right atrium may harden the X-ray beam and lead to inaccurate measurement of CT numbers in the right coronary artery, mimicking non-calcified plaque. The potential for this artefact is again reduced by using a saline flush after main contrast bolus delivery to reduce contrast within the right heart. Several software interpolation algorithms exist to minimize the streak artefacts which result from metallic objects such as surgical clips or pacemaker wires.

Other causes of streak artefact

- Aliasing—inadequate data sampling per rotation results in streak artefacts during reconstruction.
- Partial volume effect (see 📖 Partial volume effect, p. 154).
- Patient motion (see 📖 Motion artefact, p. 156).

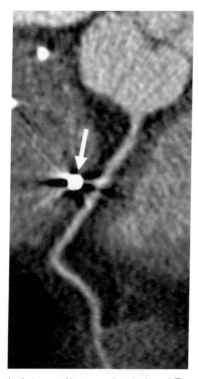

Fig. 11.1 Beam hardening caused by a pacemaker wire (arrow). The wire is surrounded by dark areas indicating low attenuation values as a result of beam hardening. In this case, the artefact crosses the adjacent right coronary artery, giving the appearance of severe stenosis. There is further streak artefact from the pacemaker wire, which appears as radial lines emanating from the wire affecting the whole image. This is likely to be the result of aliasing.

Partial volume effect

This occurs when a voxel represents an area containing two or more tissues with differing attenuation coefficients. The attenuation value assigned to the voxel is the weighted average of the different attenuation values. When a voxel is only partially filled by a structure of very high attenuation (e.g., calcium or metal), a high attenuation value is assigned to the complete voxel, which will ∴ appear bright on the image (Fig. 11.2). Because small but highly attenuating objects have their attenuation value averaged over an entire voxel, the size is overestimated. This effect is often seen with coronary calcification and stents, producing 'blooming artefact'. This may lead to overestimation of the severity of calcified lesions (Fig. 11.3) and interfere with visualization of the coronary lumen.

Blooming artefact may be reduced partially through the use of appropriate window settings (see 📖 CT numbers and windowing, p. 138). This is particularly important for the correct interpretation of any high-density structure such as coronary calcium (Fig. 11.4) or intravascular stents.

Tricks and tips

- Broad windowing for CT coronary angiography minimizes blooming artefact, reducing overestimation of the stenosis severity of calcified plaques or within stents. Ideally, the window level should be set at the CT number of calcification.

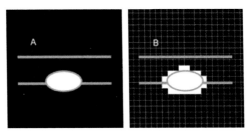

Fig. 11.2 Partial volume effect and 'blooming artefact'. (A) shows a schematic long-axis view of a coronary vessel containing a calcified plaque in its wall. When the vessel is imaged (B), pixels may be partially filled by calcium, with the high attenuation value averaged over the whole pixel, leading to overestimation of the extent of calcification.

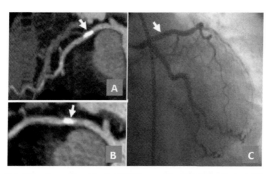

Fig. 11.3 Blooming artefact. On the MSCT images, the calcification in the LAD (A and B, arrows) obscures most of the coronary artery lumen due to the partial volume effect (blooming' artefact). The conventional angiogram (C) shows instead a patent LAD.

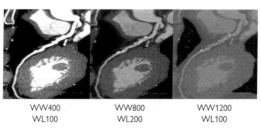

| WW400 | WW800 | WW1200 |
| WL100 | WL200 | WL100 |

Fig. 11.4 The effects of windowing on blooming artefact. Increasing the window width (left to right) minimizes blooming and the likelihood of overestimation of coronary stenosis. WW, window width; WL, window level (see 📖 CT numbers and windowing, p. 138).

Motion artefact

The most common artefacts relate to patient movement (Fig. 11.5) and respiratory motion (Fig. 11.6) during image acquisition. Motion artefacts usually appear as streaks arising tangentially to the edge of the moving object. This is due to inconsistencies in the reconstruction of the moving object as it moves during the scan.

In practice, motion artefacts may lead to areas of low attenuation that may be confused with soft plaque or stenoses. In CT coronary angiography, the right coronary artery is most commonly affected, with obvious 'steps' crossing the whole dataset. Motion artefact should be suspected if stenoses appear at the same level in more than one vessel.

Tricks and tips
- Patient instruction is key.
- Practising breath-holding prior to scanning increases the likelihood of success during scanning.
- The dataset should always be rotated through 360° to allow complete assessment.
- True non-calcified plaque stenoses often have a characteristic pattern with smooth and gradual tapering of the vessel.

Motion artefact:

If the acquisition of data varies between beats such that the different phases of the R-R interval are combined, i.e. in AF, or multi-phase reconstruction (📖 p. 31), then "Steps" may also be created as with motion artefact.

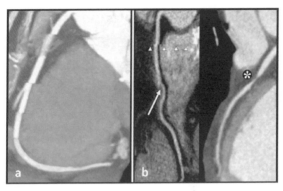

Fig. 11.5 Motion artefacts are often represented by obvious misregistration (a) but may be more subtle and suggested by their linear nature (b, arrowheads) and very abrupt appearance compared to a true soft plaque stenosis. Artefact through branch origins (white arrow) can also lead to apparent stenosis when viewed from one orientation only (asterisk).

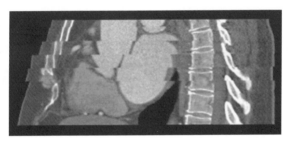

Fig. 11.6 Respiratory motion aretefact may be recognized by the misregistration of both the heart and sternum.

Data gaps and interpolation errors

These are seen as one or more heavily blurred slices between relatively normal slices. This is mainly caused by the use of either *inappropriate pitch* or *poor ECG tracking*.

Inappropriate pitch

Pitch is defined on (see 📖 Scan pitch, p. 24). In retrospectively gated studies, a scan pitch that is too high leads to data gaps because the projection data are too spread out in space to allow accurate interpolation. This is usually only a problem with excessive bradycardia. Data gaps may be inappropriately interpolated to create apparent abnormalities (Fig. 11.7).

Poor ECG tracking

An ECG trace that is noisy or has small QRS complexes may lead to failure of the tracking software to recognize and allocate data to the appropriate parts of the cardiac cycle (Fig. 11.8). In certain cases, a QRS complex may be ignored altogether. This produces a situation similar to excessive bradycardia, where the relatively high pitch leads to the creation of data gaps and resulting interpolation errors on the final image.

Tricks and tips

- Ensure a high-quality ECG trace by shaving the chest, where appropriate, and placing electrodes close to the heart to reduce transthoracic impedance.
- The raw and axial datasets should be thoroughly examined if the VR image appears abnormal.
- In patients with excessive bradycardia, table pitch should be adjusted to ensure complete z-axis coverage.

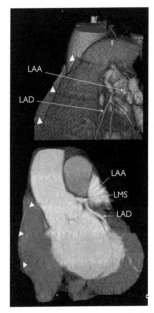

Fig. 11.7 Data gap (arrowheads) as a result of bradycardia in a patient with a heart rate of 32bpm. Inaccurate interpolation of data has led to merging of the left atrial appendage (LAA) to the LAD, although the MIP image from a different phase clearly shows the normal origin of the LAD from the left main stem (LMS). A review of the axial data readily confirms a normal LMS to LAD configuration.

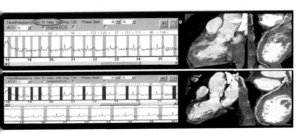

Fig. 11.8 Poor-quality ECG trace with variable baseline and poor R-wave amplitude (top left), causing errors in triggering of acquisition. The heart rate is sensed as between 51 and 199bpm. The subsequent MPR images show significant artefact (top right). ECG editing (bottom left) eliminates much of this artefact (bottom right). (▢ Plate 1 for colour version).

ECG interpretation errors

A stable, regular heart rate (Fig. 11.9) is essential for images of adequate diagnostic quality. A highly variable R–R interval leads to assignment of imaging data from consecutive heart beats to different phases of the cardiac cycle. This results in either *stair-step* artefact (Fig. 11.10) or blurring of image data, with a resultant limitation of image interpretability and decrease in diagnostic accuracy.

Although some patients with predictable heart-rate irregularity, such as atrial fibrillation, can be identified before scanning and excluded from cardiac CT, others exhibit less predictable heart-rate irregularity, e.g. ectopic beats. A further cohort have a controlled heart rate intially, but show increases during acquisition. In such cases it may be possible to restore the diagnostic adequacy of a study through ECG editing in the post-processing phase.

ECG editing

ECG editing involves review of the ECG trace after acquisition to identify ectopics and assess R–R variability. If the R–R variability remains within an acceptable range, no additional editing is needed. Where R–R variability exists, the position of the temporal windows within the cardiac cycle on the ECG trace can be modified by:

- Deleting certain temporal windows completely (e.g. after an ectopic beat) and inserting additional windows in the succeeding compensatory beat (Fig. 11.8)
- Inserting additional temporal windows throughout, if contiguous R–R intervals exhibit long pauses
- Manually adjusting the synchronization point back onto the R-wave, if mis-triggering of the acquisition occurred due to improper detection of the R-wave, allowing reconstructions to be matched to the appropriate cardiac phase.

ECG editing is an important tool for improving images derived from 64-slice CT scanners. However, scanners with higher numbers of detector rows and dual-source technology may ultimately limit the need for heart rate and rhythm control. For example, single-beat CT acquisitions obviate the need for regular R–R intervals. Newer scanners may also track the R–R interval and operate the X-ray tube only when an interval of appropriate duration is detected.

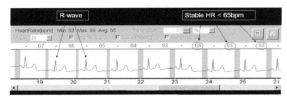

Fig. 11.9 A stable heart rate of <65bpm with an electrocardiogram (ECG) with good R-wave amplitude is essential for good-quality image acquisition. This allows the R-wave to be clearly distinguished from the other components of the ECG trace.

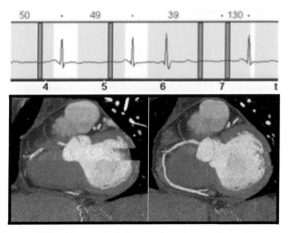

Fig. 11.10 ECG with ectopics (top). Prior to editing, there is a clear stair-step artefact in the right coronary artery (left). After editing, this artefact has almost disappeared (right).

Artefacts that mimic coronary stenoses

Pseudostenosis

A difficult (and not uncommon) problem is that of a stenosis seen on a single phase reconstruction that is not apparent in another phase (Fig. 11.11). The exact cause of this phenomenon is unclear, but it may represent a phase where a combination of torsion and movement in three dimensions gives the impression of stenosis.

Tricks and tips
* An isolated non-calcified stenosis should be assessed in three or more phases to determine whether it is real or artefactual.

Overlying structures

Another common cause of artefactual stenoses is a small partially opacified vein crossing the artery being examined. This can cause a loss of attenuation within the vessel of interest, which may mimic soft plaque (Fig. 11.12).

Tricks and tips
* Removal of the vein on the VR image may reveal the normal artery underneath the adjacent venous structure.

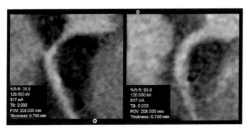

Fig. 11.11 Pseudostenosis of the right coronary artery ostium seen in the 35% R–R interval phase (left). There is no evidence of stenosis on review of the same segment in a different phase (95% R–R interval, right).

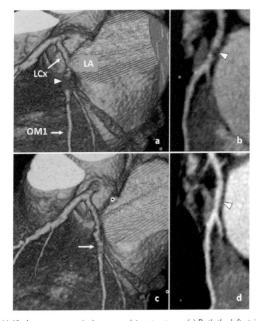

Fig. 11.12 Apparent stenosis due to overlying structures. (a) Both the left atrium (LA) and great cardiac vein (arrowhead) cross the left circumflex (LCx), artery leading to a loss of attenuation within the artery (b, arrowhead), mimicking a soft plaque stenosis. (c) Cropping of both the LA and vein reveals a normal coronary artery lumen (d, arrowhead).

Centreline tracking errors

This is an aretfact that arises during post processing. A potential problem when using automated vessel centreline tracking software is that the system may jump from artery to vein or *vice versa* if they are closely related (Fig. 11.13). Often affected are the:

- Left circumflex with the oblique vein of the left atrium and great cardiac vein
- Right coronary artery with the small cardiac vein proximally and coronary sinus distally
- Posterior descending artery PDA with the middle cardiac vein.

Careful assessment of the automated tracking must also be undertaken in areas of calcification or poor luminal contrast. The automated vessel centreline may loop within the artery or otherwise deviate from the centre, causing artefact (Fig. 11.14). This may be misinterpreted as muscle bridging or lead to overestimation of stenosis severity.

Tricks and tips

- Artefact due to a centreline tracking error should be suspected in any vessel where there is:
  - An abrupt change in luminal diameter
  - A sudden change in attenuation within the luminogram
  - Repetition of a coronary plaque on cMPR.

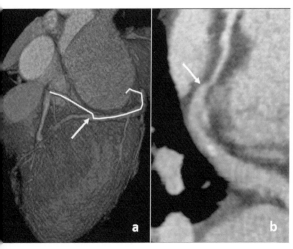

Fig. 11.13 Centreline tracking error. (a) The centreline tracks the proximal left circumflex artery but then exits into the coronary sinus (arrow). (b) On cMPR there is a marked change in vessel diameter where the centreline enters the coronary sinus (arrow).

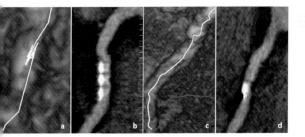

Fig. 11.14 Centreline tracking error causing a repeat artefact of a calcified lesion. (a) The centreline loops within the coronary artery in the region of a calcified plaque. (b) This causes repetition of the plaque on cMPR. (c) Manual adjustment of the centreline eliminates this artefact on cMPR (d), although some tracking artefact remains.

Cross-sectional anatomy of the thorax

Introduction

Competency in cardiovascular CT (CCT) includes the requirement for an understanding of the anatomy of the thorax when viewed in cross-section. This includes not just the heart and coronary vessels but the whole wide field of view, including pulmonary, mediastinal, and upper abdominal structures. Raw image data are reconstructed into a series of transaxial images. Other image formats (e.g. MPR, cMPR, MIP, etc.) require further post processing. Transaxial images ∴ represent the 'purest' form of reconstructed data. Familiarity is essential when reviewing CCT data, but this is often not the case for non-radiologists.

The following sections show axial CT images of the chest with emphasis on the mediastinum (see Figs 12.1 to 12.12). The highlighted line on the scout view (top left-hand corner) corresponds to the axial section at which the images are acquired. Specific anatomy of the heart, great vessels, lungs, and other mediastinal structures are dealt with in later sections.

Cross-sectional anatomy of the thorax

Trachea
The trachea bifurcates into the right and left main stem bronchi. The location of this bifurcation is found at about the level of the arch of the aorta or T5. The right main stem bronchus takes a more vertical course at the carina.

Left brachiocephalic vein
The left brachiocephalic vein is formed by the union of the left internal jugular and left subclavian vein. It joins with the right brachiocephalic vein and drains into the superior vena cava (SVC).

Left common carotid artery
The left common carotid originates directly from the arch of the aorta.

Right common carotid artery
This vessel arises from the *brachiocephalic artery/trunk*, which also gives rise to the *right subclavian artery*.

Left subclavian artery
This artery is the third branch of the ascending aorta.

Superior vena cava
The SVC is formed by the junction of the right and left brachiocephalic veins, at the lower border of the right first costal cartilage.

Ascending aorta
This is the fhe first part of the aorta. The ascending aorta gives rise to the brachiocepahalic artery/trunk, left common carotid artery, and left subclavian artery.

Descending aorta
This is a continuation of the arch of the aorta. The descending aorta becomes thoracic at T4. It gives off nine paired posterior intercostal branches to the thoracic and abdominal wall. These run in the 3rd to 11th rib interspaces. The 10th paired branch is the subcostal artery. It also gives small branches to bronchi and oesophagus.

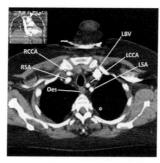

Fig. 12.1 Right common carotid artery (RCCA), right subclavian artery (RSA), oesophagus (Oes), left brachiocephalic vein (LBV), left common carotid artery (LCCA), left subclavian artery (LSA).

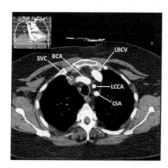

Fig. 12.2 Superior vena cava (SVC), brachiocephalic artery (BCA), left brachio-cephalic vein (LBCV), left common carotid artery (LCCA), left subclavian artery (LSA).

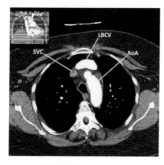

ig. 12.3 Superior vena cava (SVC), left brachiocephalic vein (LBCV), aortic arch AoA).

Oesophagus

Lies initially posterior to the trachea and aorta in the upper part of the thorax but moves forward and left to enter the diaphragm 2.5cm left of the midline at T10.

Right pulmonary artery

This travels inferior to the arch of the aorta and posterior to the SVC. It is also related posteriorly to the right pulmonary vein at the right hilum.

Left pulmonary artery

The left pulmonary artery is found anterior to the descending aorta. It is also connected to the arch of the aorta by a connection called the ligamentum arteriosum. The left main pulmonary artery passes to the left of and then superior to the bronchus.

Azygos vein

Ascends in the posterior mediastinum on the right side to T4/5, where it arches forward above the root of the right lung and drains into the SVC.

Pulmonary veins

There are inferior and superior sets of pulmonary veins, which drain into the left atrium.

Left hilar point

This is where the superior pulmonary vein crosses anterior to the left main pulmonary artery. The left hilar point is approximately 1cm higher than the right.

Right atrium

The right atrium receives blood from the coronary sinus, SVC, and inferior vena cava (IVC).

Right ventricle

This forms the front of the heart and is the most anterior chamber of the heart. There are three papillary muscles in the right ventricle. The tricuspid valve has anterior, posterior, and septal leaflets.

Left atrium

This is the most posterior compartment of the heart and is intimately related posteriorly to the left lobe bronchus and oesophagus. It receives pulmonary veins at its upper and lower posterolateral margins.

Left ventricle

The left ventricle long axis is in the left anterior oblique plane and forms most of the left heart border, although the major portion of its external surface is posterolateral.

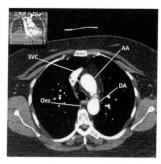

Fig. 12.4 Superior vena cava (SVC), ascending aorta (AA), descending aorta (DA), oesophagus (Oes).

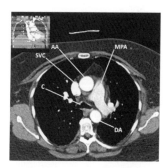

Fig. 12.5 Superior vena cava (SVC), ascending aorta (AA), main pulmonary artery (MPA), carina (C), descending aorta (DA).

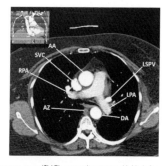

Fig. 12.6 Superior vena cava (SVC), ascending aorta (AA), left superior pulmonary vein (LSPV), left pulmonary artery (LPA), right pulmonary artery (RPA), azygous vein (AZ), descending aorta (DA).

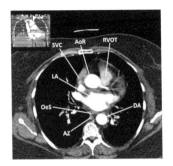

Fig. 12.7 Superior vena cava (SVC), aortic root (AoR), right ventricular outflow tract (RVOT), left atrium (LA), oesophagus (Oes), azygous vein (AZ), descending aorta (DA).

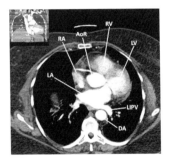

Fig. 12.8 Left atrium (LA), right atrium (RA), right ventricle (RV), left ventricle (LV) left inferior pulmonary vein (LIPV), descending aorta (DA).

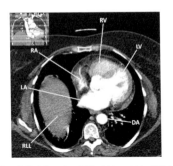

Fig. 12.9 Left atrium (LA), right atrium (RA), right ventricle (RV), left ventricle (LV) right lobe of liver (RLL), descending aorta (DA).

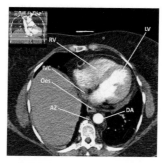

Fig. 12.10 Right ventricle (RV), left ventricle (LV), azygous vein (AZ), descending aorta (DA) oesophagus (Oes), inferior vena cava (IVC).

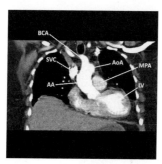

Fig. 12.11 Sagittal section of mid thorax. Left ventricle (LV), ascending aorta (AA), superior vena cava (SVC), brachiocephalic artery (BCA), aortic arch (AoA), main pulmonary artery (MPA).

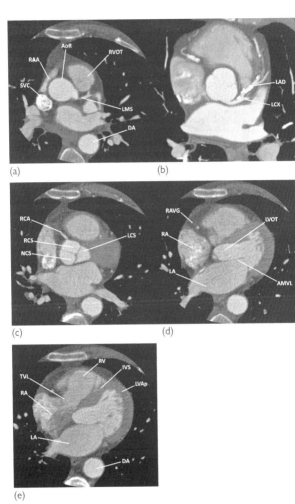

(a) (b) (c) (d) (e)

Fig. 12.12 a–e Caudal-cranial axial reconstructions of cardiovascular and coronary anatomy (above the level of the inferior thorax). Superior vena cava (SVC), aortic root (AoR), right ventricular outflow tract (RVOT), right atrial appendage (RAA), left main stem coronary artery (LMS), descending aorta (DA), left anterior descending artery (LAD), left circumflex artery (LCx), left coronary sinus (LCS), right coronary sinus (RCS), non-coronary sinus (NCS), right coronary artery (RCA), left atrium (LA), right atrium (RA), right atrio-ventricular groove (RAVG), anterior mitral valve leaflet (AMVL), interventricular septum (IVS), left ventricular apex (LVAp), tricuspid valve leaflets (TVL).

The coronary arteries and cardiac veins

The coronary arterial circulation

The myocardium is supplied by the left and right coronary arteries. The former supplies the majority of the left ventricle, whilst the latter supplies the right ventricle and usually the inferior surface of the left ventricle. This anatomy is relatively predictable in humans, although anomalous variations exist (see 📖 Anomalous coronary arteries, p. 338). Branching patterns are more variable. It is particularly important in CT coronary angiography to describe the coronary arteries consistently so that subsequent testing either of myocardial perfusion (e.g. MPS) or anatomy (e.g. invasive coronary angiography, ICA) can be appropriately guided.

A note on anatomical terminology

The heart and its associated structures are described according to the so-called 'Valentine' position—standing on its apex. Descriptions do not ∴ reflect true orientation in the body. For example, the left ventricle lies behind the right ventricle and would be more properly termed the posterior ventricle. However, the nomenclature is now established. Although this may seem a trivial issue, it is especially relevant in patients with congenital heart disease (CHD), where the usual relationships between the coronary arteries and the heart are absent (see 📖 Anomalous coronary arteries, p. 338).

Coronary dominance

The inferior surface of the heart is supplied by the posterior descending coronary artery (PDA). This is a branch artery that arises from the right coronary artery (RCA) in 85–90% of individuals and the left circumflex artery in 10–15%. The artery from which the PDA arises is said to be 'dominant'. In ~1%, both arteries supply a PDA branch and are said to be 'co-dominant'.

Dominance is important when reviewing tests of myocardial function or perfusion. Ischaemic abnormalities in the inferior wall may reflect obstructive coronary artery disease (CAD) in either the left circumflex or RCA depending on dominance. Furthermore, obstructive disease may be treated conservatively if seen in a small non-dominant RCA that supplies only a small amount of left ventricular myocardium. Coronary dominance should ∴ be reported in all cases.

The coronary ostia and left coronary artery

Coronary ostia

Both coronary ostia should arise within 10mm of the sinotubular (ST) junction; variations within this distance are considered normal. Ostia >10mm above or below the ST junction are considered to have high or low take-off, respectively.

The coronary arteries arise from the aortic sinuses closest to the pulmonary artery. The left and right coronary arteries are defined by imagining that one is sitting in the aortic sinus furthest from the pulmonary trunk, facing the pulmonary artery. The artery that arises from the side of the observer's left hand is the left coronary artery and the other the right. This convention (the *Leiden convention*) is used even in CHD (see 🔲 Anomalous coronary arteries, p. 338), where the terms left and right may have no particular meaning. The Leiden convention ensures consistent definitions in these circumstances.

Left coronary artery

The *left main coronary artery*, or LMS, typically arises from the left coronary aortic sinus in a plane that is inferior to that of the origin of the RCA. It usually runs between the left atrial appendage and the pulmonary trunk, typically for a distance of ~1–2cm, before bifurcating into the LAD, which runs in the anterior interventricular groove down to the apex of the heart (Fig. 13.1), and the *left circumflex artery* (LCx), which runs posteriorly within the left atrioventricular groove (LAVG; Fig. 13.2).

The anterolateral region of the left ventricle is supplied by branches of the LCx via *obtuse marginal branches* and the LAD artery via *diagonal branches*. Branches are ordered numerically, with the most proximal branch termed 'first' (e.g. first diagonal branch) and so on distally.

In around a quarter of individuals, the left main stem trifurcates to give a third branch in between the LAD and LCx, termed an *intermediate* (or *ramus intermedius*) *branch*, which supplies the anterolateral region.

The LAD artery also gives off *septal branches* that supply the anterior two-thirds of the interventricular septum.

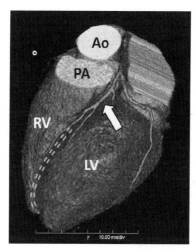

Fig. 13.1 The LAD coronary artery (arrow) arises from the bifurcation of the LMS and travels in the anterior interventricular groove (dashed lines) to supply the anterior wall, apex, and majority of the septum. Ao, aorta; PA, pulmonary artery; RV, right ventricle; LV, left ventricle.

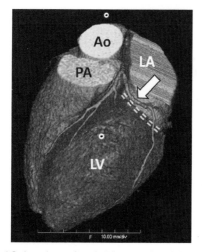

Fig. 13.2 The LCx (arrow) arises from the bifurcation of the LMS and travels in the LAVG (dashed lines) to supply the lateral wall. Ao, aorta; PA, pulmonary artery; RV, right ventricle; LV, left ventricle.

The right coronary artery

The RCA typically arises anteriorly from the right coronary aortic sinus and travels forwards and then downwards within the right atrioventricular groove (RAVG) to reach the posterior surface of the heart (Figs 13.3 and 13.4).

An early branch of the RCA is the *conus branch*, which wraps around the right ventricular outflow tract. The conus branch and *sinus node artery*, another early branch, supply the right ventricular outflow tract, right atrium, and sino-atrial node. Occasionally, these branches may have their own orifice in the right coronary sinus.

At the margin of the right ventricle, the RCA typically gives off an artery known as the *acute marginal branch*, which supplies the anterior (or free) wall of the right ventricle.

When dominant, the RCA continues in the inferior portion of the RAVG to give off the *posterior descending artery* in the inferior interventricular groove. Fifty per cent of those with RCA dominance will also have a significant *posterolateral branch* that passes along the inferior portion of the LAVG to supply the inferolateral left ventricle. The identification of this branch is important as it is likely to supply the inferoseptal papillary muscle of the mitral valve.

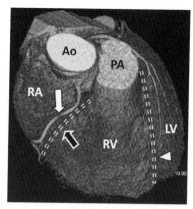

Fig. 13.3 The RCA (white arrow) arises from the anterior aspect of the aorta and travels in the RAVG (black arrow). In this projection, the LAD artery may also be seen in the anterior interventricular groove (arrowhead). Ao, aorta; PA, pulmonary artery; RA, right atrium; RV, right ventricle; LV, left ventricle.

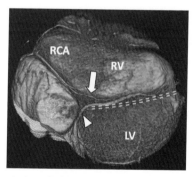

Fig. 13.4 When dominant, the RCA travels around the margin of the right heart and exits the inferior aspect of the RAVG to give off the posterior descending artery (arrow) in the inferior interventricular groove (dashed lines). The middle cardiac vein (arrowhead) also runs within this groove. RCA, right coronary artery; RV, right ventricle; LV, left ventricle.

The cardiac venous system

Knowledge of cardiac venous anatomy is often considered 2° to the corresponding arterial anatomy, as the latter is usually the focus for coronary interventions. However, knowledge of the venous anatomy of the heart is becoming increasingly important, particularly in patients being considered for biventricular pacemaker implantation. CCT is increasingly used to plan the placement of the left ventricular pacing electrode within a suitable cardiac vein. Although the CT coronary angiogram is timed for the arterial phase of contrast injection, the cardiac veins can usually be visualized without difficulty as they are often large in diameter and lie within epicardial fat.

In contrast to the coronary arteries, the cardiac veins exhibit significant anatomical variation. The following description should ∴ be used as guidance only when naming the cardiac veins seen in individual patients.

Anatomical classification

The variability of the cardiac venous system ensures that more than one classification system exists. A straightforward method is to divide the cardiac veins as follows:

- *Coronary sinus and its tributaries*—drain the left ventricle and inferior part of the right ventricle.
- *Anterior cardiac veins*—drain the anterior and anterolateral walls of the right ventricle and open into the right atrium either directly as individual veins or as one or more confluences.
- *Thebesian veins*—drain the subendocardial portions of the myocardium, opening directly into any of the four cardiac chambers.

In short, veins are described according to whether they drain the subepicardial left (coronary sinus and tributaries) or right (anterior cardiac veins) ventricles or the subendocardium (Thebesian veins).

CCT is most commonly used to assess the coronary sinus and its tributaries. It has no clear role in the imaging of anterior cardiac or Thebesian veins.

Coronary sinus and its tributaries

Anatomy
- Continuation of the great cardiac vein (Fig. 13.5).
- Arises (by definition) in the LAVG at either the:
  - junction of the left atrial oblique and great cardiac veins
  - valve of Vieussens—venous valve dividing the great cardiac vein and coronary sinus, typically located where the vein crosses the margin of the left ventricle.

Both of these may be hard to identify in practice, and the margin of the left ventricle may then be used to define the start of the coronary sinus.
- Drains into the right atrium via the coronary os.
- Variable size, although usually oval in shape.
- Enlarged in heart failure.

Clinical importance
The coronary sinus is the focus for insertion of the left ventricular lead during biventricular pacemaker implantation. It may also be the site of ablation during electrophysiological procedures (see 📖 Left atrium and pulmonary veins, p. 276). The size and location of the coronary sinus should be assessed, along with its relation to adjacent coronary arteries.

Great cardiac vein
- Continuation of the anterior interventricular vein.
- Courses within the LAVG (Figs 13.6 and 13.7).
- Most commonly runs superior to the left circumflex artery, although a deep course is possible.
- Drains into the coronary sinus.

Anterior interventricular vein
- Originates in the anterior interventricular groove (AIVG), usually at the apex (Fig. 13.6).
- Leaves the AIVG at a variable position, although usually passes between the pulmonary trunk and left atrial appendage.
- Courses left into the LAVG, whereupon it becomes the great cardiac vein.
- Receives blood from the distal left ventricular myocardium.

Middle cardiac vein
- Runs within the posterior (inferior) interventricular groove (PIVG) (Figs 13.5, 13.7, and 13.8).
- Receives blood from the inferior surface of the heart, as well as a large part of the interventricular septum.
- Usually drains into the coronary sinus, although direct communication with the right atrium may occur.

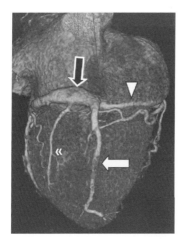

Fig. 13.5 Inferior surface of the heart showing the coronary sinus (black arrow) receiving the inferior left ventricular vein (double arrow). The middle cardiac vein (white arrow) runs along the inferior interventricular groove to drain into the coronary sinus. The small cardiac vein is also visible in the RAVG (arrowhead).

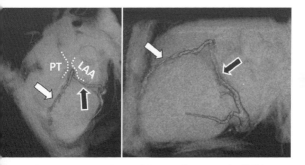

Fig. 13.6 Anterior interventricular vein (white arrow) running in the AIVG from the left ventricular apex up to the base. It passes between the pulmonary trunk (PT) and the left atrial appendage (LAA) to enter the LAVG, becoming the great cardiac vein (black arrow).

Small cardiac vein
- Runs within the inferior part of the RAVG (Figs 13.7 and 13.8).
- Receives blood from the diaphragmatic surface of the right ventricle.
- Drains into the coronary sinus.

Cardiac venous branches
- Wide anatomical variation.
- The *left (or obtuse) marginal vein* is the most common, collecting venous blood from the anterolateral part of the left ventricle and draining into the great cardiac vein (Fig. 13.6).
- The *inferior left ventricular vein* drains the inferolateral portion of the left ventricle and terminates in either the coronary sinus (usual) or great cardiac vein (occasional) (Fig. 13.7).
- The *left atrial oblique vein* passes along the inferolateral wall of the left atrium, usually between the left pulmonary veins and left atrial appendage. Clinically, union of the left atrial oblique vein and the great cardiac vein defines the start of the coronary sinus (Fig. 13.6). However, the vein is a remnant of the embryonic left SVC system, and may thus manifest as a persistent left SVC.

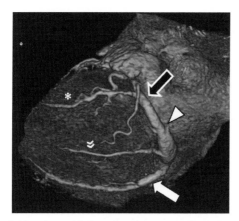

Fig. 13.7 Left lateral view of the heart showing the great cardiac vein (black arrow) receiving the left marginal vein (asterisk). The insertion of the left atrial oblique vein (arrowhead) defines the start of the coronary sinus, which receives blood from the inferior left ventricular vein (double arrow) and the middle cardiac vein (white arrow).

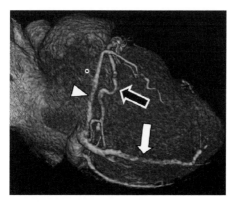

Fig. 13.8 The small cardiac vein is seen in the RAVG (arrowhead) adjacent to the RCA (black arrow). The middle cardiac vein (white arrow) is also seen in the inferior interventricular groove.

Imaging atherosclerotic plaque

Pathology of atherosclerosis

The complications of atherosclerosis, such as myocardial infarction and stroke, remain the most common cause of death in Western Europe, with increasing importance in the developing world.

- The core pathology of atherosclerosis is an accumulation of lipid in the arterial subendothelial space.
- The endothelium becomes 'leaky', probably in response to the presence of cardiovascular risk factors combined with a multifactorial genetic predisposition.
- As lipid accumulates, it becomes oxidized; this makes it an attractive target for ingestion by inflammatory cells from the bloodstream and adventitia.
- An inflammatory cycle is established, with smooth muscle cells forming a fibrous cap over the enlarging lipid core of the plaque.
- This cap can rupture or erode due to ingestion of the collagen structure by inflammatory cells.
- Calcification is thought to be a feature of 'mature' plaques, along with the appearance of adventitial new vessels.
- These vessels are prone to leaking and may lead to intraplaque hemorrhage.

It is now understood that the composition of an atherosclerotic plaque is more important than the degree of luminal obstruction it causes in determining the likelihood of it rupturing and causing an acute ischaemic event. High-risk features include:

- Infiltration by inflammatory cells, usually macrophages and T-cells
- Thin fibrous cap (65µm or less)
- Large lipid-rich core
- Evidence of positive vessel (Glagov) remodelling:
  - The external diameter of the coronary artery (i.e. measured from the epivascular surface [external elastic membrane]) should be measured for both the stenosed segment and a normal reference segment
  - If the external diameter of the stenosed segment is ≥1.05 times greater than that of the reference area, it has positively remodelled
  - Micro-calcification of the artery wall.

Coronary artery calcium scoring (1)

In the earliest days of CCT, technical limitations made accurate quantification of coronary artery stenoses impossible. However, the development of electron beam CT (see 📖 Electron beam CT, p. 6) with ECG-gated image acquisition allowed coronary artery calcification to be imaged as a surrogate marker of atherosclerosis.

- CT provides good visualization of vascular calcification because of the marked X-ray attenuation properties of calcium.
- The main clinical application of this capability has been the quantification of coronary calcification by means of the coronary calcium score (CCS)—sometimes called the Agatston score after its pioneer, Arthur Agatston.
- Calcium scoring is straightforward, the radiation burden is low (1–2mSv), and there is no need for iodinated contrast administration.

Defining coronary calcium

A calcified plaque is defined as a hyperattenuating lesion (>130HU) at least 1mm^2 in size (Fig. 14.1). The threshold of 130HU represents approximately two standard deviations above the attenuation value of blood. This cut-off value ensures that CT measures of calcium are similar to those measured histologically, and may be reproduced reliably across different scanner vendors.

Scoring coronary calcium

- Several software packages are available for evaluating CCS.
- Most highlight pixels >130HU on the unenhanced CCS images (see 📖 Fig. 14.1, p. 195), although this may be adjusted in the software settings if desired.
- Highlighted pixels considered to be within a coronary artery are selected by the operator.
- The calcium score is calculated by assigning each identified pixel a weighting factor that depends on HU value (higher HU values have higher weighting and result in higher CCS) and then summing the values that result. CCS is ∴ affected by both the density and total area of calcification in the coronary arteries.
- CCS has been categorized in several ways. A suggested scoring system is shown in Table 14.1.

Absolute vs demographically adjusted CCS

- CCS increases with age and is generally higher in men.
- This has been used as a rationale for quoting CCS in terms of age and gender centiles to identify how an individual compares to people of the same age and gender.
- For example, a 60-year-old male with CCS of 100 lies on approximately the 50th centile for age and gender; in contrast, a female with the same age and CCS lies on the ~75th centile.
- In the Multi-Ethnic Study of Atherosclerosis (MESA),[1] no further effect was shown over absolute CCS by stratifying scores according to age, gender, and ethnicity, suggesting that absolute scores alone are sufficient.

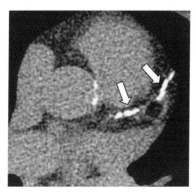

Fig. 14.1 Coronary calcification in the LAD (arrows) on a non-contrast coronary calcium study.

Table 14.1 Suggested categories for CCS and their interpretation

Score	Plaque burden
0	None identifiable
1–10	Minimal
11–100	Mild
101–400	Moderate
>400	Extensive

Further reading

Budoff MJ, Nasir K, McClelland RL, *et al.* (2009) Coronary calcium predicts events better with absolute calcium scores than age-sex-race/ethnicity percentiles: MESA (Multi-Ethnic Study of Atherosclerosis). *J Am Coll Cardiol* **53**(4), 345–352.

Coronary artery calcium scoring (2)

Clinical implications

- Pathological studies have shown that the extent of coronary calcification is directly proportional to the overall extent of atherosclerosis.
- CCS correlates well with the total extent of coronary atherosclerosis and has important prognostic value.
- Several large well-designed studies have demonstrated that patients without calcium in the coronary arteries can expect very low cardiovascular event rates (<1% per year).
- In contrast, the risk of events compared to those with zero CCS is ↑ approximately:
  - Seven-fold for scores 101–300
  - Ten-fold for scores >300.
- This prognostic information is independent of all other cardiovascular risk factors.
- The adverse prognosis associated with coronary calcification is related to accompanying high-risk non-calcified plaques, which constitute ~80% of the total atherosclerotic plaque burden.

Limitations

- The major prognostic data for CCS come from large *asymptomatic* populations.
- Up to 10% of *symptomatic* patients with a calcium score of zero will have non-calcified lesions, causing more than 70% stenosis.
- An individual's calcium score does not usually decrease with lipid-lowering therapy; in light of several negative regression studies, repeat calcium scoring is not recommended.

CCS in diabetes and renal failure

- Risk stratification by CCS is equally valid in asymptomatic patients with diabetes; those with zero CCS have a similar mortality to non-diabetics.[1]
- Intimal coronary calcium is seen in both non-renal and renal patients and is linked to renal function and traditional risks; medial calcification occurs only in patients with chronic renal dysfunction.[2]
- CCS progression has been linked to poorer control of mineral metabolism in patients with chronic renal dysfunction.[3]

Screening

- Indiscriminate use of calcium scoring is not recommended because of the lack of prospective studies demonstrating improved outcomes.
- There may be a role in screening asymptomatic patients with an intermediate Framingham risk level, where the Agatston score might allow reclassification into either a higher or lower category of risk. However, this approach remains controversial.
- A systematic review carried out for the UK NHS in 2006 concluded that CCS did not meet National Screening Criteria.[4]

Current clinical guidelines

- CCS is recommended by the UK National Institute of Health and Clinical Excellence (NICE) guidelines for the investigation of chest pain (see 📖 Guidelines, accreditation, and certification, p. 455) in patients with a 10–29% pre-test likelihood (PTL) of CAD.

Further reading

1 Elkeles RS, Godsland IF, Feher MD, *et al.* (2008) Coronary calcium measurement improves prediction of cardiovascular events in asymptomatic patients with type 2 diabetes: the PREDICT study. *Eur Heart J* **29**(18), 2244–2251.

2 Nakamura S, Ishibashi-Ueda H, Niizuma S, *et al.* (2009) Coronary calcification in patients with chronic kidney disease and coronary artery disease. *Clin J Am Soc Nephrol* **4**(12), 1892–1900.

3 Bellasi A, Kooienga L, Block GA, *et al.* (2009) How long is the warranty period for nil or low coronary artery calcium in patients new to hemodialysis? *J Nephrol* **22**(2), 255–262.

4 Waugh N, Black C, Walker S, *et al.* (2006) The effectiveness and cost-effectiveness of computed tomography screening for coronary artery disease: systematic review. *Health Technol Assess* **10**(39), 1–90.

Imaging non-calcified plaque

In the absence of calcification, the coronary artery wall cannot be reliably discerned using unenhanced CT, and administration of an intravenous iodine-based contrast agent is required.

- Plaque characterization with contrast CT relies on differences in the X-ray attenuation values of the individual plaque components.
- Lipid-rich areas generally have lower HU values than fibrous regions, with both of these lower than calcified plaque (Fig. 14.2).
- Several studies have demonstrated mean attenuation values in the range 30–50 HU for lipid-rich non-calcified plaques, with higher mean values (90–120 HU) for fibrous non-calcified lesions.
- However, there is considerable overlap in the HU values for different plaque components, making accurate distinction challenging in practice.
- Currently, quantification of non-calcified plaque is subject to considerable inter- and intra-observer variability and tends to show adequate reproducibility in large proximal vessels only.

Implications for prognosis

Any degree of coronary atherosclerosis on a cardiac CT bestows an adverse prognosis, even if the plaques are non-calcified. However, several plaque features have been advanced as confering a particular risk of cardiac events, including:

- A speckled pattern of calcification (Fig. 14.3)
- The presence of lipid-rich plaque
- Outward remodelling of the arterial wall (Glagov remodelling).

Clinical data

- Patients who have either a positively remodelled artery or an area of <30 HU plaque are at ↑ risk of acute coronary syndromes.
- The combination of positive remodelling and lipid-rich plaque confers a hazard ratio of 20 compared with normal studies.
- The presence of non-calcified plaque is an independent risk factor for adverse cardiac events over and above the presence of stenoses on CTA and inducible ischaemia on myocardial perfusion scintigraphy.
- If CCT is normal, the 1- and 3-year event rates are as low as 0.6% and 1.2%, respectively.

Future considerations

- Technical developments, such as dual- and multienergy CT, may improve the separation of energy spectra of the important plaque elements and allow more accurate quantification.
- 'Smart' contrast agents, targeted to plaque components of biological significance such as macrophages, may be able to identify vulnerable plaques likely to cause acute coronary syndromes; these plaques could then be targeted for pre-emptive stenting or drug delivery.

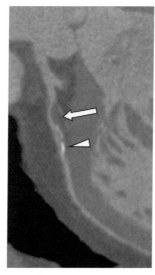

Fig. 14.2 Non-calcified plaque (arrow) with lower attenuation values than adjacent (and eccentric) calcified plaque (arrowhead).

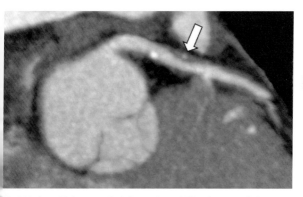

Fig. 14.3 A speckled pattern of calcification (arrow). This plaque morphology is linked with a higher likelihood of acute coronary syndrome.

Quantifying luminal stenosis

Introduction

Over two million invasive coronary angiograms are performed worldwide each year to investigate causes of chest pain, but only a third of these lead to coronary revascularization. Consequently there is the potential for CT coronary angiography (CTA) to replace those procedures that do not demonstrate significant obstructive CAD.

Such a strategy is contingent on demonstrating the diagnostic accuracy of CTA against both anatomical and functional techniques. CTA has been extensively validated against both ICA and functional tests such as myocardial perfusion scintigraphy and fractional flow reserve. A consistent finding has been that CTA has a very high negative predictive value (generally >95%) for the exclusion of CAD. However, values for positive predictive power have been poorer.

Poorer performance in the presence of CAD may be the result of technical factors such as heavy coronary calcification. However, several aspects of study design should also be considered when interpreting published data.

Factors affecting diagnostic accuracy

Several studies have reported that the diagnostic accuracy of CT is impaired in patients who have:
- BMI >30 (although ACCURACY (see 📖 Comparison with invasive coronary angiography, p. 204) is a notable exception)
- High or irregular heart rate—heart rate control is key (see 📖 Heart-rate control, p. 78)
- Heavy coronary calcification (coronary calcium score >400).

Tips and tricks

Positive CCT results are more reliable when the effects of CT artefacts on the assessment of luminal stenosis are borne in mind. The following should be sought specifically:
- Blooming artefact (see 📖 Partial volume effect, p. 154) with calcified lesions
- Beam hardening (see 📖 Beam hardening, p. 152) with mixed lesions or coronary stents
- Step artefact and pseudostenoses (see 📖 Motion artefact, p. 156) with non-calcified plaques.

The following may help during post processing:
- Always adjust window settings to minimize blooming (see 📖 CT numbers and windowing, p. 138).
- The presence of any contrast alongside a purely calcified plaque makes it unlikely that there will be a >50% stenosis on invasive angiography.
- All wholly non-calcified plaques should be assessed in multiple planes and phases.

Diagnostic performance

To date, there have been 50+ studies evaluating the performance of CTA against ICA for the detection of CAD. There have been three multicentre studies (see 📖 Comparison with invasive coronary angiography, p. 205) and several systematic reviews (see 📖 Comparison with invasive coronary angiography, p. 205). Several considerations must be kept in mind when interpreting published data evaluating the diagnostic performance of CTA.

Pre-test likelihood of significant coronary artery disease

- Many studies recruit symptomatic patients in whom a clinical decision had been made already to refer for ICA. The PTL of significant CAD in these populations is ∴ high.
- The effect of PTL on post-test likelihood of significant CAD has been demonstrated (see box), with patients at intermediate likelihood having the most to gain from CTA.
- Current US and European guidelines advocate CTA in patients at low or intermediate (~<70%) PTL of CAD (see 📖 Guidelines, accreditation, and certification, p. 455).
- The median age in the CORE64 multicentre CTA trial (see 📖 Comparison with invasive coronary angiography, p. 204) was 59 years and the prevalence of angina 60%. Given that a 60-year-old male with angina has ~80–90% PTL of significant CAD, some enrolled patients would probably not have been eligible for clinical CTA according to current appropriateness criteria (see 📖 Appropriate use criteria for cardiovascular CT, p. 458).

Prevalence of coronary artery disease in study populations

- Although linked to PTL of CAD, disease prevalence has further effects on statistics generated by intertest comparisons.
- Data derived from populations with high or low CAD prevalence tend to underestimate negative or positive predictive values, respectively.
- Positive and negative likelihood ratios may be better than positive and negative predictive values. The likelihood ratio for a test result compares the likelihood of that result in patients with disease to the likelihood of that result in patients without disease and may be independent of disease prevalence.
- In very general terms, positive and negative likelihood ratios of >10 and <0.1 are most likely to lead to conclusive changes from pre- to post-test probabilities.

Highly selected patient populations

- Early studies in CTA excluded 'non-evaluable' coronary segments from analysis, biasing data in favour of better results. This was a feature mainly of 16-slice CT studies.
- Patients with dysrhythmia, poorly-controlled heart rates, significant obesity, and renal dysfunction are often excluded from studies.
- Some studies have excluded patients with high calcium scores.
- All of the above may reduce the applicability of CTA study results to 'real-world' patient groups.

Effect of pre-test probability[1]

	Low		Intermediate		High	
	CT+	CT−	CT+	CT−	CT+	CT−
Pre-test likelihood		13		53		87
Post-test likelihood	68	0	88	0	96	17

The effects of a positive or negative CTA (CT+ and CT−, respectively) on post-test likelihood of significant CAD are dependent on pre-test likelihood. In this study, 254 patients underwent both CTA and ICA, with any stenosis >50% classed significant. Patients were grouped according to pre-test likelihood [high (>70%), intermediate (30–70%), and low (<30%)]. Assuming that likelihoods of approximately >90% and <10% represent diagnostic certainty for the presence or absence of significant CAD, the data suggest that patients at intermediate pre-test likelihood are stratified most appropriately, although a negative scan in a low-likelihood patient is equally reassuring. Conversely, no outcome in high-likelihood patients is useful as the pre-test likelihood is high enough to be certain of significant CAD without needing to perform CTA whilst a negative scan does not adequately exclude the condition. This is the rationale for current CTA appropriateness criteria (see 📖 Chapter 30, p 458).

Further reading

1 Meijboom WB, van Mieghem CA, Mollet NR, *et al.* (2007) 64-slice computed tomography coronary angiography in patients with high, intermediate, or low pretest probability of significant coronary artery disease. *J Am Coll Cardiol* **50**, 1469–1475.

Comparison with invasive coronary angiography

Multicentre studies

To date, three multicentre studies have evaluated the diagnostic performance of 64-slice CTA against ICA.[1-3] Each used a ≥50% cut-off to determine stenosis significance and studied symptomatic patients already referred clinically for ICA. Summary results are shown in Table 14.2.

CORE64[1]

- 291 symptomatic patients; median age 59; ~60% had angina.
- Prevalence of significant stenosis 56%.
- By design, CCS<600 in all patients.
- Poorer negative predictive value (NPV) than shown in previous single-centre studies but positive predictive value (PPV) relatively high.
- CTA and ICA were similar in predicting need for revascularization.

ACCURACY[2]

- 230 symptomatic patients; mean age 57.
- Prevalence of significant stenosis 25%.
- Comparisons for detection of both ≥50% and ≥70% stenoses—results similar.
- High NPV (99%) but poorer PPV, although low prevalence of CAD.
- CCS > 400 significantly reduced specificity.

Meijboom WB et al. (2008) JACC 52, 2135–2144[3]

- Multisite, multivendor study.
- 360 patients (aged 50–70); ~40% had angina.
- Prevalence of significant stenosis 68%.
- High NPV (>97%), lower PPV.
- Specificity was poorest in segments with calcification obscuring >50% of the coronary lumen.

Systematic reviews

Recent systematic reviews of 64-slice CTA have shown similar results.[4-6] Each evaluated >20 studies with >2000 patients and a median CAD prevalence of ~60%. Results are summarized in Table 14.3.

Conclusions

Results of both multicentre studies and systematic reviews indicate that CTA has high NPV but poorer PPV for the detection of >50% stenosis on ICA. Heavy calcification has the greatest effect on accurate interpretation. Given the potential of CAD prevalence to confound results, the values for positive and negative predictive likelihoods (see 📖 Diagnostic performance, p. 202) are encouraging and indicate that CTA has a strong influence on the post-test likelihood of significant CAD.

Table 14.2 Summary results for the three multicentre trials comparing CTA with ICA[1–3]

Analysis	Trial	Sens	Spec	PPV	NPV	PLR	NLR
Patient	CORE64[1]	85	90	91	83	8.5	0.17
	ACCURACY[2]	95	83	64	99	5.6	0.07
	Meijboom et al.[3]	99	64	86	97	2.7	0.02
Vessel	CORE64[1]	75	93	82	89	10.7	0.26
	ACCURACY[2]	84	90	51	99	8.4	0.17
	Meijboom et al.[3]	95	77	59	98	4.1	0.06
Segment	Meijboom et al.[3]	88	90	47	99	8.8	0.13

Sens, sensitivity; Spec, specificity; P/NPV, positive/negative predictive value; P/NLR, positive and negative likelihood ratio.

Table 14.3 Summary results for systematic reviews comparing CTA with ICA[4–6]

Analysis	Trial	Sens	Spec	PPV	NPV	PLR	NLR
Patient	Mowatt et al.[4]	99	89	93	100	9.3	0.02
	Stein et al.[5]	98	88	93	96	8.0	0.03
	Sun et al.[6]	97	88	94	95	8.1	0.03
Segment	Mowatt et al.[4]	90	97	76	99	26.1	0.10
	Stein et al.[5]	90	96	73	99	20.6	0.10
	Sun et al.[6]	90	96	75	98	22.5	0.10

Sens, sensitivity; Spec, specificity; P/NPV, positive/negative predictive value; P/NLR, positive and negative likelihood ratio.

Further reading

1 Miller JM, Rochitte CE, Dewey M, et al. (2008) Diagnostic performance of coronary angiography by 64-row CT. N Engl J Med **359**, 2324–2336.

2 Budoff MJ, Dowe D, Jollis JG, et al. (2008) Diagnostic performance of 64-multidetector row coronary computed tomographic angiography for evaluation of coronary artery stenosis in individuals without known coronary artery disease: results from the prospective multicenter ACCURACY (Assessment by Coronary Computed Tomographic Angiography of Individuals Undergoing Invasive Coronary Angiography) trial. J Am Coll Cardiol **52**, 1724–1732.

3 Meijboom WB, Meijs MF, Schuijf JD, et al. (2008) Diagnostic accuracy of 64-slice computed tomography coronary angiography: a prospective, multicenter, multivendor study. J Am Coll Cardiol **52**, 2135–2144.

4 Mowatt G, Cummins E, Waugh N, et al. (2008) Systematic review of the clinical effectiveness and cost-effectiveness of 64-slice or higher computed tomography angiography as an alternative to invasive coronary angiography in the investigation of coronary artery disease. Health Technol Assess **12**, iii–143.

5 Stein PD, Yaekoub AY, Matta F, et al. (2008) 64-slice CT for diagnosis of coronary artery disease: a systematic review. Am J Med **121**, 715–725.

6 Sun Z, Lin C, Davidson R, Dong C, and Liao Y (2008) Diagnostic value of 64-slice CT angiography in coronary artery disease: a systematic review. Eur J Radiol **67**(1), 78–84.

Comparison with other techniques

CTA has been compared to a number of other techniques, most prominently SPECT MPS and fractional flow reserve (FFR) on ICA. For better or worse, results from these studies have been used to comment on the adequacy of CTA. Vital to interpreting results from these studies is an understanding that CTA is an anatomical technique that determines the presence of atherosclerosis and its effects on the diameter of the coronary lumen. In contrast, MPS and FFR measure the functional consequences of coronary stenoses and are influenced by several other factors beyond the stenosis itself, including coronary flow reserve and collateralization. Given the different parameters under evaluation, perfect agreement between techniques is neither expected nor desired.

With this in mind:

- There is moderate correlation between CCT and both histology and intravascular ultrasound (IVUS) for the quantification of plaque size
- Agreement is better in proximal, large arteries but falls significantly in smaller vessels
- Compared with FFR and MPS, CTA has a negative predictive value >95%, suggesting that stenoses causing <50% reduction in luminal diameter are rarely functionally significant.
- For stenoses ≥50%, CTA tends to overestimate the likelihood of functional significance when compared to invasive measures (e.g. FFR)
- The likelihood of inducible ischaemia on MPS arising from a ≥50% stenosis on CTA is ~50–60%
- When using a stenosis cut-off of ≥70% to predict functional significance, CTA specificity improves at the expense of sensitivity.

Conclusions

Based on these results, a pragmatic approach should be adopted to classifying lesion severity. In a clinical report, lesions should be characterized as causing <50, 50–70, and >70% reduction in luminal diameter. This has the following clinical implications:

- For those with <50% stenosis, medical management is usual
- For those with stenoses causing 50–70% reduction in luminal diameter, functional imaging should be recommended
- For those with >70% stenosis, invasive angiography with a view to percutaneous coronary intervention is recommended provided that this is deemed clinically appropriate and acceptable to the patient
- The presence of ≥50% stenoses in >1 coronary artery should prompt referral for functional imaging in order to guide revascularization.

Prognostic performance

There is relatively little data concerning the impact of CTA on prognosis. Most available results are from single-centre studies; large multicentre trials are underway.

Stable chest pain

- In the largest study to date,[1] the presence of >50% stenosis on CTA was an independent predictor of major adverse cardiac events (MACE).
- CTA and myocardial perfusion scintigraphy results were synergistic in predicting outcomes.
- In other studies, potential predictors of MACE include stenosis severity, the number of coronary areries affected, and the presence of atherosclerotic plaque in the LMS.

Acute chest pain

The majority of studies have evaluated CTA in the emergency department setting and in patients with ECG findings and/or cardiac enzymes that are indeterminate.

- Diagnostic accuracy in this cohort is generally similar to that previously described (see 📖 Comparison with invasive coronary angiography, p. 204).
- CTA generally reduces time to discharge or diagnosis of acute coronary syndrome.
- Normal CTA is associated with a good prognosis and low likelihood of future cardiac events.

Further reading

1 van Werkhoven JM, Schuijf JD, Gaemperli O, *et al.* (2009) Prognostic value of multislice computed tomography and gated single-photon emission computed tomography in patients with suspected coronary artery disease. *J Am Coll Cardiol* **53**, 623–632.

Coronary stent imaging

Introduction

Background

Percutaneous coronary intervention (PCI) with stent implantation is now the most common form of coronary revascularization. Prior to stenting, coronary stenoses were relieved by balloon angioplasty alone ('plain old balloon angioplasty', POBA). Although immediate results were good, restenosis was a particular problem. This limitation was reduced substantially by the introduction of stents deployed within the coronary artery by balloon inflation. Stents are constructed from a variety of materials, including stainless steel, cobalt-chromium, and tantalum, and maintain coronary artery patency through a scaffolding effect. Broadly, two forms exist: bare-metal stents (BMS) and stents coated with a drug-eluting polymer (drug-eluting stents, DES).

In-stent restenosis

Stent implantation results in injury to the vessel wall, which in turn leads to a healing response with inflammation and proliferation of smooth muscle cells (*neo-intimal hyperplasia*). An excessive healing response can cause restenosis of the stent lumen that may lead to recurrence of symptoms. The similarities between neo-intimal proliferation and tumour growth led to the development of stents coated with a drugs designed to retard the restenotic process (DES). The most common antiproliferative drugs used in DES are sirolimus (e.g. Cypher™ stents) and paclitaxel (e.g. TAXUS™ stents). DES have reduced the rate of in-stent restenosis compared to BMS, although the problem has not been entirely abolished.

Role of CCT

Stent images are often affected by the partial volume effect (see 🔲 Partial volume effect, p. 154), which can be problematic for CCT interpretation. The severity of this artefact depends in part on the metal from which the stent is constructed (see 🔲 The blooming effect, p. 212). Despite this limitation, CCT can be useful for evaluating stents in the LMS and proximal coronary arteries.

PCI is increasingly performed on the unprotected LMS in the DES era. As in-stent re-stenosis is a particularly dangerous complication in this setting, routine angiographic surveillance is recommended within 6 months. CCT has been shown to be safe and reliable in excluding in-stent re-stenosis in patients with LMS and proximal coronary stents, and is now often used as an alternative to conventional invasive angiography. In this setting, CCT is able to define:

• Stent patency (Fig. 15.1a)
• Neo-intimal hyperplasia, defined as <50% diameter narrowing (Fig. 15.1b)
• In-stent restenosis, defined as 50–99% diameter narrowing (Fig. 15.1c)
• Stent occlusion, defined as total (100%) luminal obliteration (Fig. 15.1d).

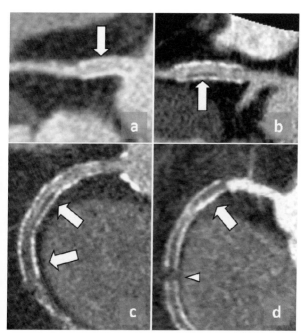

Fig. 15.1 (a) Patent stent implanted in the LMS coronary artery. No filling defects are seen within the stent. (b) Neo-intimal hyperplasia (arrow) is displayed as a dark rim of tissue within this stent implanted in the proximal LAD. This condition is mostly asymptomatic. (c) In-stent restenosis (arrows) appears as a thicker filling defect in a stent implanted in the RCA. This condition can be associated with recurrent chest pain. (d) Stent occlusion (arrow). There is total obliteration of the in-stent lumen. Note also the gap (arrowhead) between two stents implanted in the RCA.

The blooming effect

Coronary stents can be difficult to assess by CCT due to the partial volume effect (see 📖 Partial volume effect, p. 154), making stent struts appear larger than they actually are.

- Structures with a very bright appearance (e.g. the stent struts) may obscure adjacent structures (e.g. the stent lumen).
- This phenomenon may hinder assessment of the in-stent lumen and is referred to as the 'blooming effect'.
- The finding of contrast-enhancement distal to the stent is not sufficient to confirm stent patency as retrograde filling of the vessel may occur via collateral pathways.
- If the stent is being evaluated for the presence of non-occlusive in-stent restenosis, direct visualization of the in-stent lumen becomes mandatory.

The blooming effect (Fig. 15.2) is particularly problematic in:

- Smaller stents (<3.0mm), where the in-stent lumen can be completely obscured
- Stents with thick struts (e.g. ≥0.15mm)
- Stents made of steel, cobalt-chromium, or tantalum, compared with those made of magnesium stents: magnesium stents exhibit a lumen visibility of 90%, compared with 50–59% for most other stents
- Overlapping (stent-in-stent) and bifurcation stenting

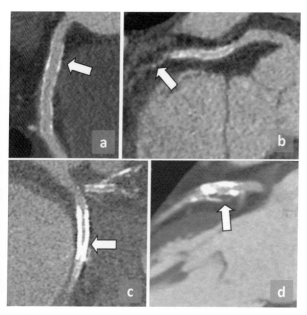

Fig. 15.2 (a) A 3-mm stent implanted in the RCA shows minimal blooming effect, allowing the exclusion of in-stent restenosis. (b) In a 2.25-mm stent implanted in the LCx, the blooming effect is more detrimental and hinders assessment of the in-stent lumen. In this case, the lumen appears misleadingly patent in spite of the absence of distal runoff (arrow), which indicates restenosis. (c) The blooming effect from a 3-mm tantalum stent implanted in the LCx is very marked and prevents visualization of the in-stent lumen. (d) In the event of a stent-in-stent configuration or pre-existing heavy calcification of the vessel wall, the blooming effect is exacerbated by multiple layers of metal and/or calcium.

Technical requirements

In order to compensate for the blooming effect, some technical refinements
are required for coronary stent imaging:

- High spatial resolution (see 📖 Spatial resolution, p. 26), i.e. thin
  detectors (minimum requirement is 64-slice CCT scanners or higher)
- High temporal resolution (see 📖 Temporal resolution, p. 28) is
  necessary because the blooming effect is exacerbated by motion
  artefacts (blurring) (see 📖 Sources of artefact, p. 151)
- Heart rate control with β-blockers is advisable
- Reconstruction of the raw dataset with dedicated (sharp) convolution
  kernels (see 📖 Convolution filters and kernels, p. 134) may decrease
  blooming and is ∴ recommended (Fig. 15.3)

Dual-energy acquisition modes (application of two different kilovoltages,
e.g. 80 and 140kV, see 📖 X-ray tube voltage, p. 23) may improve the
assessment of coronary stents in the near future.

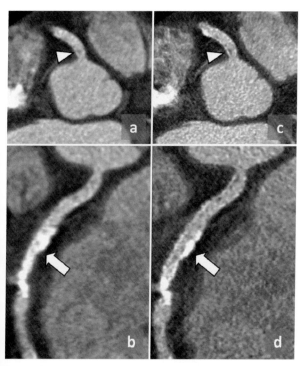

Fig. 15.3 Coronary artery stent evaluation on images reconstructed using medium-smooth (a, b) and sharp (c, d) kernels. Smoothing of the image reduces noise but obscures proximal coronary plaque (a, arrowhead) and worsens blooming artefact in the stented region (b, arrow). Using a sharp kernel results in higher image noise but spatial resolution improves such that proximal coronary plaque can be identified (c, arrowhead) and stent assessment is more straightforward (d, arrow).

Diagnostic performance

Several clinical studies have compared CCT to conventional angiography for the detection of in-stent restenosis, defined as ≥50% luminal narrowing (Table 15.1). These studies consistently demonstrate that:

- CCT has a high negative predictive value
- Stent diameter is the most important predictor of in-stent luminal visibility: cut-off diameters of 2.75 or 3mm were identified for patient selection
- In patients with stent diameters ≥3mm, the sensitivity of DSCT for the detection of in-stent re-stenosis was found to be significantly higher than that of a traditional diagnostic work-up based on the combination of exercise electrocardiography, myocardial perfusion scintigraphy, and dobutamine-stress echocardiography (98% versus 65%)
- Stents implantated in the left main artery and proximal LAD/LCx arteries are the most appropriate for the use of CCT to rule out in-stent restenosis due to the larger stent sizes (Fig. 15.4); this part of the coronary tree is also relatively protected from motion artefacts.

Recent systematic review of nine published studies showed the sensitivity, specificity, positive, and negative predictive values of CT for the detection of in-stent stenosis to be 88, 92, 74, and 97%, respectively[1].

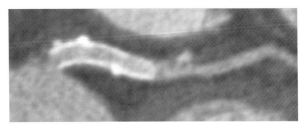

Fig. 15.4 Stent within the LMS coronary artery.

Further reading

1 Stein PD, Yaekoub AY, Matta F, et al. (2008) 64-slice CT for diagnosis of coronary artery disease: a systematic review. *Am J Med* **121**, 715–725.

Table 15.1 Detection of in-stent restenosis—diagnostic performance of CT compared with conventional angiography.[1–11]

64-Slice CT	Unevaluable stents (%)	Sensitivity (%)	Specificity (%)	PPV (%)	NPV (%)
Rixe[1]					
All diameters	42	86	98	86	98
>3mm	22	100	100	100	100
3mm	42	83	96	83	96
<3mm*	92	—	100	—	100
Ehara[2]					
All diameters	12	92	81	54	98
Cademartiri[3]					
All diameters	7	90	86	44	98
Das[4]					
All diameters	3	97	88	78	99
Schuijf[5]					
All diameters	14	100	100	—	—
Carbone[6]					
All diameters	28	75	86	83	79
≥3mm	3	85	97	94	95
Hecht[7]					
All diameters	0	94	75	39	99
Carrabba[8]					
All diameters	0	84	97	92	97
Manghat[9]					
All diameters	10	85	86	61	96
≥3mm	0	100	94	81	100
DSCT					
Pugliese[10]					
All diameters	5	94	92	77	98
≥3.5mm	0	100	100	100	100
3mm	0	100	97	91	100
≤2.75mm	22	84	64	52	90
Oncel[11]					
All diameters	0	100	94	89	100

*Only 1 stent available, without in-stent restenosis.

Conclusion

Although no guidelines have yet been published, the available clinical data suggest that CCT is likely to be appropriate in:

• Follow-up of asymptomatic patients after unprotected LMS
• Patients with symptoms, but low clinical probability of in-stent re-stenosis.

The appropriateness of CCT should be carefully considered in the context of unfavourable stent characteristics such as:

• Diameter <2.75mm
• Hyper-dense metal, thick struts, and/or underdeployed stent
• Stent-in-stent configuration
• Heavily calcified underlying vessel wall.

Non-invasive assessment of disease progression in the native coronary tree is an appealing application of CCT, but only if a diagnostic study is likely. Tissue prolapses, stent malapposition, and underdeployment are generally beyond the resolution of CCT.

It is conceivable that the next generation of stents—thinner struts, absorbable, non-metallic—will be less affected by the blooming effect. The introduction of these new devices may increase the applicability of CCT in patients after PCI.

Further reading

1 Rixe J, Achenbach S, Ropers D, *et al.* (2006) Assessment of coronary artery stent restenosis by 64-slice multi-detector computed tomography. *Eur Heart J* **27**, 2567–2572.

2 Ehara M, Kawai M, Surmely JF, *et al.* (2007) Diagnostic accuracy of coronary in-stent restenosis using 64-slice computed tomography: comparison with invasive coronary angiography. *J Am Coll Cardiol* **49**, 951–959.

3 Cademartiri F, Schuijf JD, Pugliese F, *et al.* (2007) Usefulness of 64-slice multislice computed tomography coronary angiography to assess in-stent restenosis. *J Am Coll Cardiol* **49**, 2204–2210.

4 Das KM, El-Menyar AA, Salam AM, *et al.* (2007) Contrast-enhanced 64-section coronary multidetector CT angiography versus conventional coronary angiography for stent assessment. *Radiology* **245**, 424–432.

5 Schuijf JD, Pundziute G, Jukema JW, *et al.* (2007) Evaluation of patients with previous coronary stent implantation with 64-section CT. *Radiology* **245**, 416–423.

6 Carbone I, Francone M, Algeri E, *et al.* (2008) Non-invasive evaluation of coronary artery stent patency with retrospectively ECG-gated 64-slice CT angiography. *Eur Radiol* **18**, 234–243.

7 Hecht HS, Zaric M, Jelnin V, Lubarsky L, Prakash M, AND Roubin G. (2008) Usefulness of 64-detector computed tomographic angiography for diagnosing in-stent restenosis in native coronary arteries. *Am J Cardiol* **101**, 820–824.

8 Carrabba N, Bamoshmoosh M, Carusi LM, *et al.* (2007) Usefulness of 64-slice multidetector computed tomography for detecting drug eluting in-stent restenosis. *Am J Cardiol* **100**, 1754–1758.

9 Manghat N, Van Lingen R, Hewson P, *et al.* (2008) Usefulness of 64-detector row computed tomography for evaluation of intracoronary stents in symptomatic patients with suspected in-stent restenosis. *Am J Cardiol* **101**, 1567–1573.

10 Pugliese F, Weustink AC, Van Mieghem C, *et al.* (2008) Dual source coronary computed tomography angiography for detecting in-stent restenosis. *Heart* **94**, 848–854.

11 Oncel D, Oncel G, Tastan A, and Tamci B (2008) Evaluation of coronary stent patency and in-stent restenosis with dual-source CT coronary angiography without heart rate control. *Am J Roentgenol* **191**, 56–63.

Coronary artery bypass graft imaging

Introduction

Background

Coronary artery bypass grafting (CABG), introduced in the 1960s, allows revascularization of the myocardium by providing an alternative route for blood flow around coronary artery stenoses. It is possibly the most intensively investigated surgical procedure in existence. Advances in the pharmacological treatment of CAD mean that revascularization (PCI or CABG) is mostly reserved for those patients who remain symptomatic despite optimal medical therapy. The choice between PCI and CABG for revascularization has become blurred, particularly with the increasing use of LMS PCI. However, the most recent guidelines suggest that patients with more severe CAD have higher survival rates and less need for repeat revascularization after CABG.[1]

Grafts

Vessels used for grafting include the great saphenous vein ('vein grafts') left and right internal mammary arteries (LIMA and RIMA, respectively) radial artery and, rarely, the gastro-epiploic artery. In general, arterial grafts have superior patency rates when compared to vein grafts as they are better able to tolerate systemic arterial haemodynamics.

The LIMA and RIMA arise from their respective subclavian arteries and travel down the inner surface of the ribcage approximately 1cm lateral to the sternum. When used as bypass grafts, the subclavian origin is left intact whilst the rest of the artery is mobilized. The distal end is anastomosed to the relevant coronary artery (typically the LAD). Side branches are obstructed using surgical clips, whose density can occasionally cause problematic artefacts on CCT images.

Other grafts are harvested from their usual positions and prepared. One end is anastamosed to the ascending aorta whilst the other is grafted to the relevant coronary artery. As both ends require anastamosis, these grafts are sometimes referred to as interrupted grafts.

Typical anatomy of interrupted grafts

- RCA grafts usually arise from the right anterior surface of the aorta and travel vertically downwards, often to the inferior surface of the heart.
- Obtuse marginal grafts mostly arise from the left anterior aspect of the aorta and travel towards the lateral wall. (NB: The LCx is difficult to graft due to its location within the LAVG).
- Grafts to the LAD and its branches arise from the anterior surface of the aorta and run downwards towards the AIVG (LAD) or anterolateral surface of the heart (diagonals).

Role of CCT

The aim is to provide information on graft patency and graft anatomy. The native coronary vessels, in particular distal run-off, should also be evaluated, although heavy calcification and stents affect assessment.

- Coronary grafts are often larger than native coronary vessels and are less susceptible to motion artefact, allowing high diagnostic accuracy for the detection of stenoses.
- Cardiac imaging workstations have 3D volume-rendering capabilities that allow excellent demonstration of the course and position of grafts (Fig. 16.1a).
- Interrupted grafts (vein grafts, radial artery grafts) pursue a varying course from the ascending aorta to their distal insertions.
- Anatomical detail is particularly relevant prior to repeat cardiac surgery; grafts frequently occupy a retro-sternal position, rendering them susceptible to injury during repeat sternotomy (Fig. 16.1b).
- The right ventricle is also located anteriorly within the thorax. This may partially adhere to the sternum in the post-surgical patient and can be injured during repeat surgery.

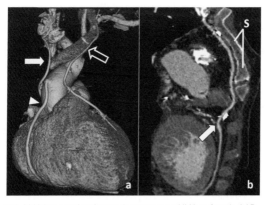

Fig. 16.1 (a) Volume-rendered image demonstrating a LIMA graft to the LAD (white outline arrow), a RIMA graft to the lateral obtuse marginal artery (white arrow) and a saphenous vein graft (SVG) to the RCA (arrowhead). (b) Curved multi-planar reformat showing good distal run-off from the LIMA to LAD (white arrow marks the anastomosis). Note the blooming of the surgical clips and the close proximity of the LIMA to the sternum (S). (📖 Plate 2 for colour version).

Further reading

Wijns W, Kolh P, Danchin N, et al. (2010) Guidelines on myocardial revascularization: The Task Force on Myocardial Revascularization of the European Society of Cardiology (ESC) and the European Association for Cardio-Thoracic Surgery (EACTS). *Eur Heart J* **31**(20), 2501–2555.

Scan acquisition

Scan acquisition for graft imaging (see 📖 CT coronary angiography, p. 108) is similar to standard CTA, as native coronary information is also usually required.

- Any conventional CCT scanning technique may be used, with the choice depending on the patient's heart rate and rhythm, and the need for functional information (i.e. prospective or retrospective studies, with or without tube modulation).
- Coronary artery grafts are generally less susceptible to motion artefact than native coronaries, increasing the chance of diagnostic image quality in patients with ↑ heart rates or dysrhythmias.
- Graft positions are relatively fixed when compared to native vessels, again reducing motion artefact and improving image quality.
- Vein grafts are the easiest to evaluate by virtue of their larger calibre compared to distal native coronary arteries (Fig. 16.2).

Although similar in principle to standard CTA acquisition (Fig. 16.2), there are some special requirements for graft studies.

- Scan coverage needs to be extended cranially to cover proximal graft insertions into the ascending aorta.
- Internal mammary graft visualization requires cranial extension to include the subclavian arteries. This can be achieved by initiating the scan just above the clavicles.

Increasing scan coverage increases both scanning time and radiation dose

- The prolongation of scan acquisition is dependent on the z-axis coverage of the scanner (see 📖 Detector terminology, p. 16), e.g. prospectively gated axial acquisitions would take longer on a 64-slice compared with a 320-slice CT— the entire chest could be covered in two steps (2 × 16~32cm) with 320 slices but eight steps (8 × 4~32cm) with 64 slices.
- There is a dramatic increase in radiation exposure in studies gated retrospectively without tube current modulation (see 📖 ECG gating, p. 34). Exposure may be reduced either by modulating the tube current (mAs) during retrospective acquisitions or by acquiring images prospectively.
- Graft studies require a longer breath hold to maximize image quality— patients with significant underlying cardio-respiratory disease may find this difficult if the scan time is prolonged.

Increasing scan time may impact on contrast timing.

- A graft study commencing above the clavicles may demonstrate suboptimal contrast opacification of the distal graft insertions unless the contrast parameters are adjusted.
- This risk is minimized by increasing the total volume of contrast or injection speed, thereby ensuring prolonged vessel enhancement.

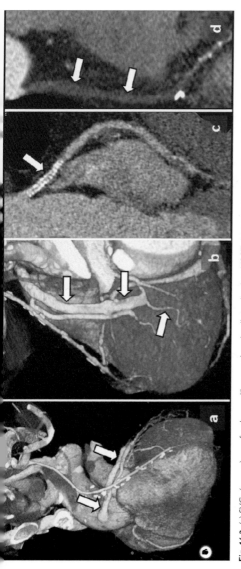

Fig. 16.2 (a) SVGs (arrows) are often large caliber vessels and well visualized on MSCT. (b) It is important to assess both the graft and the vessel it supplies (arrows), in this case an obtuse marginal branch of the left circumflex artery. Volume-rendered images should not be used to assess the coronary lumen. SVGs may be stented (c) and are more prone to occlusion (d) than arterial grafts.

Image analysis and interpretation

Metallic streak artefact (see 📖 Beam hardening, p. 152) is a common occurrence in graft studies, and can be caused by sternal wiring, surgical graft clips, valve prostheses, or pacing wires.

- The appearances are of light/dark streaks radiating from the edges, with ill-defined object margins.
- These artefacts occur at abrupt transitions of attenuation with hyperdense objects (such as surgical clips) with Hounsfield unit values beyond the processing capacity of CT electronics.
- Diagnostic image quality is reduced when areas of interest (such as the graft itself) are obscured, for example by surgical clips (Fig. 16.3b).
- Tilting the CT gantry (not available on all scanners) may exclude smaller metallic objects from the imaging plane, or at least throw any resulting artefact away from the region of interest.
- Image processing algorithms may minimize the streaking effect, but these are manufacturer dependent.

Partial volume (blooming), beam hardening, and motion artefacts (see 📖 Sources of artefact, p. 151) should all be considered in CABG studies.

Diagnostic performance

64-slice CT is able to obtain diagnostic images of grafts in almost all cases depending on heart rate and dysrhythmias.

- Diagnostic accuracy for identification of significant stenoses (>50%) in the body of grafts is high.
- A recent National Institute of Health Research Health Technology Appraisal of 64-slice CT subjected four studies involving 543 patients with CABG published between 2002 and 2006 to meta-analysis.[1] Pooled sensitivity, specificity, PPV and NPV for the detection of >50% graft stenosis were 99, 96, 93, and 99%, respectively.
- More recent studies, including those using DSCT, have yielded similar results.
- The high NPV allows reassurance of patients with a negative examination.
- 2010 American College of Cardiology appropriateness criteria (see 📖 Appropriate use criteria for cardiovascular CT, p. 458) rate CCT as an appropriate indication for the assessment of grafts in symptomatic patients.
- Distal graft anastamoses in small target vessels can be hard to analyse, which can significantly reduce diagnostic confidence.
- Results for the evaluation of native coronary arteries are poorer as they are likely to be diseased and heavily calcified. Although the NPV of CCT remains high, the PPV is only ~80%.

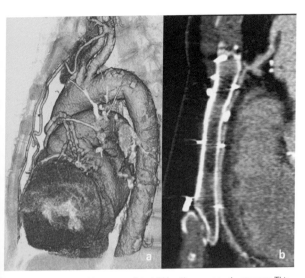

Fig. 16.3 Assessment of the course of the LIMA with respect to the sternum. This is an important factor when considering redo sternotomy in a patient with a healthy LIMA graft. (a) Volume-rendered images allow 3D assessment of the course with respect to the sternum, allowing surgeons to assess the most appropriate surgical approach. (b) Curved MPR of the same patient showing blooming of surgical clips and sternal wires (arrows) and the close proximity of the LIMA to the sternum. (📖 Plate 3 for colour version).

Further reading

1 Mowatt G, Cummins E, Waugh N, et al. (2008) Systematic review of the clinical effectiveness and cost-effectiveness of 64-slice or higher computed tomography angiography as an alternative to invasive coronary angiography in the investigation of coronary artery disease. *Health Technol Assess* **12**(17), iii–iv, ix–143.

Conclusions

Cardiac CT imaging after CABG allows evaluation of graft patency, anatomy, distal runoff, and native coronary vessels.

- Coronary grafts are larger and less susceptible to motion artefact than native coronary vessels.
- ↑ scan coverage leads to ↑ radiation dose and prolonged breath hold, and may affect contrast requirements and timings.
- Metallic streak artefact is largely unavoidable at present.
- Partial volume artefact contributes to calcium and stent bloom.
- Beam hardening and step artefacts may mimic stenosis.
- Vessel analysis using multiple views is essential in distinguishing true pathology from exaggerating or mimicking artefacts.
- Despite these potential pitfalls, the diagnostic accuracy of CCT for the detection of graft stenosis is high, with sensitivities and specificities reported as consistently >95%.
- Small distal graft anastamosis can be difficult to evaluate.
- Native coronary vessels are likely to be diseased and heavily calcified, reducing interpretative accuracy.

Evaluation of ventricular and atrial function

Introduction

For retrospectively gated studies, data obtained during the MSCT coronary angiogram can also be used to assess left ventricular (LV) function. Furthermore, extended scan protocols allow right ventricular (RV) function to be assessed. It should be remembered that LV functional information comes for 'free' with the CCT coronary angiographic dataset. As CT is a cross-sectional technique it allows accurate assessment of both LV and RV function if required, and this chapter will discuss both LV and RV volumetric assessment and the necessary protocols.

Anatomy

The terms right and left, when applied to a cardiac chamber, refer to morphology, not position. This is particularly important in patients with CHD (see 🕮 Congenital heart disease, p. 331).

Relevant morphological features include:
- Right ventricle—usually heavily trabeculated, lacks fibrous continuation between the inlet and outlet valves, and has most apically attached atrio-ventricular valve annulus.
- Left ventricle—smooth walled with no attachment of the inlet valve leaflet to the septum.

CT acquisition

For left ventriculography there is no requirement to amend the standard CCT coronary angiography protocol.
- The use of iodinated contrast for CT coronary angiography allows clear delineation of the LV endocardium from the iodinated blood pool.
- LV functional information comes for 'free' with a retrospectively gated MSCT coronary angiogram.
- Extended scan protocols allow RV function (see 🕮 Combined CT coronary and pulmonary angiography, p. 432).
- For RV studies, iodinated contrast is required in the RV blood pool to distinguish it from the RV endocardium.
- This may present problems when performing concurrent CT coronary angiography, as streak artefact may inhibit the interpretation of the proximal RCA.
- Reconstruction of the datasets at multiple phases of the cardiac cycle (usually every 5 or 10%) allows calculation of both end-diastolic and end-systolic volumes.
- Stroke volume, cardiac output, and ejection fraction can then be calculated.

Assessment of global left ventricular function

Assessment of LV global and regional systolic function is possible on all retrospectively gated CT coronary angiography studies.

- This is not possible using prospectively gated studies; alternative techniques such as transthoracic echocardiography (TTE), may be necessary.
- With modern post-processing software, calculation of global LV function is quick and should be included as part of a standard CCT report.
- There are no guidelines on the number of retrospective phases that should be used to evaluate LV function, but a minimum of eight to ten should be processed to ensure accurate identification of end-systole.
- The size of the dataset increases significantly with each phase reconstructed, as each phase usually contains 200–300 axial slices.

Volumes and mass

Calculation of LV volumes is usually based on the attenuation of the blood pool and is derived using a threshold technique (Fig. 17.1). This distinguishes between the higher attenuation of the blood pool and the lower attenuation of the myocardium.

- Good LV contrast opacification (as is required in any case for CT coronary angiography) is necessary for accurate LV analysis.
- LV mass is calculated from the product of the myocardial volume and the specific gravity of heart muscle (1.05g/mL).
- There are no multicentre trials or meta-analyses evaluating ≥64-slice MSCT for the evaluation of global LV function.
- MSCT has been validated in small, single-centre studies against cardiovascular magnetic resonance (CMR), TTE and SPECT MPS; limits of agreement tend to be wide.
- In general, LV volumes calculated by MSCT are typically higher than those seen on CMR and MPS. This overestimation is systematic for both systolic and diastolic volumes, and ∴ has a smaller impact on LV ejection fraction values.
- Inter- and intra-observer reproducibility is generally good (Table 17.1).

Global function

- The most commonly measured parameter is LV ejection fraction (LVEF); global function should always be assessed visually as well.
- LVEF is related to the end-diastolic (LVEDV) and end-systolic (LVESV) volumes according to the following equation:

$$LVEF = \frac{LVEDV - LVESV \times 100\%}{LVEDV}$$

- As a general rule, LVEF >50% is normal, 40–50% mildly impaired, 30–40% moderately impaired, and <30% severely impaired.
- Large trials comparing techniques are lacking, particularly in patients with LV dysfunction.

- In general, MSCT shows excellent agreement with CMR and TTE, usually with mean difference in LVEF of ~1–2%. However, as with calculation of LV volumes, limits of agreement tend to be quite wide.
- Inter- and intraobserver variabilities in MSCT-derived LVEF are typically in the region of ±3%[1] (Table 17.1).

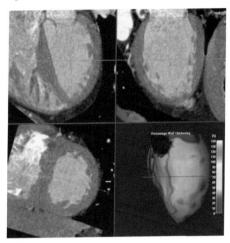

Fig. 17.1 Left ventriculography using a threshold technique. (📖 Plate 4 for colour version)

Table 17.1 Inter- and intraobserver variabilities for CCT-derived LV volumes, global function, and mass.[1] SD, standard deviation

	Interobserver variability		Intraobserver variability	
	Mean	**SD**	**Mean**	**SD**
LVEDV (mL)	12	18	4	11
LVESV (mL)	5	13	2	6
LVEF (%)	1	3	−1	2
LV mass (g)	3	15	2	12

Further reading

Nicol E, Stirrup J, Roughton M, *et al.* (2009) 64-Channel cardiac computed tomography: intraobserver and interobserver variability (Part 2): Global and regional ventricular function, mass and first pass perfusion. *J Comp Assist Tomogr* **33**(2), 169–174.

Assessment of regional left ventricular function

Although regional abnormalities can occur in cardiomyopathies, the most common cause of regional LV dysfunction is CAD. Assessment of regional abnormalities of ventricular function is usually done by eye and depends on operator experience. The key to reporting regional dysfunction is to use a standard system to segment the heart. The American Heart Association 17 segment model (which includes a true apical segment) is encouraged to allow similar segment models between imaging techniques.

Measures of regional function

- LV regional diastolic wall thickness, wall motion, and wall thickening can also be derived from the CCT dataset.
- LV regional function may be assessed using the standard 17-segment model for the left ventricle (Fig. 17.2) and described in terms of the motion and thickening of each segment.
- Wall motion is generally described as normal, hypokinetic (reduced movement), akinetic (no movement), or dyskinetic (movement in the wrong direction). Hypokinesis may be mild, moderate, or severe.
- Assessment of wall motion in isolation is insensitive for the detection of dysfunctional segments as they may move passively as a result of normally functioning adjacent segments. Assessment of wall thickening is ∴ mandatory.
- Wall thickening may be described as normal (>50% thickening between diastole and systole), reduced (to a degree that may be mild, moderate, or severe), or absent.
- The likely affected coronary territory may be predicted using the 17-segment model (Fig. 17.3) and by correlation with CTA.
- MSCT shows good agreement with TTE and CMR for normal, akinetic, and dyskinetic wall motion, but only a moderate agreement in the assessment of hypokinetic segments. This is most likely due to the difference in spatial resolution between these modalities.
- DSCT shows excellent agreement with invasive left ventriocuolography for the detection of regional wall motion abnormalities.[1]
- Inter- and intraobserver agreement is generally good,[1,2] although the majority of published data come from patient populations with a low incidence of regional LV dysfunction.
- In those with reperfused acute myocardial infarction, interobserver agreement for the detection of regional dysfunction is similar for both MSCT and CMR.[3]

Resting perfusion

It is advisable to assess regional LV perfusion (see 📖 Evaluation of myocardial perfusion, p. 270) as part of the overall assessment of LV function, as the combination of a perfusion defect with a regional wall motion abnormality is a more specific finding than isolated hypoattenuation or the first-pass study.

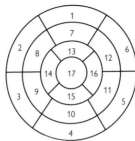

1. Basal anterior	7. Mid anterior	13. Apical anterior
2. Basal anteroseptal	8. Mid anteroseptal	14. Apical septal
3. Basal inferoseptal	9. Mid inferoseptal	15. Apical inferior
4. Basal inferior	10. Mid inferior	16. Apical lateral
5. Basal inferolateral	11. Mid inferolateral	17. Apex
6. Basal anterolateral	12. Mid anterolateral	

Fig. 17.2 17 segment model. Reproduced with permission from Sabharwal N, Loong CY, and Kelion A (2008). *Nuclear Cardiology*. Oxford University Press.

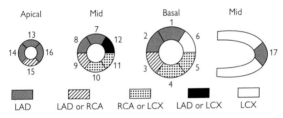

Fig. 17.3 Typical coronary artery distribution for the 17-segment model, assuming RCA dominance.[4] American Heart Association 17-segment model of the human heart. Copyright 1997 with permission from Elsevier.

Further reading

1 Pflederer T, Ho KT, Anger T, *et al.* (2009) Assessment of regional left ventricular function by dual source computed tomography: interobserver variability and validation to laevocardiography. *Eur J Radiol* **72**(1), 85–91.

2 Nicol E, Stirrup J, Roughton M, *et al.* (2009) 64-Channel cardiac computed tomography: intraobserver and interobserver variability (Part 2): Global and regional ventricular function, mass and first pass perfusion. *J Comp Assist Tomogr* **33**(2), 169–174.

3 Sarwar A, Shapiro M, Nasir K, *et al.* (2009) Evaluating global and regional left ventricular function in patients with reperfused acute myocardial infarction by 64-slice multidetector CT: A comparison to magnetic resonance imaging. *J Cardiovasc Comput Tomogr* **3**, 170–77.

4 Pereztol-Valdés O, Candell-Riera J, Santana-Boado C, *et al.* (2005) Correspondence between left ventricular 17 myocardial segments and coronary arteries. *Eur Heart J* **26**, 2637–2643.

Right ventriculography

Assessment of RV global and regional systolic function is possible using any protocol that allows delineation of the RV blood pool from the RV myocardium. This includes a retrospectively gated CTPA study or a combined, retrospectively gated CT coronary and pulmonary angiography study (see 📖 Combined CT coronary and pulmonary angiography, p. 432).

- Right ventriculography is not possible with prospectively gated or ungated studies.
- In contrast to LV analysis, which is usually straightforward, analysis of RV function is usually time-consuming and is not a routine part of reporting in standard cardiac CT.
- Recently vendors have started to include semi-automated RV analysis tools in their software, but these are not widely validated and the results should be interpreted with caution.
- Generally, the pool of data validating RV function is smaller than that for LV function and comes from cohorts with either CHD or pulmonary hypertension.

Volumes and mass

RV volumes are based on the attenuation of the RV blood pool and derived using a threshold technique (Fig. 17.4). This has an advantage over tracing techniques as the heavy trabeculations of the RV are excluded from the volumetric analysis. This should be borne in mind when comparing volumetric data using different methods.

- Correlation between MSCT and CMR is moderate; MSCT slightly overestimates volumes.[1]
- RV mass is calculated from the product of the myocardial volume and specific gravity of heart muscle (1.05g/mL), but assessment of the thin-walled RV is challenging.

Function

It is possible to assess both global and regional RV function using a retrospectively gated combined coronary and pulmonary angiography protocol.

- Global function is described using the RV ejection fraction (RVEF).
- RVEF is related to the end-diastolic (RVEDV) and end-systolic (RVESV) volumes according to the following equation:

$$RVEF = \frac{RVEDV - RVESV \times 100\%}{RVEDV}$$

- As a general rule, RVEF > 50% is normal, 40–50% mildly impaired, 30–40% moderately impaired, and <30% severely impaired.
- There is good agreement between MSCT and CMR for RV ejection fraction, with a mean difference typically 1–2%.[1]
- RV regional wall motion can also be derived from the dataset, but is assessed visually as there is no standard segmentation model for the right ventricle.

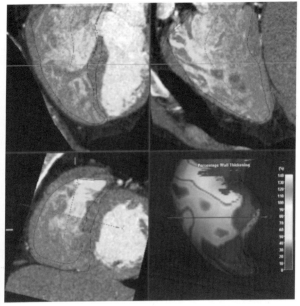

Fig. 17.4 Right ventriculography using a threshold technique. (☐ Plate 5 for colour version.

Further reading

1 Nicol ED, Kafka H, Stirrup J, et al. (2009) A single, comprehensive non-invasive cardiovascular assessment in pulmonary arterial hypertension: combined computed tomography pulmonary and coronary angiography. *Int J Cardiol* **136**(3), 278–288.

Atrial assessment

Introduction

As with ventriculography, the opacification of the atrial blood pool allows volumetric analysis to be performed using CT angiographic datasets. Assessment of the left atrium requires no change to the standard CT coronary angiography protocol; evaluation of the right atrium requires extended or specific contrast protocols, e.g. a gated CTPA protocol (see Gated CT pulmonary angiogram, p. 110). There has been increasing interest in atrial volumes as an independent predictor of cardiac events such as heart failure, myocardial infarction, AF, stroke, and cardiovascular death.

Anatomy

Relevant morphological features of the atria include:
- Left atrium—usually receives the pulmonary venous return with a tubular-based ('finger-like') atrial appendage
- Right atrium—usually receives systemic venous return and has a broad-based atrial appendage.

Assessment of atrial volumes

Right and left atrial volumes are based on the attenuation of the atrial blood pool and derived using either a threshold technique or a modified Simpson's method.
- Normal ranges have not yet been specified for MSCT.
- There is good correlation between MSCT and CMR and 3D echocardiography for left atrial volumes.
- Inter- and intraobserver variability is low.[1]
- Reproducibility is better for MSCT than TTE.
- MSCT volumes are systematically greater than with 2D echocardiography.

Assessment of atrial function

It is possible to assess the function of both atria using a retrospectively gated combined coronary and pulmonary angiography protocol (see Combined CT coronary and pulmonary angiography, p. 432), although the technique has yet to find widespread use clinically.

Further reading

1 Wolf F, Ourednicek P, Loewe C, *et al.* (2010) Evaluation of left atrial function by multidetector computed tomography before left atrial radiofrequency-catheter ablation: Comparison of a manual and automated 3D volume segmentation method *Eur J Radiol* **75**(2), e141–e146.

Ventricular pathology

Introduction

The most common requests for cardiovascular CT are to exclude coronary disease, and usually LV function will be entirely normal. However, in patients with coronary stenoses that are equivocal (i.e. 50–70%) or significant, assessment of both global and regional LV function is valuable and may improve reporting specificity.

Occasionally, patients referred for assessment of the coronary arteries will turn out to have unsuspected ventricular disease. Additionally, some patients are referred for cardiovascular CT to monitor ventricular function in the setting of known pathology, such as those who have previously had cardiac MRI follow-up but have had a pacemaker or implantable defibrillator inserted. This section will highlight the most common pathologies where assessment of LV, RV, or biventricular function is required.

Ventricular pathologies include:
- Ischaemic LV dysfunction
- Cardiomyopathies
- Infiltrative diseases
- Tumours.

Investigating ischaemic left ventricular dysfunction

General considerations

Hibernating myocardium

In some patients with LV dysfunction $2°$ to coronary disease, systolic impairment may not be entirely due to previous infarction (scar). A variable amount of the dysfunctional myocardium may be 'hibernating', i.e. viable but dysfunctional due to impaired coronary flow.

Hibernating myocardium is a clinical concept; the underlying pathophysiology remains controversial. Two mechanisms are proposed:

- Reduced resting perfusion leads to down-regulation of contractile function without the development of metabolic ischaemia
- Resting perfusion is virtually normal, but absence of vasodilator reserve leads to demand ischaemia on minimal exertion with repetitive post-ischaemic stunning which never has the opportunity to recover.

It is probable that revascularization is beneficial for patients with significant hibernating myocardium, but not for those with scar.

- A number of studies have shown that patients with impaired LV function and little viable myocardium are at high risk (17%) of cardiac events whether revascularized or not.
- Those with significant viable myocardium are at similarly high risk if managed conservatively (20%), but at lower risk following revascularization (7%).
- However, all studies to date have been retrospective and non-randomized, and ∴ vulnerable to important selection biases.

Roles of imaging in ischaemic left ventricular dysfunction

Imaging in known or suspected ischaemic LV dysfunction has two roles:

1 In patients *with* documented coronary disease, to identify those with significant amounts of hibernating myocardium who are likely to benefit from revascularization

2 In patients *without* known coronary disease, to distinguish between ischaemic LV dysfunction, with the potential to benefit from revascularization and cardiomyopathy.

All imaging modalities (SPECT, PET, echo, MRI) offer protocols to distinguish between scar and viable myocardium in patients with known coronary anatomy and are widely used for the first indication. For those with symptoms due to LV dysfunction but no background of coronary disease, these investigations have also been used diagnostically for the second indication, relying on regional dysfunction or evidence of sub-endocardial or transmural scarring as criteria for ischaemic LV dysfunction.

However, some patients with dilated cardiomyopathy can have relatively regional dysfunction, whilst some patients with ischaemic LV dysfunction, indeed those with most to gain from revascularization, can have global dysfunction with little or no scar but extensive hibernation. There is ∴ no reliable alternative to the assessment of coronary anatomy in distinguishing ischaemic from myopathic LV dysfunction.

The role of cardiac CT

Distinguishing ischaemic left ventricular dysfunction from dilated cardiomyopathy

CCT is the only non-invasive imaging modality able to define coronary anatomy reliably, making it an attractive technique for ruling out significant coronary disease in patients presenting with LV impairment of undefined cause. A number of studies have demonstrated an excellent performance for this indication, using initially 16-slice and more recently 64-slice scanners.

In a single-centre study of 132 patients presenting with apparent dilated cardiomyopathy, two were excluded for atrial fibrillation and the others underwent both CCT and ICA.[1]

- 88 had normal coronary arteries, whilst 42 had coronary disease at invasive angiography (number of vessels: one 11, two 13, three 18).
- For the detection of >70% stenosis in any vessel, CCT had an NPV of 99.4% and a PPV of 99.9%.
- All patients with coronary disease except one were correctly classified by CCT according to the number of diseased vessels.

It is probable that the PPV of CCT will fall as it is rolled out into routine clinical practice across centres, but it is likely that the NPV will remain high. Thus CCT may become an increasingly important screening tool to rule out significant coronary disease in patients presenting with heart failure.

Cardiac CT to distinguish between scar and viable myocardium

Currently, CCT cannot be recommended as an alternative to the other imaging modalities in the routine assessment of hibernating myocardium in patients with ischaemic LV dysfunction. However, where it has been used to identify coronary disease in patients with LV dysfunction of hitherto unknown aetiology, it may provide useful clues to the state of the myocardium:

- Diastolic wall thinning (<6mm) suggests loss of viability
- Regional myocardial hypoperfusion at rest suggests microvascular damage (i.e. infarction); transmural extent can be assessed
- Myocardial hyperenhancement on delayed imaging post contrast injection (see 📖 Image interpretation, p. 266) indicates scar, analogous to late gadolinium enhancement on cardiac MRI; transmural extent can be assessed.

Myocardial hyperenhancement has been validated against SPECT, low-dose dobutamine echo, and MRI in patients scanned immediately post invasive angiography in the setting of acute myocardial infarction. Whether this technique is valuable in the chronic setting for distinguishing between scar and hibernating myocardium has yet to be established.

Further reading

1 Andreini D, Pontone G, Bartorelli AL, et al. (2009) Sixty-four-slice multidetector computed tomography. An accurate imaging modality for the evaluation of coronary arteries in dilated cardiomyopathy of unknown etiology. *Circulation: Cardiovasc Imaging* **2**, 199–205.

Cardiomyopathies and myocardial infiltration

Definitions

The World Health Organization defines cardiomyopathies as 'diseases of the myocardium associated with cardiac dysfunction'.[1] Irrespective of any identifiable 2° cause, they are classified morphologically and physiologically as:

- Dilated cardiomyopathy
- Hypertrophic cardiomyopathy
- Restrictive cardiomyopathy (rare)
- Arrhythmogenic RV cardiomyopathy
- 'Unclassified' cardiomyopathies, including:
  - LV non-compaction
  - Takotsubo cardiomyopathy.

Myocardial infiltrations, such as amyloidosis and sarcoidosis, can present with features of one or more of the cardiomyopathies.

Role of imaging

Imaging has a number of roles in the evaluation of patients with possible cardiomyopathy or myocardial infiltration:

- Establish and quantify the fact of ventricular dysfunction
- Identify treatable 2° causes of ventricular dysfunction, such as coronary or valvular disease
- Provide additional pathophysiological information to guide prognostication and management, such as the degree of fibrosis or the presence of infiltrative material.

All imaging modalities provide valuable information in each of these categories. Echocardiography is the first-line investigation for almost all patients, and usually provides a good assessment of LV function and valve structure and function. Second-line imaging may be required to provide more reproducible quantification of LV function, to image the right ventricle more reliably, to exclude significant underlying coronary disease, and to examine myocardial thickness and structure in more detail. Cardiac MRI is excellent in this role, but is unsuitable for a significant minority of patients, e.g. those unable to lie flat for a prolonged period, or with a pacemaker or implantable defibrillator. Moreover, MRI provides only limited information about underlying coronary disease.

Cardiovascular CT is increasingly important where:

- Cardiac MRI is contraindicated
- It is necessary to distinguish between ischaemic LV dysfunction and a myopathic process
- Unexpected abnormalities of ventricular function are identified on routine CCT scans for coronary disease.

Further reading

1 Report of the 1995 World Health Organization/International Society and Federation of Cardiology Task Force on the definition and classification of cardiomyopathies (1996) *Circulation* **93**, 841–842.

Cardiac CT appearances in cardiomyopathies

Dilated cardiomyopathy

- Dilated cardiomyopathy is the dilatation and impaired contraction of the left ventricle or both ventricles.
- The degree of dysfunction is disproportionate to any abnormality of loading conditions.
- The degree of dysfunction is disproportionate to any coronary disease.
- Normal or reduced myocardial thickness.
- Mitral annulus may be dilated, with leaflet tethering.

Hypertrophic cardiomyopathy

- LV hypertrophy (>15mm end-diastolic) in the absence of ↑ afterload.
- Often asymmetrical, classically affecting the interventricular septum (Fig. 18.1) or sometimes apex (apical hypertrophic cardiomyopathy).
- Myocardial thickness ≤30mm is a risk factor for sudden death.
- Non-dilated LV cavity with hyperdynamic function (except in the end-stage).
- May have LVOT narrowing with systolic anterior motion of the anterior mitral valve leaflet.
- May have RV hypertrophy.
- Late myocardial hyper-enhancement has been described on CCT, suggesting fibrosis: this is known to be an adverse prognostic marker on MRI.[1]

Restrictive cardiomyopathy

- Restrictive filling and reduced diastolic volume of the left ventricle or both ventricles.
- Normal or near-normal systolic function and myocardial thickness.
- Dilated atria.
- Late myocardial hyperenhancement suggesting fibrosis would be expected, although this has not yet been reported in the literature.

Arrhythmogenic right ventricular cardiomyopathy

- When performing CCT, aim to optimize contrast in right heart.
- CCT findings in arhythmogenic right ventricular cardiomyopathy (ARVC) based on Johns Hopkins series[2] (Table 18.1).

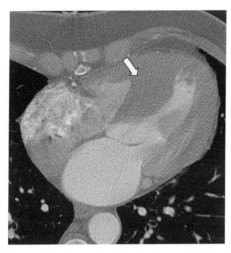

Fig. 18.1 Hypertrophic cardiomyopathy with marked asymmetrical hypertrophy of the interventricular septum (arrow) but with concurrent significant lateral wall hypertrophy. Note the mid cavity obliteration in this early systolic phase.

Table 18.1 CCT criteria for the diagnosis of arrhythmogenic right ventricular cardiomyopathy2

CCT criterion	ARVC (n = 17)	Not ARVC (n = 14)
Fat in RV free wall (−50 to −150HU)	76%	7%
Dilated RV (EDV mean±SD)	224±49mL	163±30mL
Scalloping of RV free wall	76%	7%
RV wall motion abnormalities	47%	7%
Conspicuous low-attenuation RV trabeculae	100%	21%

Edv, end diastolic volume.

Further reading

1. Shiozaki AA, Santos TSG, Artega E, Rochitte CE (2007) Myocardial delayed enhancement by computed tomography in hypertrophic cardiomyopathy. *Circulation* **115**, e430–431.
2. Bomma C, Dalal D, Tandri H, *et al.* (2007) Evolving role of multidetector computed tomography in evaluation of arrhythmogenic right ventricular dysplasia/cardiomyopathy. *Am J Cardiol* **100**, 99–105.

Cardiac CT in 'unclassified' cardiomyopathies and myocardial infiltrations

Left ventricular non-compaction[1]
- Prominent spongy/trabeculated inner myocardial layer.
- Particularly affects apical and mid segments of inferior and lateral walls.
- Ratio of non-compacted: compacted myocardium >2.3:1.

Takotsubo cardiomyopathy[2]
- Transient apical ballooning with akinesia/dyskinesia, resolving over a few days.
- Hyperdynamic basal myocardial segments.
- Myocardium viable.
- Coronaries unobstructed.

Amyloidosis
- Thickened myocardium.
- Hypodynamic systolic function without cavity dilatation.
- Impaired diastolic function.
- Dilated atria.
- May have thickened valve cusps/leaflets.
- Circumferential biventricular subendocardial late hyperenhancement, with atrial involvement, has been described with SCT.[3]

Sarcoidosis
- Wall thinning.
- Late hyperenhancement in basal septum and lateral wall, affecting any myocardial layer, has been described with SCT.[4]

Further reading
1 Carlson DW, Sullenberger LE, Cho KH, et al. (2007) Isolated ventricular noncompaction. *J Cardiovasc Comput Tomogr* **1**, 108–109.
2 Hara T, Hayashi T, Izawa I, and Kajiya T (2007) Noninvasive detection of Takotsubo cardiomyopathy using multidetector row computed tomography. *Int Heart J* **48**, 773–778.
3 Marwan M, Pflederer T, Ropers D, et al. (2008) Cardiac amyloidosis imaged by dual-source computed tomography. *J Cardiovasc Comput Tomogr* **2**, 403–405.
4 Muth G, Daniel WG, and Achenbach S (2008) Late enhancement on cardiac computed tomography in a patient with cardiac sarcoidosis. *J Cardiovasc Comput Tomogr* **2**, 272–273.

Cardiac masses

Cardiac tumours are rare (0.1–0.3% at autopsy) and presentation is variable. Benign tumours are by far the most common. Malignant cardiac tumours are most likely to represent metastatic disease from an extracardiac 1°.

The differential diagnosis of benign and malignant tumours of the heart may be compiled on the basis of demographic and CCT features. True diagnoses are often made only after histological examination after operation. However, CCT may define and delineate the mass, and potentially provide detail as to the best interventional or surgical approach from the broader 3D CCT dataset.

Benign cardiac tumours

Myxoma

Myxomas are the most common 1° cardiac tumour (30% of all 1° cardiac tumours), often presenting in middle age with symptoms of left heart obstruction or malaise. They are associated with emboli in 50% of cases. They may also be asymptomatic, discovered incidentally on cardiac imaging performed for other indications. CCT features include:

- 75% left atrium (Fig. 18.2), 20% right atrium, 5% ventricular.
- Usually attached to fossa ovalis (thick or thin stalk).
- Variable size.
- Combination of myxoid and fibrous tissue, giving a heterogeneous appearance with low density and foci of calcification.
- Contrast enhancement may be heterogenous (little in areas of necrosis, intense in areas of inflammation) or homogenous.
- Differential diagnosis includes:
  - Myofibroblastic sarcomas
  - Malignant fibrous histiocytoma (MFH)
  - Leiomyosarcoma
  - Fibrosarcoma
  - Myxosarcoma.
- Consider Carney syndrome if multiple/recurrent myxomas.

Papillary fibroelastoma

Papillary fibroelastomas (Fig. 18.3) are the second most common 1° benign tumour in adults, accounting for 75% of true valve tumours (i.e. excluding vegetations). They have a predilection for left-sided heart valves (particularly the mitral valve), and may lead to tumour or thrombus embolisation. On CCT, papillary fibroelastomas are usually:

- Small (<2cm) endocardial papillomas, usually on the valve surfaces of older patients
- Non-invasive—unlike infective vegetations, they do not cause valve destruction.

Lipoma

Lipomas account for 10% of benign 1° tumours and can present at any age. They may present with symptoms of chamber obstruction/dysrhythmia, or may be asymptomatic. Characteristic CCT features include:

- Solitary
- May be large
- Often epicardial, but may arise in myocardium and interatrial septum
- Characteristically well-defined homogenous fat density, with no contrast enhancement
- May contain soft tissue strands.

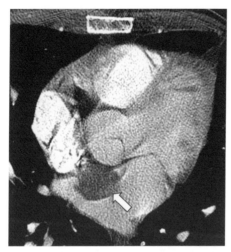

Fig. 18.2 Left atrial mxyoma in a patient who presented with breathlessness. Cine images may demonstrate functional mitral stenosis 2° to partial obstruction by the prolapsing myxoma.

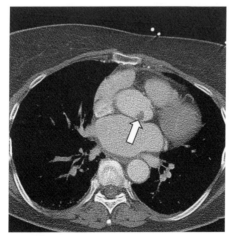

Fig. 18.3 Papillary fibroelastoma affecting the aortic valve (arrow).

Rhabdomyoma

Rrhabdomyomas may be considered a non-neoplastic hamartoma. They are the most common benign childhood cardiac tumour (90%), with 75% occurring in babies <1 year. They are rare in adults. Most patients are asymptomatic, although presentation may include dysrhythmia, murmur, or heart failure. Fifty per cent of patients with cardiac rhabdomyoma have tuberose sclerosis; spontaneous tumour regression is common. On CCT they are:

- Frequently multiple
- Usually found either within ventricular myocardium or as pedunculated masses extending into the cavity
- Associated with diffuse myocardial thickening if multiple
- Low density on contrast-enhanced CT.

Fibroma

Fibromas are the second most common 1° benign childhood cardiac tumour, but may present in adults. They usually present with heart failure, dysrhythmia, and sudden death. They are associated with Gorlin syndrome (nevoid basal cell carcinoma syndrome). On CCT they:

- Typically involve ventricular myocardium, extending into the LV cavity
- May be large
- Have a homogenous low-density appearance, with foci of calcification and homogenous enhancement with contrast.

Haemangioma

Haemagiomas are benign vascular tumours that may affect any chamber and present at any age. They are usually asymptomatic, but may cause chest pain, dyspnoea, pericardial effusion, heart failure, and dysrhythmia. If multiple, consider Kasabach–Merritt syndrome. They are:

- Heterogeneous tumours with intense enhancement after contrast.

Intracardiac paraganglioma

Paraganglionomas (phaeochromocytomas) may, very rarely, be found in the heart. Patients present in adulthood with symptoms typical fo phaechromocytoma. Twenty per cent have additional extracardiac para gangliomas. Identification usually follows biochemical diagnosis and a neg ative adrenal CT/MRI. Whole-body iodine-131 metaiodobenzylguanidine (MIBG) scintigraphy is used to determine presence and location. On CCT they are:

- Often large
- Associated with bone metastases in 5%
- Mostly epicardial, in the roof of the left atrium
- Heterogenous tumours which may contain calcification and central necrosis; may be infiltrative and require wide excision
- Often iso-dense to myocardium on unenhanced studies, but enhance intensely after contrast administration.

⚠ There is a risk of hypertensive crisis during administration of iodinate contrast, so full α- and β-blockade is required; MRI may be preferable.

Malignant cardiac tumours

Metastases

Cardiac metastases are far more common than 1° cardiac tumours and are found in ~12% of cancer patients at autopsy. Most are probably asymptomatic. The most common 1° sites are lung, breast, lymphoma, and malignant melanoma. Melanoma (~50%) and leukaemia (~30%) are particularly likely to metastasise to the heart. On CCT:

- The epicardial surface and myocardium are most commonly affected (Fig. 18.4)
- Pericardial effusions are common
- Metastasis suggested in the presence of multiple lesions, nodular pericardial thickening, and pericardial effusion.

Sarcomas

Sarcomas, although rare mesenchymal tumours, are the most common malignant 1° cardiac tumour. They usually have a very poor prognosis a metastases (especially to the lungs) are often widespread at presentation Dyspnoea is the most common symptom. On CCT, sarcomas are typically enhancing masses often with pericardial involvement.

Any type may affect the heart:

- Angiosarcoma (33%) is the most common, occurring mostly in males; mainly right atrial, although may diffusely affect the pericardium only
- Undifferentiated sarcoma (25%)
- Malignant fibrous histiosarcoma
- Leiomyosarcoma: usually left atrial; may interfere with mitral valve
- Osteosarcoma: usually left atrial, occasionally calcified
- Rhabdomyosarcoma: may affect any chamber (and sometimes more than one); often large, broad-based and infiltrative.

Sarcomas may be occasionally confused with myxoma, especially those that may have a myxoid stroma (MFH, leiomyosarcoma, osteosarcoma).

Primary cardiac lymphoma

1° cardiac lymphomas are typically non-Hodgkin type. By definition they only involve the heart or pericardium at diagnosis. They are more common in immunocompromised individuals, and may present with unresponsive progressive heart failure, chest pain, caval obstruction tamponade, and dysrhythmia. They are usually diagnosed shortly before death; early diagnosis improves prognosis. On CCT:

- Pericardial effusions are common and may be very large
- Right atrium is most commonly involved
- Two chambers are often involved
- Hypo- or iso-dense (to myocardium) soft tissue mass, with heterogeneous enhancement with contrast.

Immunosuppression-related tumours post transplantation

- Eight per cent lymphomas.
- Related to Epstein–Barr virus and cyclosporin.

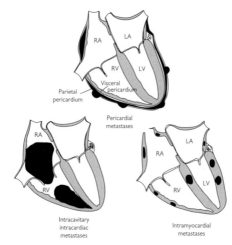

Fig. 18.4 Cardiac locations for metastases. Reproduced from Roberts WC (1997) Primary and secondary neoplasms of the heart. *Am J Cardiol* **80**: 671–682, copyright 1997 with permission from Elsevier.

Cardiac pseudotumours

Lipomatous hypertrophy of the interatrial septum

Lipomatous hypertrophy (LPH) is a pseudotumour leading to thickening of the interatrial septum but sparing the fossa ovalis. It is often seen in obese elderly patients and is usually asymptomatic. It is more common with chronic atrial fibrillation.

• CT shows its characteristic position and fat density (Fig. 18.5).
• If atypical features consider liposarcoma.

Thrombus

Thrombus in the left ventricle is usually associated with wall motion abnormalities, typically an apical aneurysm after an infarct. It is also seen in other conditions such as endomyocardial fibrosis and Loeffler's syndrome. CCT findings include:

• left ventricle—associated wall motion abnormality
• left atrium—typically posteriorly or in the appendage (Fig. 18.6) and associated with atrial fibrillation
• Thrombus is homogenous and low density, attached to wall.

Calcification

Occasionally, mass-like calcification may be seen, typically in the posterior mitral valve annulus (Fig. 18.7).

Granulomatous disease

Sarcoidosis and tuberculosis may produce focal mixed attenuation enhancing nodules.

Echinococcal disease (hydatid)

Cardiac hydatid disease is rare. Cyst rupture may lead to sudden death due to anaphylaxis or tamponade. CCT demonstrates:

• Thin-walled fluid-filled cyst(s)
• Usually univesicular.

Amyloidosis (see ☐ Cardiac pseudotumours, p. 256)

Hypertrophic cardiomyopathy (see ☐ Cardiac CT appearances in cardiomyopathies, p. 246)

Vegetations (see ☐ Aortic regurgitation, p. 297)

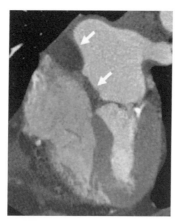

Fig. 18.5 LPH of the interatrial septum (arrows). Note that the density of the atrial septum is similar to that of fat.

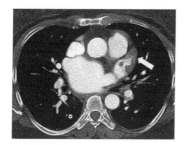

Fig. 18.6 Large left atrial appendage thrombus (arrow) in a patient with paroxsysmal atrial fibrillation.

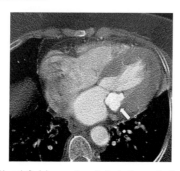

Fig. 18.7 Mass-like calcified degeneration of mitral valve annulus (arrow).

Evaluation of myocardial scarring and perfusion

Introduction

Evaluation of global and regional LV function by CCT allows identification of impaired myocardial function. However, of particular interest is the ability of CCT to detect myocardial scarring and, by implication, myocardial viability. The extent of myocardial scarring is an important indicator of prognosis. Many techniques may be used to demonstrate myocardial viability, including CMR and gated SPECT MPS, but the role of CCT in this setting remains undefined. Recent work has demonstrated that conventional iodinated X-ray contrast media show delayed uptake and washout in areas of myocardial scar. If this were a consistent finding, it would be possible to perform coronary angiography and assess myocardial viability during the same imaging session. There is further potential to assess coronary flow reserve during stress. This capability would greatly enahnce a technique whose 1° weakness is overestimation of coronary artery stenosis severity.

At the time of writing, both the assessment of myocardial scarring and perfusion by CCT are techniques predominantly within the research domain. It is possible that in the next few years they will enter mainstream clinical use. However, it should be remembered that these techniques will have to compete clinically with well-established techniques, some with decades of experience and validation data to support them (e.g. SPECT MPS).

Contrast pharmacokinetics

Properties of iodinated contrast

- Iodinated X-ray contrast agents are water soluble, do not undergo metabolism, and are excreted unchanged by the kidneys.
- Vascular endothelium has ubiquitous coverage by 12-nm pores which allow transit of molecules up to 20,000Da.
- The small size of iodinated contrast molecules (~770Da for Iomeprol) coupled with their water solubility permits free distribution of contrast across the vascular endothelium, and thus between the intravascular extracellular space (blood pool) and the extravascular extracellular space (interstitium).
- There is no accumulation within intact cells.
- Contrast distribution may be described simply according to a two-compartment model (Fig. 19.1).

Contrast kinetics in infarcted myocardium

After myocardial infarction, alterations in inflow and outflow constants (Fig. 19.1B) and the extravascular extracellular space (Fig. 19.1C) may be exploited for the purposes of imaging.

Acute myocardial infarction

- Characterized by *microvascular plugging and dysfunction*, *myocyte membrane rupture* and *interstitial oedema* in variable proportions and extent, depending on the delay in institution and adequacy of reperfusion therapy.
- Microvascular dysfunction may be present in a significant proportion of patients, even after successful restoration of perfusion.
- *Microvascular plugging and dysfunction*—impairment of contrast exchange between the blood pool (Fig. 19.1A) and extravascular extracellular space (Fig. 19.1C) such that both inflow and outflow of contrast (Fig. 19.1B) is delayed: an initial delay in contrast enhancement is followed by hyperenhancement as the contrast is retained in the extravascular extracellular space.
- *Myocyte membrane rupture*—exposes the previously closed intracellular space to the extracellular environment, effectively increasing the volume of the extravascular extracellular space (Fig. 19.1C) into which contrast can distribute.
- *Interstitial oedema*—expands the extravascular extracellular space, increasing the volume of contrast distribution and promoting accumulation within the zone of myocardial necrosis.

Chronic myocardial infarction

- Maturation of the myocardial infarct is characterized by a reduction in functional capillary density and replacement of ruptured myocytes by collagenous scar.
- Reduction in functional capillary density—the lack of viable myocardium leads to a dramatic fall in functional capillary density, which in turn delays the inflow and outflow of contrast in infarcted myocardium (Fig. 19.1B).

- Collagenous scar—although the interstitial oedema which characterizes acute infarction has resolved, the extravascular extracellular space remains expanded as collagenous scar is less densely packed than myocardium (Fig. 19.1C): the volume of contrast distribution remains relatively higher than in normal myocardium, although wall thickness diminishes as the collagenous scar contracts.

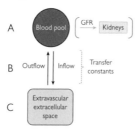

Fig. 19.1 Two-compartment model of iodinated contrast distribution.

Enhancement patterns

- Despite differing underlying microvascular and ultrastructural changes, contrast kinetics within acute and chronic myocardial infarcts are similar.
- On arterial phase images, **hypo**-enhancement may be seen due to the delay in wash-in of contrast (Fig. 19.2).
- On delayed pass images, **hyper**-enhancement is seen, due to a combination of ↑ volume of contrast distribution and delayed wash-out of contrast compared to areas of healthy myocardium (Fig. 19.2).
- In animal models, delayed enhancement typically occurs around 5min after contrast injection and persists for around 40min.
- In humans, a scan delay of 7–10min after contrast bolus administration is usually sufficient.

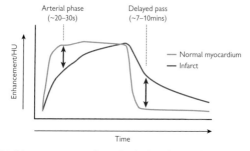

Fig. 19.2 Enhancement patters of normal and infarcted myocardium.

Scan acquisition: technical aspects

Scan parameters

Delayed pass imaging is performed solely to identify areas of ↑ contrast enhancement that indicate myocardial scarring. Details of coronary artery anatomy and ventricular function are obtained from images acquired in the arterial phase. It is necessary to adjust the acquisition parameters for a delayed pass scan because of the additional radiation burden, coupled with the limited information required from the study.

X-ray tube voltage

Delayed enhancement patterns may be subtle. Chronic myocardial scar may enhance in the range 150–190HU, whilst normal myocardium may be in the range 60–120HU, depending on tube voltage. To facilitate detection with such a narrow window of difference, the peak energy of the X-ray beam can be adjusted to maximize its relative attenuation by enhanced tissue. This may be achieved by *reducing* the voltage. The lower energy X-ray beam is attenuated more by tissues that are relatively enhanced, improving image contrast. A tube voltage of 80–100kVp is preferred in this setting, in contrast to the 120kVp typically used in standard CTA.

X-ray tube current

Even though image contrast is enhanced by reducing the tube voltage, the X-ray beam is globally attenuated to a greater degree due to its lower peak energy. Signal-to-noise ratio is ∴ reduced (see 📖, X-ray tube current, p. 22). This may be offset by increasing the tube current. Although this will not change the spectrum of X-ray energies within the beam, it will increase the absolute number of photons emitted, increasing the total number reaching the detectors. Increasing tube current has no specific benefits for delayed pass imaging *per se*, but improves the signal-to-noise ratio in the final image.

Dual-energy imaging

DECT (see 📖 Dual-source CT, p. 44) may be the technique of choice in the future for myocardial perfusion imaging. The technique takes advantage of the fact that tissues attenuate X-ray beams of different energies to differing degrees depending on their density. Thus DECT can be used to map the iodine content of tissues with differing levels of contrast enhancement, potentially increasing the accuracy of the scan for the detection of delayed enhancement within myocardial scar. Although proven in concept, the technology remains relatively new and further validation is required.

Retrospective versus prospective gating

There is no firm consensus on the most appropriate phase of the cardiac cycle to assess delayed enhancement, although an end-diastolic phase is typically used. Artefacts mimicking both arterial phase hypoenhancement and delayed hyperenhancement may occur in any phase of the cardiac cycle, and review of additional phases is useful for confirmation or exclusion. Prospective gating offers the opportunity to perform delayed pass scanning with reduced X-ray exposure but, as for CT coronary angiography, should only be undertaken in those with controlled heart rates.

Contrast protocols

Most data regarding delayed enhancement CT protocols comes from scans acquired either immediately after ICA (in the acute setting) or after the use of standard CTA contrast protocols (see 📖 CT coronary angiography, p. 108). However, a modified scan protocol may be used where the main contrast infusion is followed by a low-volume slow-flow infusion of contrast (30mL over 5min) which runs between the initial and delayed pass scans (Fig. 19.3). There is some evidence that this results in improved characterization of myocardial scarring taking CMR as a gold-standard.[1] However, in the clinical setting it is imperative that arterial phase contrast enhancement be kept optimal for CTA, and there is not enough data to support a change in protocol at this time.

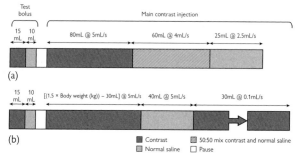

Fig. 19.3 (a) Standard CTA contrast protocol. (b) Modified contrast protocol.

Further reading

1 Brodoefel H, Reimann A, Klumpp B, et al. (2007) Assessment of myocardial viability in a reperfused porcine model: evaluation of different MSCT contrast protocols in acute and subacute infarct stages in comparison with MRI. *J Comput Assist Tomogr* **31**(2), 290–298.

Image interpretation

General approach

- The end-diastolic phase (typically around 65% R–R interval) should be selected for initial evaluation, although other phases may be useful if available, particularly in the presence of artefact.
- Images are best viewed as multiplanar reformats (see 📖 Multiplanar reformatting, p. 142), with planes set to represent horizontal and vertical long and short axes of the left ventricle.
- Window width and level should be set to maximize the contrast between enhanced and relatively unenhanced myocardium: for an 80kVp scan, a good starting window width and level (see 📖 CT numbers and windowing, p. 138) is 175HU, although each case is likely to require some adjustment to achieve optimum images.
- If a reduced X-ray tube voltage is used, the ↓ signal-to-noise ratio (see 📖 X-ray tube voltage, p. 23) may cause difficulty in interpretation of sub-millimetre multiplanar reformatted images. It may ∴ be necessary to increase the slice width to improve the quality of the image: a slice width of 5mm is usually sufficient.
- The extent of delayed enhancement should be expressed according to the 17-segment model of the left ventricle (see 📖 Assessment of regional left ventricular function, p. 235), with an approximation of the total percentage infarcted myocardium presented in the final report (e.g. 4/17 segments ≈20% original myocardium) (see Fig. 19.4).
- The depth of infarction may be characterized as transmural if >50% of the thickness of the myocardial segment shows delayed enhancement; note that this definition will cause underestimation of residual viability in certain circumstances, but evidence from MPS suggests that the amount of segmental viability that is clinically relevant in hibernating myocardium is at least 50–60%.
- Partial thickness myocardial scarring should be reported if <50%; this is likely to be the cause if the delayed enhancement is primarily subendocardial.

⚠ Delayed enhancement patterns on CCT in cardiomyopathies have yet to be characterized.

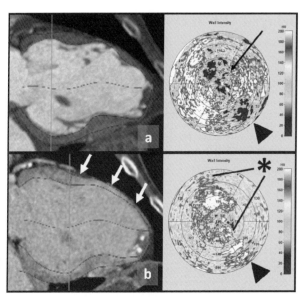

Fig. 19.4 Enhancement patterns of myocardial scarring on CCT. (a) Arterial phase images of the left ventricle (left) and 17-segment polar plot of absolute Hounsfield units (HU, right) showing hypoenhancement at the apex (arrow) and inferolaterally. A calcified apical thrombus is also visible. (b) Delayed pass imaging in the same patient shows extensive enhancement in the anterior wall and apex (arrows, left and asterisk, right) and also inferolaterally (arrowhead). (📖 Plate 6 for colour version).

Delayed CCT in clinical practice

Following acute myocardial infarction

Delayed myocardial enhancement has been studied widely in patients immediately following 1° percutaneous coronary intervention for acute myocardial infarction. Delayed enhancement in the area of acute infarction is usually substantial and correlates well with other techniques such as myocardial perfusion scintigraphy.[1] The depth and extent of delayed enhancement correlate with the likelihood of functional recovery. Larger areas of delayed hyperenhancement predict higher rates of short- and medium-term adverse cardiovascular events, and a higher likelihood of adverse LV remodelling.

Although attractive, the role of CCT in the acute setting is not well defined. Clinically it is usually more relevant to request imaging to define residual ischaemia in the infarcted territory or in remote territories supplied through anatomically significant but non-culprit coronary stenoses. These questions cannot yet be answered by CCT, although adenosine-stress CCT may allow this in the future. Other tests, such as stress echocardiography or MPS, are currently better placed to offer this information, in addition to quantifying the depth and extent of myocardial scarring, and should be considered as first-line treatment.

Assessment of chronic myocardial scarring

In contrast to the delayed enhancement seen in acute myocardial infarction, that seen in the chronic setting is usually much more subtle. This probably reflects the lack of interstitial oedema and replacement of ruptured myocytes with collagenous scar. Nonetheless, in the chronic setting, delayed hyperenhancement implies myocardial scarring and thus irreversible dysfunction. Delayed enhancement on CCT correlates well with gadolinium-enhanced CMR, as well as with fixed perfusion abnormalities on MPS. Absence of delayed enhancement correlates with viability on MPS. However, whilst CMR and MPS are underpinned by an extensive literature, there is currently very little prognostic data regarding delayed enhancement on CCT.

Conclusion

There is undoubtedly a potential role for CCT in the assessment of acute and chronic myocardial scarring. However, at present the data are too limited to allow the technique to be recommended for routine clinical practice.

Further reading

1 Sato A, Hiroe M, Nozato T, *et al.* (2008) Early validation study of 64-slice multidetector computed tomography for the assessment of myocardial viability and the prediction of left ventricular remodelling after acute myocardial infarction. *Eur Heart J* **29**(4), 490–498.

Evaluation of myocardial perfusion

Myocardial scar assessment on CCT is a resting technique that identifies only one aspect of myocardial status and gives no information on the state of myocardial perfusion or coronary flow reserve (see 📖 Comparison of multimodality imaging, p. 465). A major limitation of CT coronary angiography at present is its poor positive predictive value, with lesion severity consistently overestimated in clinical studies (particularly when a >50% cut-off is used to predict significance). The ability to evaluate stress and resting myocardial perfusion on CCT could potentially circumvent this weakness.

In theory, this should be straightforward. Delivery of iodinated contrast and thus enhancement of a tissue is proportional to blood flow. Regions receiving relatively reduced flow should enhance poorly compared to those served by unobstructed coronary arteries, leading to heterogeneity of myocardial contrast enhancement. Despite this apparent simplicity, the assessment of myocardial perfusion using CCT is still at an early stage, primarily because of poor temporal resolution (until very recently).

Method of cardiovascular stress

In order to evaluate coronary flow reserve (see 📖 Comparision of multimodality imaging, p. 465), some form of cardiovascular stress must be used. Both exercsie and dobutamine stress lead to increases in heart rate that exceed the temporal resolution of current scanners (and probably those to come for some years), rendering them useless as CCT stress agents. However, adenosine (see 📖 Cardiac stress for functional imaging, p. 470) results in only modest rises in heart rate. Although these rises are manageable for 64-slice CT scanners, they may still result in suboptimal images in many patients. The improved temporal resolution of dual-source and >64-slice CT scanners offers the potential to scan patients during adenosine infusion with relatively little impact on diagnostic image quality.

⚠ It may be preferable to avoid the use of β-blockers prior to adenosine-stress CCT. β-blockade has been shown to lead to a small but meaningful underestimation of ischaemia on both adenosine-stress SPECT and PET MPS. It is possible that the same effect may result for CCT measures of perfusion, although this remains to be proved.

Clinical data

- In a study of 34 patients, CCT and SPECT MPS showed similar diagnostic accuracy for the detection of both >50% and >70% stenoses on ICA.[1]
- More recently, dynamic perfusion adenosine-stress CCT has been used to evaluate myocardial blood flow; preliminary results show encouraging agreement with CMR.[2]
- Radiation exposure using modern scanners appears to be equivalent to SPECT MPS (~12mSv), provided the resting study is prospectively gated.

Conclusion

It is likely to be several years before stress CCT enters the clinical domain. Early data have demonstrated proof of concept and feasability, but the decades of diagnostic and prognostic validation that already underpin techniques such as MPS and stress echocardiography make these first-line for the foreseeable future.

Further reading

1 Blankstein R, Shturman I.D, Rogers IS, *et al.* (2009) Adenosine-induced stress myocardial perfusion imaging using dual-source cardiac computed tomography. *J Am Coll Cardiol* **54**(12), 1072–1084.

2 Bastarrika G, Ramos-Duran L, Rosenblum MA, Kang DK, Rowe GW, and Schoepf UJ (2010) Adenosine-stress dynamic myocardial CT perfusion imaging: initial clinical experience. *Invest Radiol* **45**(6), 306–313.

Evaluation of the left atrium and pulmonary veins

Introduction

Clinical cardiac electrophysiology (EP) presupposes that, for every dys-rhythmia, there is a critical anatomical region responsible for either the generation or propagation of abnormal electrical impulses. The destruction or isolation of these regions should prevent the recurrence of that dysrhythmia. There are ∴ there are two broad aims in EP:

1 Identification, characterization and localization of the dysrhythmia
2 Ablation of the focus of the dysrhythmia.

Catheter ablation

When first introduced in 1982 for the treatment of atrial fibrillation with rapid ventricular response, catheter ablation was performed using high-energy DC shocks delivered under general anaesthetic. Unsurprisingly, the technique was associated with a relatively high complication rate. The development of radiofrequency (RF) ablation and suitable electrode catheters allowed the identification and focal destruction of arrhythmogenic substrates.

The full range of catheter ablation approaches is beyond the scope of this book. In broad terms, the technique involves:

- Identification of the focus of dysrhythmia
- Positioning of an ablation catheter adjacent to the focus
- Application of RF energy (often at 50–55°C for up to 1min) to destroy the myocardium and hence the aberrant electrical circuit.

RF current is passed from the electrode into the underlying tissue and dissipated as heat.

- The magnitude of heating within the tissue is inversely proportional to the fourth power of the distance from the catheter.
- The depth of myocardium affected is ∴ small, allowing accurate, focal destruction of myocardial tissue.
- The frequencies used (typically 300–1000Hz) are well tolerated and do not result in cardiac or skeletal muscle stimulation.
- The procedure can be performed under sedation and local anaesthetic.
- RF ablation may still lead to complications such as pulmonary vein stenosis or perforation of the pulmonary veins, atrium, or adjacent structures such as the oesophagus.

Fluoroscopy has been used for the placement of ablation catheters since the first development of the technique. However, this form of imaging is limited by poor soft-tissue contrast, inaccurate definition of the transitional zone between the left atrium and pulmonary veins, and the need for the operator to extrapolate a 2D fluoroscopic image into three dimensions. The use of an alternative modality to pre-define the 3D anatomy of the left atrium and pulmonary veins is ∴ desirable.

Cardiac CT prior to electrophysiology procedures

The value of integrated imaging techniques has led to increasing use of CCT to guide EP procedures. In particular, the technique can:

- Provide high spatial resolution images of the atria and pulmonary and coronary veins
- Evaluate possible substrates for ventricular dysrhythmia, e.g. CAD, anomalous coronary arteries, ventricular dysfunction, or CHD
- Highlight the proximity of extracardiac structures, e.g. the oesophagus, which might be affected by complications of the EP procedure.

CCT is unable to provide real-time data during the invasive procedure as there is no capacity at present to image during catheter placement. This has led to the development of image fusion software, which can merge CCT data, electro-anatomical mapping data, and fluoroscopic images to provide real-time 3D delineation of the atria and pulmonary veins.

Scan parameters

Pre-EP CCT data can be acquired from a standard CT coronary angiography dataset without alteration of tube settings or contrast dose.

- If there is no requirement to study the coronary arteries, a prospectively gated study may be acquired.
- If a substrate for dysrhythmia is being sought, a retrospectively gated acquisition is preferable as the presence of dysrhythmia increases the likelihood that multiple phases will be required to assess coronary anatomy adequately.

Viewing CCT data

CCT images may be viewed as transaxial slices or epicardial and intra-atrial volume-rendered 3D reconstructions.

Transaxial slices have the benefit of representing all of the acquired CCT data without contamination by further post-processing.

- This view is useful for identifying the relationship of organs which may be close to the pulmonary veins and left atrium, such as the oesophagus.
- It is possible to make inaccurate measurements in this view if the target is measured out of plane.
- A lack of familiarity may preclude use of this format, especially for clinicians inexperienced in cardiac imaging.

Epicardial volume-rendered 3D reconstructions are useful for delineating the number and anatomy of the pulmonary veins as they enter the left atrium, as well as estimating left atrial shape and size.

Intra-atrial volume-rendered 3D reconstructions require special reconstruction software algorithms and allow assessment of the pulmonary vein ostia from a viewpoint within the left atrium. This allows accurate measurement of the ostia and identification of relevant intervenous saddles and endocardial ridges.

Left atrium and pulmonary veins

Left atrium

- Dimensions may be assessed from both transaxial slices and volume-rendered 3D reconstructions.
- As the left atrium is not perfectly spherical, maximum and minimum cross-sectional diameters in orthogonal planes should be quoted.
- Measurements should be made between the external surface of the posterior aortic root and the internal surface of the left atrial wall.
- Left atrial size should not exceed 5.5cm in its maximum dimension.

Pulmonary veins

- Highly variable anatomy.
- Typically, the left atrium receives one superior and one inferior vein from each lung, each of which enters through a separate orifice (Fig. 20.1).
- Deviation from this arrangement is seen in at least 40% of patients.
  - The most common variation is the joining of two pulmonary veins to form a common vein prior to entering the left atrium, resulting in a single ostium; this variant is most common on the left side, which is in turn more commonly the site of RF ablation
  - Another common variant is the presence of one or more accessory pulmonary veins, which are named after the lobe of the lung that they drain; this variant occurs most commonly on the right side, typically with a right middle lobe vein or superior branch of the right lower lobe vein
- Typically, the superior veins are larger than the inferior veins.

Pulmonary vein ostia

- Myocardial fibres extend as a muscular cuff from the left atrium into the pulmonary veins.
- These cuffs, more prominent in the superior than in the inferior pulmonary veins, are an important focus for atrial tachycardias and fibrillation and are often targets for ablation.
- Ablation of these areas may result in either *de novo* pulmonary vein stenosis or worsening of pre-existing stenoses, probably as a result of scarring and contraction of the venous wall after injury.
- Documentation of the dimensions of the pulmonary vein ostia is ∴ important to serve as a baseline measurement should subsequent complications occur (Figs 20.2 and 20.3).
- Pulmonary vein ostia are oval in shape, with the supero-inferior usually greater than the antero-posterior dimension; the clinical report should ∴ include orthogonal dimensions.

It is unusual to see abnormalities of lung perfusion as a result of pulmonary vein stenosis until the stenosis exceeds 70%, although symptoms may develop earlier. There is no definitive cut-off which defines pulmonary vein stenosis—qualitative comparison with the other pulmonary veins is sufficient.

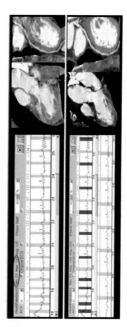

Plate 1 (📖 Fig. 11.8, p. 159).

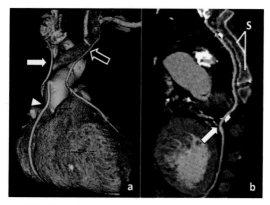

Plate 2 (📖 Fig. 16.1, p. 221).

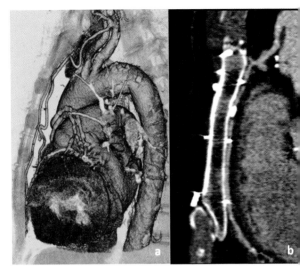

Plate 3 (📖 Fig. 16.3, p. 227).

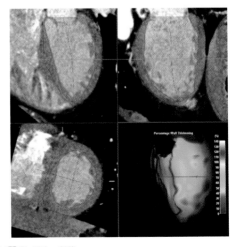

Plate 4 (📖 Fig. 17.1, p. 233).

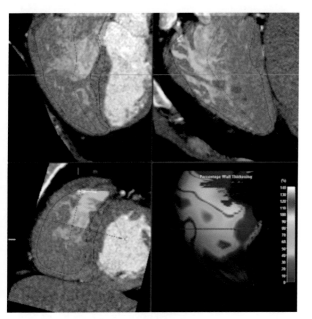

Plate 5 (Fig. 17.4, p. 237).

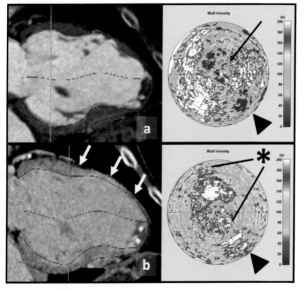

Plate 6 (Fig. 19.4, p. 267).

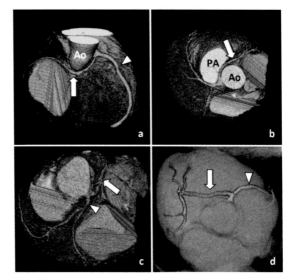

Plate 7 (📖 Fig. 23.1, p. 339).

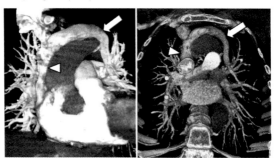

Plate 8 (📖 Fig. 23.14, p. 361).

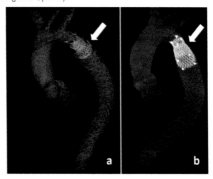

Plate 9 (📖 Fig. 25.6, p. 407).

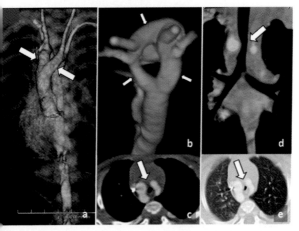

Plate 10 (📖 Fig. 25.7, p. 409).

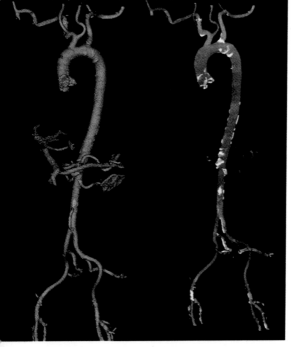

Plate 11 (📖 Fig. 28.1, p. 435).

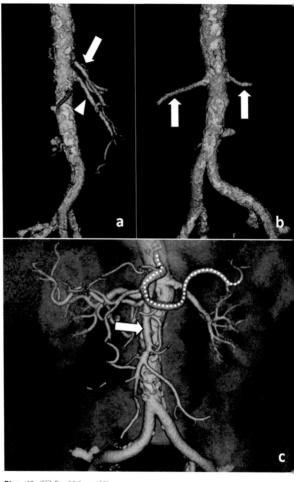

Plate 12 (Fig. 28.2, p. 439).

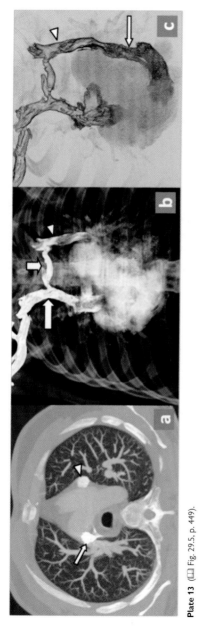

Plate 13 (□ Fig. 29.5, p. 449).

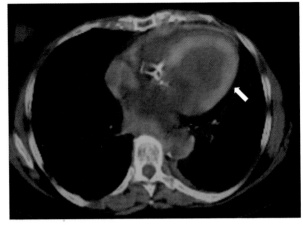

Plate 14 (📖 Fig. 31.2, p. 479).

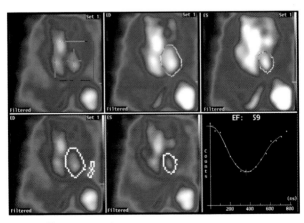

Plate 15 (📖 Fig. 31.3, p. 480).

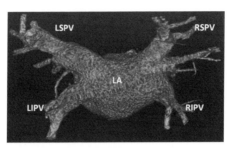

Fig. 20.1 Volume-rendered reconstruction of the pulmonary veins and left atrium. LA, left atrium; LSPV, left superior pulmonary vein; LIPV, left inferior pulmonary vein; RSPV, right superior pulmonary vein; RIPV, right inferior pulmonary vein.

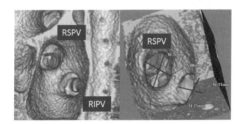

Fig. 20.2 Right pulmonary vein ostia as seen from within the left atrium. 3D reconstruction of CT datasets allows accurate measurement of the pulmonary vein ostial diameters. RSPV, right superior pulmonary vein; RIPV, right inferior pulmonary vein.

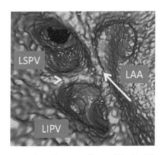

Fig. 20.3 Left pulmonary vein ostia as seen from within the left atrium. Here, the left superior pulmonary vein (LSPV) and left inferior pulmonary vein (LIPV) are separated by an intervenous saddle (arrow-head). The entrance to the left atrial appendage (LAA) is separated from the pulmonary vein ostia by a prominent endocardial ridge (arrow).

Other relevant anatomy

Coronary sinus
- Formed by the confluence of the great cardiac and left atrial oblique veins (see 📖 The coronary arteries and cardiac veins, Fig. 13.6, p. 187 and Fig. 20.4).
- Drains into the right atrium.
- The inferoposterior interatrial pathway lies in the region of the coronary sinus ostium and may contain abnormal foci within it (which often lead to atrio-ventricular nodal re-entrant tachycardia (AVNRT).
- Ablation may result in stenosis of the coronary ostium, although this is often clinically insignificant.
- Of greater importance is the possibility of coronary artery damage, as the distal dominant coronary artery (right or circumflex) may pass underneath the coronary sinus.
- It is ∴ important to assess the relationship of the coronary sinus to surrounding structures, in particular its proximity to the coronary arteries on the inferior surface of the heart (Fig. 20.4).

Oesophagus
- Passes in close proximity to the posterior wall of the left atrium and left pulmonary veins (Fig. 20.5).
- Ablation in these areas is associated with a small risk of left atrium or pulmonary vein (PV) perforation with extension into the oesophagus, resulting in the formation of a cardio-oesophageal fistula.

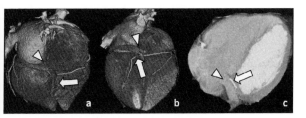

Fig. 20.4 Relationship of the coronary sinus to the coronary arteries. (a) Only a small branch of the distal RCA (arrow) runs beneath the coronary sinus (arrowhead). (b) A much larger posterolateral branch of the RCA (arrow) runs beneath the confluence of the middle cardiac vein and the coronary sinus (arrowhead). (c) Trans-axial image of the same patient, where the RCA (arrow) can be seen closely approximate to the ostium of the coronary sinus (arrowhead).

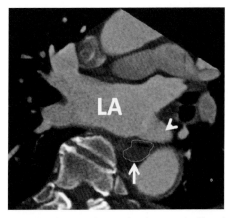

Fig. 20.5 Relationship of the oesophagus to the pulmonary veins. Here, the oesophagus (arrow, white outline) can be seen closely approximate to the left inferior pulmonary vein (arrowhead). LA, left atrium.

Substrates for ventricular dysrhythmia

Anomalous coronary artery

The majority of anomalous coronary arteries (see 📖 Anomalous coronary arteries (1), p. 338) are clinically silent and most are probably never discovered. The prevalence in the general population is ~1% but 4–15% in young patients who suffer sudden cardiac death. Coronary anomalies most associated with dysrhythmia include:

- Anomalous left coronary artery arising from the right sinus of Valsalva and taking a pre-aortic course between the aortic and pulmonary trunks
- Anomalous RCA arising from the left sinus of Valsalva and taking a pre-aortic course between the aortic and pulmonary trunks.

(The incidence of either of these anomalies is around 0.08% in patients up to the age of 21.)

- Coronary artery hypoplasia or atresia
- High take-off coronary artery

All are readily identifiable on the standard CTA dataset (see 📖 CT coronary angiography, p. 108). The presence of pre-existing dysrhythmia is an important indicator of the likely functional significance of the coronary artery anomaly. Where doubt exists, further investigation such as dynamic exercise stress testing is warranted.

Coronary artery disease

- Ischaemia is an important stimulus for dysrhythmia and previous myocardial scarring increases the likelihood of abnormal ventricular foci.
- Evidence of concomitant CAD on the CCT dataset should be sought.
- Evaluation of myocardial contrast enhancement may indicate myocardial scarring.

Cardiomyopathy

- Evaluation of global and regional LV function on CCT can allow diagnosis of cardiomyopathy.
- Idiopathic dilated cardiomyopathy may be suspected when there is no evidence of CAD on CTA but evidence of impaired ventricular function on functional assessment.
- Hypertrophic cardiomyopathy may be suspected in the presence of asymmetric ventricular hypertrophy.

Congenital heart disease

- Around 25% of patients with CHD have dysrhythmias.
- This is especially the case in patients who have undergone previous corrective surgery.
- Up to half of patients with Ebstein's anomaly may suffer from supraventricular tachycardia.

Template report for pre-electrophysiology CT

Review wide field of view
- Lung findings.
- Mediastinum, in particular relationship of oesophagus to the left atrium.
- Anatomy of aorta and pulmonary vessels.

Gross anatomy of the heart
- Pulmonary venous anatomy and ostial dimensions.
- Left atrial anatomy.
- Anatomy of left ventricle, including mitral valve, septum, and outflow tract.
- Right atrial and ventricular anatomy, including tricuspid valve, where possible.

Coronary venous anatomy
- In particular, relationship of the coronary sinus to the distal dominant coronary artery.

Coronary artery assessment
- Presence of anomalous coronary arteries.
- Evidence of coronary artery stenosis.

Ventricular function
- LV volumes and ejection fraction.
- Regional LV wall motion and thickening.
- Assessment of myocardial contrast enhancement.

Valve imaging

Introduction

Background
- Valvular heart disease (VHD) is common.
- Rheumatic heart disease, previously the most common cause of VHD, is now much less common in the developed world.
- Degenerative valve disease is now increasingly common as a result of ↑ life expectancy.
- Calcific aortic stenosis and mitral regurgitation are the most common valve pathologies.
- Particular issues in the management of VHD include:
  - Aging population at ↑ peri-operative risk
  - Recurrence of valve problems in operated patients.

Imaging
- Management strategies depend on both structural and functional assessment of the valve pathology.
- TTE is the standard technique for the evaluation of *all* valve lesions and is generally indicated in any patient with a murmur when valve disease is suspected.
- TOE (or transoesophageal echocardiography) is able to measure valve and regurgitant orifice areas as well as flow-dependent variables such as mean gradient and maximal flow velocity across the valve.
- When further imaging is required, CMR can provide additional information and is especially indicated in cases of poor acoustic windows or discrepant findings
- CMR provides a reliable method of estimating the severity of valve stenosis and regurgitation, and compares favourably with TTE.

Role of cardiac CT
- CCT has a limited role; it is only rarely indicated for the 1° assessment of cardiac valves (e.g. assessment of aortic valve calcification and/or valve area when poor TTE windows preclude accurate assessment).
- It is not possible to evaluate valve haemodynamics on CCT.
- Valve assessment is usually indicated as part of a wider analysis of the CTA dataset when valve disease is suspected.
- CTA may be used particularly in patients with bacterial endocarditis to evaluate an aortic root abscess or the coronary arteries prior to valve replacement.
- CCT is particularly strong at quantifying valve calcification, which correlates with both severity of valve disease and prognosis.
- Valve planimetry is also possible with CCT.
- Although some parameters have been compared with TTE and CMR, CCT is much less well validated in general.

⚠ It is worth reiterating that CCT remains a second-line investigation for VHD, with the majority of assessments occurring opportunistically as part of a wider CCT assessment.

Acquisition for valve imaging

Valve assessment with CCT requires multiphase image reconstruction to create a cine image of the valve in either systole or diastole, depending on the valve lesion in question.

- Either retrospective protocols or prospective protocols with an enlarged acquisition window can be used for examination of the cardiac valves.
- For left-sided valves, no specific alteration to contrast timing is necessary.
- For right-sided valves, contrast timing must be adjusted to achieve RV blood pool attenuation, either alone or in combination with the LV blood pool (see 📖 Right ventriculography, p 236; see 📖 Gated CT pulmonary angiogram, p 110).

Aetiology, associated lesions, and consequence of the valve pathology can be made from a single breath-hold acquisition because a complete volume of data is acquired during the scan.

Anatomical assessment is made of the valve in question, and stenotic and regurgitant orifices are measured with planimetry of the valve area.

In contrast to echocardiography and MRI, no haemodynamic data regarding valve function are available from CCT.

Post-processing

CT images should be examined in the axial, sagittal, and coronal planes or a post-processing workstation.

- The oblique tool allows simultaneous examination of a structure in orthogonal planes in two windows.
- This is particularly valuable in valve analysis, ensuring accurate and reproducible measurements of the valves, great vessels, and cardiac chambers.
- Fine adjustments can be made in the pilot image while simultaneously examining the true image.

For assessment of the cardiac structures, it is recommended that the views examined are the equivalent to those used in echocardiography and MRI: *two-chamber*, *four-chamber* and *three-chamber plus LV outflow tract*. The following method allows consistent orientation of the CT images in these views.

Stage 1

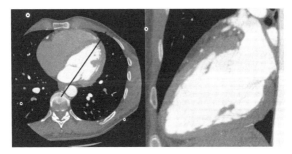

Fig. 21.1 Using the oblique tool and the axial images, a line is drawn from the centre of the mitral valve to the LV apex, giving a 'pilot' two-chamber view.

Stage 2

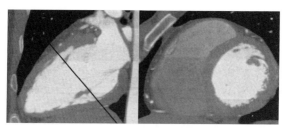

Fig. 21.2 From the 'pilot' two-chamber view, the oblique tool is placed perpendicularly to the ventricular long axis to create a 'pilot' short-axis image. All true images are reconstructed using this view.

Stage 3

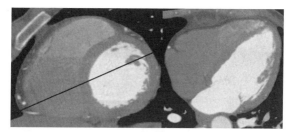

Fig. 21.3 The four-chamber view is formed with the oblique tool running from the mid-LV cavity to the anterior and inferior corner of the right ventricle.

Stage 4

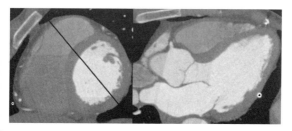

Fig. 21.4 The three-chamber view (or para-sternal long-axis equivalent) is constructed by passing the oblique tool through the mid-LV cavity to transect the RV outflow tract at 11 o'clock.

Stage 5

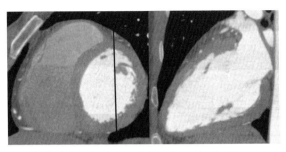

Fig. 21.5 Finally, the two-chamber view is formed by passing the oblique tool vertically within the LV cavity towards 12 o'clock.

Multiphase reconstruction

Retrospective gating (see ☐ ECG gating, p. 34) allows reconstruction of images in any phase of the cardiac cycle. Most post-processing software is capable of displaying 3D images as a cine-loop of the complete cardiac cycle. Viewing the beating heart allows choice of the phase of the cardiac cycle where the area of a given valve is at its smallest, a capability that is particularly useful for the assessment of stenotic valves.

- Examination of the cardiac valves in systole (aortic and pulmonary stenosis, mitral and tricuspid regurgitation) is best achieved between phases 5% and 30% of the R–R interval.
  - Phases should ideally be reconstructed at 5% increments (i.e. 20 total phases).
  - The best phase for aortic stenosis is 10%; for mitral regurgitation, 5% has been quoted.
- For diastolic examination (aortic and pulmonary regurgitation, mitral and tricuspid stenosis), phases between 55 and 75% should be examined, again in increments of 5%.
- Multiphase and multiplane reconstruction for each valve allows calculation of the largest or smallest valve area by planimetry, depending on the pathology of interest
- Although 65% of the R–R interval has been suggested as the best diastolic phase, multiple phases should be examined as the timing of the smallest or largest valve area may vary.

Artefacts

As with all imaging modalities which rely on ECG gating, an irregular heartbeat can cause mis-registration artefact (see 📖 Motion artefact, p. 156). Arrhythmias such as atrial fibrillation, flutter, or ectopic beats will lead to image blurring. This is of particular importance in evaluation of the cardiac valves, which relies on planimetry measurements to assess the degree of stenosis or regurgitation. As with CCT in general, sinus rhythm is preferable. If cardioversion is considered, imaging should be planned once sinus rhythm is restored. To avoid ectopic beats, β-blockers may be administered if there are no contraindications (see 📖 Partial volume effect, p. 154); particular caution is required in patients with aortic stenosis.

Degenerative valve disease is often associated with calcification of the valve leaflet or annulus. Severe calcification can lead to blooming artefact (see 📖 Heart-rate control, p. 78), resulting in an underestimation of valve area as measured by planimetry.

Prosthetic material constructed of metal alloys can lead to beam hardening (see 📖 Beam hardening, p. 152), with streaks or radial lines crossing the image. This can impair the examination of certain types of prosthetic valve. In particular, *in vitro* and *in vivo* studies have shown that the Bjork–Shiley valve causes significant beam hardening artefact, rendering accurate assessment impossible.

Aortic stenosis (1)

Background

- Most common valve lesion.
- Prevalence: 5 in 10,000 of US adults, 7% of UK adults >65 years of age.
- Most common cause of aortic stenosis: degenerative calcification of an otherwise normal valve.
- Other causes, particularly in those <60 years, include calcification of congenital bicuspid aortic valve and rheumatic valve disease.
- Usually assessed using 2D and Doppler echocardiography, with valve area estimated using the continuity equation (Table 21.1).

Consequences

Aortic stenosis results in a pressure-loaded ventricle and causes concentric LV hypertrophy. Bicuspid valves are associated with an aortopathy and progressive dilatation of the aortic root and ascending aorta. All of these anatomical sequelae can be assessed accurately using CCT.

CCT post-processing

- As a first-pass technique, CT is unable to assess transvalvar flow. Assessment of aortic stenosis is ∴ achieved by planimetry.
- From the three-chamber view (see 🕮 Post-processing, Fig. 21.4, p. 287), the oblique tool is positioned through the centre of the aortic valve to create a 'true' LV outflow tract view.
- The oblique tool is then placed perpendicular to the aorta to produce a cross-sectional image through the valve (Fig. 21.6).
- The image plane is moved cranially and caudally through the valve in multiple systolic phases to obtain an image with the smallest aortic valve area (AVA).
- The phase of the cardiac cycle during which AVA is smallest is between 5 and 30% of the R–R interval, typically at 15%.

Table 21.1 Severity of aortic stenosis as assessed by Doppler velocity, peak gradient, and continuity-derived AVA

	Mild	Moderate	Severe
Doppler			
m/s	2.5–3.0	3–4	>4
Peak mmHg	<40	40–64	>64
AVA	>1.2	0.8–1.2	<0.8

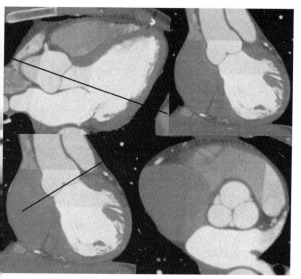

Fig. 21.6 Cut-planes for assessment of the aortic valve.

Aortic stenosis (2)

Grading of aortic stenosis

Calcification

Degenerative aortic valve disease is associated with significant calcification of the valve (Fig. 21.7).

- The degree of calcification shows limited correlation with echocardiographically derived pressure gradients and AVA calculations.
- An Agatston score equivalent (see 📖 Coronary artery calcium scoring, p. 194) of >2200 from the aortic valve is indicative of moderate to severe aortic stenosis, and further assessment is warranted.
- Other studies have found a correlation between incidental aortic valve calcification, seen on a chest CT scan, and echocardiographic assessment.
- These studies do not suggest that CCT should replace echocardiography, especially given the lack of haemodynamic data offered by the former, but an incidental finding of moderate to severe aortic valve calcification should prompt further assessment.

Planimetry

The normal AVA is 3–4 cm^2. Aortic stenosis becomes clinically relevant at <2cm^2 and severe at <0.8cm^2.

- Several studies have demonstrated a good correlation between AVA as measured by CCT compared to echocardiography.
- All compared CCT with TTE and transoesophageal echocardiography (TOE); in general, TOE and CCT showed the greatest agreement for planimetric measurements of AVA.
- However, CCT may overestimate AVA (and thus underestimate the severity of AS) compared to the Doppler-based assessment of AVA using the continuity equation.

Assessment of aetiology

Clues to the aetiology can be taken from the scan volume.

- Bicuspid aortic valves, seen in approximately 1% of the population, are readily diagnosed by CCT, with a better sensitivity than TTE.
- Bicuspid valves are associated with coarctation of the aorta (see 📖 Coarctation of the aorta, p. 406): 60–80% of coarctation patients have a bicuspid valve.
- The aortic arch can be assessed by extending the scan volume cranially thus incorporating the most common site for coarctation (immediately distal to the left subclavian artery).
- Degenerative aortic valve disease, involving progressive calcification and thus immobility of the cusps, is the most common cause in the seventh decade and beyond.
- Rheumatic disease, unlike degenerative aortic stenosis, shows commissural fusion and is invariably associated with mitral stenosis.

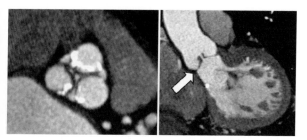

Fig. 21.7 Calcific aortic stenosis. Calcium is clearly seen in the leaflets of the aortic valve (left). There is also thickening of the valve leaflets and reduction in orifice area (right, arrow).

Aortic regurgitation

Background

- Aortic regurgitation (AR) may be caused by disease of either the aortic valve itself or the aortic root.
- *Aortic valve disease*—degeneration of a normal or bicuspid valve and infective endocarditis; rheumatic valve disease is now rare.
- *Aortic root disease*—hypertension, aortic dissection, connective tissue diseases (e.g. Marfans syndrome), and seronegative spondyloarthritides (ankylosing spondylitis, Reiter's syndrome, psoriatic arthropathy).

Cardiac CT acquisition

- For evaluation of the aortic valve and aetiology of AR, the scanning field of view should include the heart and the complete thoracic aorta, including the aortic arch and descending thoracic aorta.
- The decision to include these structures should be made before the contrast-enhanced acquisition and can be based on an assessment of the topogram (see ▢ Scan protocols, p. 100) or calcium scoring acquisition (see ▢ Coronary artery calcium scoring, p. 106).
- Although CCT cannot assess transvalvar flow, the regurgitant orifice area may be assessed by planimetry.

Cardiac CT post-processing

This is essentially the same as for aortic stenosis (see ▢ Aortic stenosis, p. 292).

- Diastolic phases (50–70%) are required for assessment of the regurgitant orifice area (ROA).
- The image plane is scrolled cranio-caudally to identify the diastolic phase with the largest ROA, which is then measured by planimetry.

Grading of aortic regurgitation

- ROA agrees well with the grade of AR on TTE.
- ROA measured by CCT correlates well with assessment by TTE for mild, moderate, and severe levels of regurgitation.
- The sensitivity and specificity for the detection of moderate to severe AR range from 85 to 95% and 88 to 100%, respectively, with PPV and NPV of 100% and 98%, respectively.
- For the detection of mild regurgitation CCT is less accurate, usually as a result of blooming artefacts from a heavily calcified valve.
- Suggested cut-off values for moderate AR are ROA >0.25–0.37mm^2 and for severe AR ROA >0.75–0.81mm^2.

Assessment of aetiology

- Valve disease such as a bicuspid aortic valve, calcific degeneration, rheumatic disease, or infective endocarditis may be readily identified; CCT is superior to TTE for the detection of bicuspid valves.
- Valvular calcification is readily identified on non-enhanced CT.
- The mitral valve can be assessed for evidence of rheumatic disease.

- Endocarditis can be diagnosed by the identification of vegetations, typically on the aortic surface of the valve; an aortic root abscess may also be seen (Fig. 21.8).
- Aortic root dilatation (see 📖 Aortic aneurysms and dilatation, p. 400) rather than 1° leaflet pathology is the most common cause of AR: the valve becomes distorted with impaired coaptation of the leaflets. A bicuspid valve is associated with a dilating aortopathy and coarctation (see 📖 Coarctation of the aorta, p. 406).
- Connective tissue diseases and hypertension cause aortic dilatation and may lead to dissection, which is readily identified by CCT (see 📖 Aortic aneurysms and dilatation, p. 400).

Consequences of aortic regurgitation

- Acute AR causes a rapid increase in LV end-diastolic pressure, resulting in pulmonary oedema; the most common causes are aortic dissection and infective endocarditis, and the definitive treatment for a valve causing such haemodynamic instability is surgery.
- Chronic AR results in a volume-loaded left ventricle, which dilates and eventually fails. For retrospectively gated acquisitions (see 📖 ECG gating, p. 34), measurement of LV volumes and ejection fraction should be routine
- Measurements of the aortic root, ascending aorta, arch, and descending aorta should be taken if aortic disease is suspected. Dilatation >4.5cm may require surgical intervention.

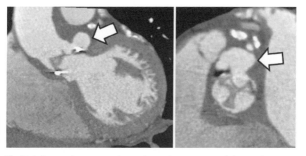

Fig. 21.8 Ruptured aortic root abscess (arrows) in a patient with bioprosthetic aortic valve endocarditis and paravalvular leak.

Mitral stenosis

Background

- Overwhelmingly the most common cause of mitral stenosis is rheumatic heart disease, although this is now uncommon in the developed world as a result of improved living conditions and widespread use of antibiotics.
- Both the mitral valve leaflets and sub-valvular apparatus are affected.
- Progressive commissural fusion, leaflet thickening, and calcification and shortening of the chordae tendineae result in a restricted and stenosed valve.
- Rarer causes include congenital mitral stenosis, mucopolysaccharidoses, endocardial fibroelastosis, and carcinoid.

Cardiac CT post-processing

- From the two- and four-chamber views (see 📖 Figs. 21.2 and 21.3), a short-axis image through the tips of the mitral leaflets should be reconstructed.
- Care should be taken to ensure a perpendicular section.
- Commisural fusion of the valve leaflets results in a funnel-shaped valve, tapering to a stenosed orifice. Measurements must be taken at the tips of the leaflets to ensure accurate assessment of the mitral valve area (MVA): measurements closer to the annulus will result in underestimation of the severity of stenosis.
- All diastolic phases should be examined to identify the phase with the smallest valve area, which should then be measured by planimetry.

Grading of mitral stenosis

Normal MVA is >4cm^2. Below 2cm^2 the stenosis becomes haemodynamically significant, resulting in a rise in left atrial pressure.

- Valve orifice areas of >1.5cm^2, 1.0–1.5cm^2, and <1.0cm^2 correspond to mild, moderate, and severe mitral stenosis, respectively.
- On TTE, mitral stenosis is usually assessed by a combination of planimetry and pulsed-wave Doppler; the Doppler tracing can be analysed to derive the mean forward pressure gradient and pressure half-time (orifice area = 220/pressure half-time).
- CCT- and TTE-derived values for MVA do not differ significantly, with good correlation across a range of mitral stenosis severities.

Assessment of aetiology

- The hallmarks of rheumatic mitral stenosis are thickening of the valve leaflets (Fig. 21.9a), commissural fusion, and shortening of the chordae; a characteristic 'hockey-stick' appearance is present, as well as bowing of the valve leaflets in early diastole (Fig. 21.9b).
- Carcinoid syndrome typically results in tricuspid and pulmonary valve pathology. Rarely, it may lead to mitral stenosis if there is a coexisting right-to-left shunt at the atrial level or in the case of a secreting pulmonary carcinoid tumour. Features include plaque deposition on the valves and sub-valvular apparatus, leading to thickening and

retraction of the leaflets: the leaflets become fixed in a semi-open position, resulting in a mixed picture of stenosis and regurgitation.

Consequences of mitral stenosis

- Mitral stenosis leads to a pressure overloaded and dilated left atrium.
- The back-pressure on the pulmonary vasculature and right heart leads to pulmonary hypertension and RV dilatation and failure, with tricuspid regurgitation.
- Particular attention should be paid to the size of the tricuspid valve annulus if the patient is referred for mitral valve surgery, as concomitant tricuspid annuloplasty is indicated if the diameter exceeds 4cm.
- Dilatation of the left atrium predisposes to atrial arrhythmias: the presence of thrombus should be sought, especially in the left atrium appendage.
- The left ventricle usually has normal size and function as it is protected from abnormal haemodynamics by the stenosed mitral valve.

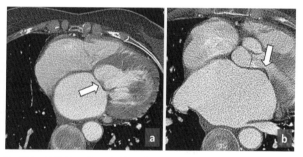

Fig. 21.9a (a) Thickened mitral valve leaflets (a, arrow) and classical systolic 'hockey-stick' appearance of mitral valve stenosis (b, arrow).

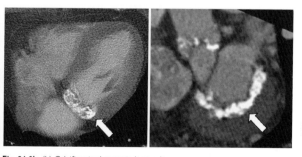

Fig. 21.9b (b) Calcific mitral stenosis (arrows).

Mitral regurgitation (1)

Background

- Second most common valve disease after aortic stenosis.
- Incidence is >20% in the sixth decade and beyond.
- Mitral regurgitation (MR) may be due to either a 1° valve abnormality or 2° dysfunction of the mitral valve apparatus ('functional' MR).
- 1° valve abnormalities are typically caused by myxomatous degeneration, rheumatic fever, and endocarditis.
- Functional abnormalities are caused by LV dysfunction (causing dilatation of the mitral valve annulus) and/or papillary muscle dysfunction due to ischaemic heart disease.
- Rarer causes include cardiomyopathy and connective tissue disorders.

Cardiac CT post-processing

Assessment of the ROA is possible with multiplane multiphase reconstruction. Geometric analyses such as leaflet angle and tenting offer clues to the aetiology of the MR.

Regurgitant orifice area

- The mitral valve should be inspected in the three-chamber view (see 📖 Fig. 21.4), either in multiple phases individually or as a cine-loop. MR is suggested by poor leaflet coaptation or prolapse. If MR is present, a perpendicular short-axis view should be obtained using the oblique tool.
- The short-axis image plane should be scrolled from apex to base in multiple systolic phases to identify the phase with the smallest ROA, which should be measured by planimetry (Fig. 21.10).

Geometric assessment

- From the two- and four-chamber views, a systolic short-axis view of the mitral valve should be obtained to assess the mitral commissures (Fig. 21.11).
- An antero-posterior plane should then be obtained perpendicular to the mitral valve coaptation line to assess the valve at the level of the central scallops.
- Using this image, the angle at which the leaflets meet the plane of the annulus should be measured (*leaflet angle*).
- The tenting height is measured as the distance between the annulus plane and the leaflet coaptation point.

Grading of mitral regurgitation

Regurgitant orifice area

- ROA shows good agreement with the grade of MR as quantified by TOE and invasive left ventriculography.
- CCT can differentiate severe MR (ROA 72 ± 37mm^2) from moderate (32 ± 16mm^2) or mild MR (21 ± 9mm^2), although mild and moderate MR are indistinguishable by ROA.

Geometric assessment

- Heart failure and LV dilatation alter the geometry of the mitral valve apparatus, with annular dilatation and ↑ traction on the chordae tendineae, limiting leaflet coaptation in systole: this causes 'functional' MR.
- Geometric assessment is useful for the quantification of MR in the context of heart failure.
- The mitral valve tenting height loosely correlates with the degree of MR as compared to echocardiographic measurements.
- A raised tenting height >6.6cm is associated with functional MR.
- The systolic leaflet angle is also ↑ in functional MR.

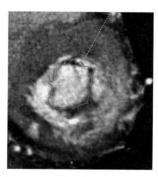

Fig. 21.10 Mitral valve planimetry in diastole in a patient with mild mixed mitral valve disease.

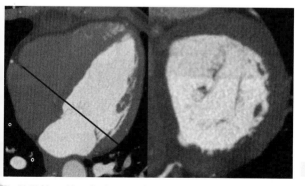

Fig. 21.11 Normal four-chamber view of mitral valve (left) with cutplane for en-face mitral valve view (right).

Mitral regurgitation (2)

Assessment of aetiology

CCT allows detailed morphological assessment of the mitral valve and subvalvular apparatus.

- The 1° indication for CCT in patients with MR is to establish the presence of CAD. An occluded vessel, particularly the dominant coronary artery (see 📖 The coronary arterial circulation, p. 178), suggests a functional or ischaemic cause for the MR.
- Thickened shortened leaflets suggest a rheumatic cause; leaflet prolapse (Fig. 21.12) or ruptured chordae tendineae suggests degenerative pathology; and vegetations suggest endocarditis (Fig. 21.13),
- The geometry of the valve and assessment of LV function may suggest functional MR 2° to heart failure.
- Mitral valve annular calcification is also readily identified on CCT, and may have important implications if surgical intervention is required: prosthetic valve implantation into calcified tissue can be difficult.

Consequences of mitral regurgitation

Chronic severe MR leads to progressive LV dilatation and failure, pulmonary hypertension, right heart failure, and tricuspid regurgitation.

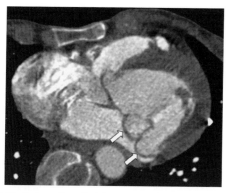

Fig. 21.12 Mitral valve prolapse. Both the mitral leaflets bow back into the left atrium (arrows).

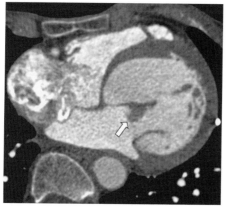

Fig. 21.13 A large vegetation (arrow) adherent to the anterior mitral valve leaflet in a patient with *Staphylococcus aureus* endocarditis.

Tricuspid regurgitation

Background

- Most commonly caused by pulmonary hypertension 2° to other pathologies (e.g. mitral or pulmonary disease).
- Functional tricuspid regurgitation (TR) also occurs in the context of RV dilatation due to failure of valve leaflet coaptation.
- Rarer causes include rheumatic heart disease, endocarditis (intravenous drug abusers), and Ebstein's anomaly.
- CCT can be anatomically informative. Regurgitation of contrast media into the IVC and hepatic veins can be a non-specific marker of right-sided heart disease, especially in pulmonary hypertension.

Cardiac CT post-processing

Regurgitant orifice area

- To delineate the right-sided valves adequately (Fig. 21.14), the scan should be timed to include contrast in the right side of the heart. This may be achieved using a gated CT pulmonary angiogram contrast protocol (see 📖 Gated CT pulmonary angiogram, p. 110).
- The valve should be inspected in the four-chamber view in multiple phases; poor leaflet coaptation and prolapse suggest TR.
- A two-chamber view through the tricuspid valve should be obtained by placing the oblique tool in the long axis through the centre of the valve whilst inspecting the valve in the four-chamber view.
- If TR is present, a perpendicular short-axis view should be obtained.
- The short-axis image plane should be scrolled from apex to base in multiple systolic phases to identify the phase with the largest ROA, which should be measured by planimetry.
- The extent of contrast reflux into the IVC and hepatic veins should be assessed from the axial image stack (Fig. 21.15).

Grading of tricuspid regurgitation

Vena cava and hepatic vein reflux

- Reflux of contrast into the IVC and hepatic veins has been semi-quantitatively compared with TR assessed on echocardiography in a cohort of patients with pulmonary hypertension.
- There is a moderately good agreement between echocardiographic grading and CT grading of the TR.
- The absence of contrast reflux into the IVC suggests no or minimal TR on echocardiography.
- Contrast reflux is a relatively non-specific sign of right heart disease, pericardial constriction, or pulmonary hypertension: it may also be present with high contrast injection rates (>3mL/s) or if the patient inadvertently performs the Valsalva manoeuvre during breath-holding.

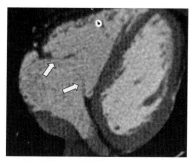

Fig. 21.14 Normal tricuspid valve anatomy.

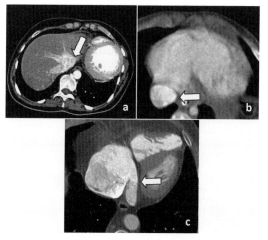

Fig. 21.15 Non-cardiac manifestations of severe TR include regurgitation of contrast medium into dilated hepatic veins (a), the inferior vena cave (b), and the coronary sinus (c).

Assessment of aetiology

One of the most common factors in the pathogenesis of tricuspid valve dysfunction is annular dilatation associated with pulmonary hypertension in the context of left-sided heart disease, particularly MR and mitral stenosis.

- CCT enables detailed morphological assessment of the tricuspid valve and sub-valvular apparatus.
- Carcinoid heart disease produces thickening and retraction of the right-sided valve leaflets/cusps: the valve becomes 'stuck' half open, resulting in regurgitation and stenosis.
- Thickening and shortening of the leaflets also occurs in rheumatic disease, invariably in association with involvement of the left-sided valves.
- Ebstein's anomaly (see 📖 Congenital valve pathology, Fig. 23.22, p 369) is a congenital abnormality caused by incomplete delamination of the posterior and septal leaflets from the ventricular wall *in utero*; the tricuspid annulus is displaced apically, resulting in atrialization of the ventricle and consequent TR.
- The lung fields should be reviewed for evidence of septic emboli suggesting infective endocarditis (Fig. 21.16).

Consequences of tricuspid regurgitation

Chronic severe TR leads to progressive RV dilatation and failure (Fig. 21.17). TR and tricuspid annular dilatation are particularly important in left-sided valve disease. The presence of TR or annular dilatation at the time of mitral valve repair or replacement has a significant detrimental impact on post-operative long-term prognosis. Concomitant tricuspid annuloplasty is indicated in this setting, irrespective of the degree of TR.

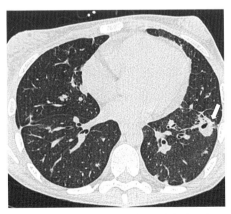

Fig. 21.16 A cavitating soft tissue mass in the left lower lobe (arrow) representing septic infarct 2° to tricuspid valve endocarditis.

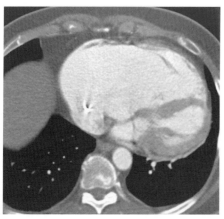

Fig. 21.17 RV dilatation in a patient with severe TR. Note pacing wire in right atrium.

Tricuspid stenosis

Background
- The most common cause of tricuspid stenosis is rheumatic valve disease, although this is now uncommon in the developed world.
- Rheumatic tricuspid stenosis is invariably associated with left-sided valve disease.
- Other causes include carcinoid and congenital tricuspid stenosis.

Cardiac CT post-processing
- Four- and two-chamber views should be obtained, as for TR (see 📖 Figs. 21.2 and 21.3), to inspect the valve leaflets and sub-valvular apparatus.
- The short-axis image plane should be scrolled from apex to base in multiple diastolic phases to identify the phase with the smallest valve area, which should be measured by planimetry.
- As with the mitral valve, care should be taken to position the image plane at the tips of the leaflets to avoid overestimating valve area on planimetry.

Grading of tricuspid stenosis
- The normal tricuspid area is 3–5cm^2; tricuspid stenosis is severe if valve area <1cm^2.
- There are no comparative studies between CCT and echocardiography in tricuspid stenosis.
- If there are features consistent with tricuspid stenosis (shortened, thickened valve leaflets and a valve area <3cm^2), referral for assessment by an alternative imaging modality, such as echocardiography, should be made.

Assessment of aetiology
- Features of rheumatic valve disease such as shortened, thickened leaflets and thickening of the sub-valvar apparatus should be recorded; left-sided valves should also be assessed.
- Carcinoid valve disease also thickens and shortens the leaflets, resulting in a mixed picture of stenosis and regurgitation; it is often associated with pulmonary valve disease.
- As the superior aspect of the liver is often within the scan field, metastatic carcinoid lesions may be identified, as well as lesions within the lung.

Consequences of tricuspid stenosis
Tricuspid stenosis results in ↑ venous pressure and features of right-sided heart failure, with ascites, pleural effusions, and peripheral oedema. Right atrial enlargement (Fig. 21.18) and subsequent arrhythmias are a common complication.

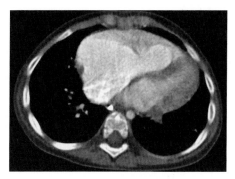

Fig. 21.18 Tricuspid stenosis with marked right atrial enlargement.

Pulmonary regurgitation

Background

- Trivial pulmonary regurgitation (PR) is a normal finding in the majority of the adult population. Isolated significant PR is uncommon.
- Common causes include pulmonary hypertension and congenital pulmonary artery abnormalities causing failure of leaflet coaptation.
- Connective tissue disorders, such as Marfan's syndrome, may also lead to arterial dilatation and valvular incompetence
- Iatrogenic causes, such as after valvuloplasty or surgical correction of tetralogy of Fallot (see 📖 Tetralogy of Fallot, p 364), are seen in the adult congenital heart disease (ACHD) population.
- Other causes: carcinoid syndrome, infective endocarditis.

Cardiac CT post-processing

- As for assessment of the tricuspid valve, contrast should be timed to provide opacification of the right heart using a gated CT pulmonary angiogram contrast protocol (see 📖 Gated CT pulmonary angiogram, p. 110).
- Using the sagittal view through the RV outflow tract and pulmonary valve, the oblique tool should be passed through the centre of the valve to create a long-axis view (Fig. 21.19).
- Orthogonal short-axis views through the valve, in multiple imaging planes and phases (usually 60–80% of the R–R interval), are used to identify the largest regurgitant orifice area.

Grading of pulmonary regurgitation

- CCT may be used to assess RV volumes and function (see 📖 Right ventriculography, p. 236) to plan timing of intervention in chronic PR; such measurements agree well with CMR.
- There are no comparative studies comparing CCT with echocardiography or CMR.
- A severely dilated valve annulus with obvious failure of cusp coaptation should prompt assessment with another imaging modality.

Assessment of aetiology

- Shortened, thickened cusps which appear to be stuck half-open suggest carcinoid heart disease.
- Vegetations may be seen on the valve in infective endocarditis.
- Dilatation of the pulmonary trunk and arteries suggest 2° PR due to annular dilatation and failure of cusp coaptation.
- ACHD patients may have relevant post-surgical changes, e.g. ventricular septal defect patch, pulmonary conduit, etc.

Consequences of pulmonary regurgitation

Chronic PR leads to a volume-overloaded right heart. The right ventricle dilates and fails, and the interventricular septum bulges into the left heart during diastole, causing a characteristic 'D'-shaped left ventricle in the short axis. TR may develop.

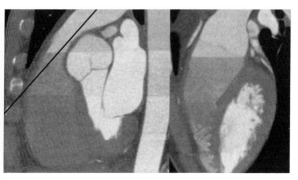

Fig. 21.19 Orientation for assessment of the pulmonary valve.

Pulmonary stenosis

Background

- Pulmonary stenosis is almost always congenital (tetralogy of Fallot, maternal rubella, Turner's syndrome, Noonan's syndrome, William's syndrome).
- Rare acquired causes include carcinoid heart disease, infective endocarditis, and rheumatic disease.
- Stenosis usually occurs at the valve level, but infundibular and peripheral stenoses do occur.
- The prognosis in mild to moderate cases is very good, with intervention rarely indicated.

CCT post-processing

- The image plane is constructed with the same method used for PR (see 📖 Pulmonary regurgitation, p. 310).
- The systolic phases (5–30% R–R interval) are examined in multiple short-axis views to identify the phase with the smallest valve area, which should be measured by planimetry.

Grading of pulmonary stenosis

- The normal pulmonary valve is tricuspid and has an area of 2.5–4.0cm^2.
- A valve area >1cm^2 corresponds to a Doppler pressure gradient of 25–49mmHg and indicates mild stenosis.
- Moderate pulmonary stenosis is defined by a valve area of 0.5–1.0cm^2 (49–79mmHg),and severe stenosis by an area <0.5cm^2 (>80mmHg).
- There are no studies comparing measurements by CCT and echocardiography.

Assessment of aetiology

- Congenital pulmonary stenosis is usually due to fusion of the valve cusps, resulting in a dome-shaped valve in systole.
- Pulmonary infundibular stenosis and peripheral pulmonary artery stenoses can be differentiated from valvular stenosis by careful inspection of the pulmonary artery branches and RV outflow tract.
- Rheumatic heart disease involves thickening and calcification of the valve cusps (Fig. 21.20): left-sided valve involvement is invariable.
- Carcinoid heart disease typically results in a mixed picture of stenosis and regurgitation.
- One or more vegetations in the context of persistent septicaemia with a typical organism suggest infective endocarditis.

Consequences of pulmonary stenosis

- Congenital pulmonary stenosis may be associated with atrial and ventricular septal defects, a patent ductus arteriosus, and tetralogy of Fallot.
- Pulmonary stenosis of any cause will result in a pressure overloaded right ventricle, hypertrophy, TR, and, if a patent foramen ovale (PFO) is present (25% of the adult population), right-to-left shunting if the pressure in the right atrium exceeds that in the left.

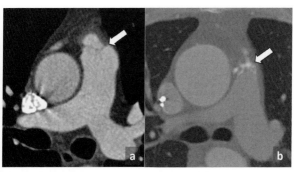

Fig 21.20 (a) Normal pulmonary valve (arrow). (b) Pulmonary valve calcification (arrow) in a patient with pulmonary stenosis.

Prosthetic valves (1)

A full discussion and summary of the indications for valve surgery is beyond the scope of this book. Comprehensive guidelines are available online ($\Diamond$ http://www.escardio.org/guidelines-surveys/esc-guidelines/Pages valvular-heart-disease.aspx). Broadly, three interventions are available:

- Replacement of the valve with a mechanical, bio-prosthetic or homograft valve
- Native valve repair
- Percutaneous valvotomy.

Aortic valve

- Valve replacement with either a mechanical or bio-prosthetic device is the most common intervention; both devices are used to treat aortic stenosis, whilst mechanical valves are more commonly used for AR.

Mitral valve

- Approximately one-third of patients with mitral stenosis will undergo percutaneous valvotomy; the remainder generally receive a mechanical prosthesis.
- Patients with MR due to leaflet prolapse (~50% of total cases) usually undergo mitral valve repair.
- Other patients with MR receive either a mechanical prosthesis (~40%) or a bio-prosthetic valve (~10%).
- Approximately one-third of patients undergoing surgery for MR have a least moderate TR requiring concomitant tricuspid annuloplasty.

Types of valve

Mechanical

- Ball-and-cage valves are now rarely used due to their noise, haemodynamic inefficiency, and higher propensity for thrombosis. However, their long-term durability ensures that they are still present in the population. A silastic ball is mounted inside a cage comprising three (aortic) or four (mitral) struts. The Starr–Edwards silastic ball valve is an example of a ball-and-cage valve. The ball and struts may be seen at fluoroscopy.
- Single tilting-disc valves superseded the ball and cage valves in the 1970s. They are made from a graphite disc with a pyrolitic carbon coating, mounted in either a stainless steel or titanium housing, with a polyester or Teflon sewing ring. The disc opening angle can be assessed by fluoroscopy and the valve gradient by Doppler echocardiography.
- Bi-leaflet valves have superior flow characteristics compared with the other mechanical valves. Two pyrolite carbon semicircular discs pivot in the centre of a housing made of either graphite or pyrolite-coated titanium. The disc opening angle can be assessed by fluoroscopy.

The accuracy of CCT for the assessment of prosthetic valves varies. For the evaluation of tilting-disc valves, CCT correlates poorly with traditional assessment techniques. In particular, the Bjork–Shiley valve causes significant beam hardening artefact, resulting in non-diagnostic images. However, bi-leaflet valve opening angle can readily be assessed using CCT. The use of contrast can help evaluate the aetiology of valve dysfunction, such as thrombosis or leaflet restriction by pannus.

Bio-prosthetic

These are xenograft tissue valves comprising porcine or bovine tissue and may be *stented* (supported by a mechanical frame) or *unstented*.

- *Stented valves* consist of three wire or polypropylene struts with the porcine or bovine material mounted on top. This arrangement is then attached to an alloy sewing ring.
- *Unstented valves* have no rigid frame, being instead supported by the aortic root. This system allows the valve to deform properly during opening and closing, and allows a larger opening orifice compared to a stented valve of similar size. The result is a more physiological flow profile. They are mostly used in the aortic position, and comprise a porcine or heterograft valve mounted on a sewing ring.

Homografts

- Cadaveric tissue valves used most commonly in the aortic position.
- When used to replace the aortic valve, most commonly comprise both the aortic valve and root, which are then implanted together (root replacement).
- Depending on the length of the homograft, coronary artery re-implantation may be necessary.
- Root replacement has the benefit of maintaining the normal geometric arrangement of the aortic valve and root.

Autografts

- Native valves that are explanted and relocated to a different position.
- Most common procedure: *Ross operation*.
  - Used to treat aortic stenosis in young children and adults.
  - The pulmonary valve is excised and implanted in the aortic position (pulmonary autograft), whilst a homograft is placed in the pulmonary position.
  - Although this has the disadvantage of being a two-valve procedure for a single-valve pathology, the haemodynamic results are excellent.
  - Most importantly, the pulmonary valve, now in the aortic position, will continue to grow with the child.

Prosthetic valves (2)

Scan acquisition

The scan should normally be performed with retrospective gating and dose-modulation disabled, giving a multiphase cine image that may be viewed without reduction in image quality in systole or diastole. This acquisition results in a high radiation dose.

Cardiac CT post-processing

To assess the opening angle of a mechanical single-disc or bi-leaflet valve, an image perpendicular to the leaflet motion is required.

- The image should be oriented so that the valve is seen in the short-axis view (Fig. 21.21).
- From this view, using the oblique tool, the valve should be transected in the mid-line, perpendicular to the straight edge of the semi-circular valve discs.
- The resulting reconstruction can be used to measure the leaflet opening angle.

Complications

Pannus and thrombus

- *Pannus* represents excessive endothelial proliferation on or around the valve; this in-growth of tissue can immobilize a valve leaflet, causing either regurgitation or stenosis depending on whether it fixes the valve in the open or closed position.
- On CCT, pannus appears as a small low-density region located on the inflow side of the prosthetic valve suture ring.
- It is important to differentiate pannus from thrombus: the latter may be successfully treated with thrombolytic therapy, whilst pannus requires surgical intervention.
- *Thrombus* may fix a semicircular disc in the open position and occlude the valve orifice, resulting in an ↑ valve gradient but minimal regurgitation.
- The fixing of the disc by thrombus can be readily identified by CCT.

⚠ Pannus and thrombus may coexist.

Endocarditis, pseudoaneurysms, and paraprosthetic leaks

- CCT features of endocarditis include the presence of vegetations on the valve leaflets, ring, or supporting struts.
- Abscess formation within the aortic root is identified by extravasation of contrast into the vessel wall at the site of the valve.
- A pseudoaneurysm is a cavity not lined by the native endothelium surrounding the prosthetic valve; the entry site of the aneurysm is caused by tearing of the native tissue by the valve sutures.
- Paraprosthetic leaks are normally identified by colour flow Doppler at echocardiography; CCT often demonstrates failure of apposition of the suture ring and adjacent structures, and contrast may be seen between the valve and native tissue.
- Non-cardiac findings may include mycotic aneurysms, commonly in the brain and lung.

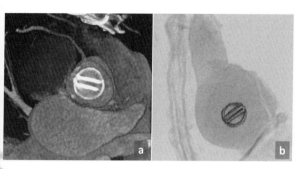

Fig. 21.21 St Jude double tilting disc prosthetic valves in the aortic (a) and mitral (b) positions.

Pericardial disease

The pericardium

Introduction

Pericardial disease is most commonly assessed with echocardiography. However, restricted acoustic windows may limit visualization of the pericardium, and posterior loculated or right-sided pericardial pathology may be extremely difficult to visualize.

CCT and CMR (see 📖 Cardiovascular magnetic resonance imaging, p. 488) offer distinct advantages over echocardiography in the imaging of pericardial disease. These include a wider FOV, allowing examination of the entire thorax, and better spatial resolution. CCT in particular offers excellent spatial (see 📖 Spatial resolution, p. 26) and temporal resolution (see 📖 Temporal resolution, p. 28), allowing motion-free imaging of the pericardium and associated pathology.

Pericardial anatomy

The pericardium is a two-layered membrane consisting of *fibrous* and *serous* components.

- The *fibrous pericardium* encloses the heart and roots of the great vessels; it fuses with the central diaphragmatic tendon and adventitia of the great vessels, and is adherent to the mediastinal pleura.
- The *serous pericardium* forms a bag lining the inside of the fibrous pericardium (parietal layer) and covering the heart and roots of the great vessels (visceral layer); this forms a potential space, where pericardial fluid may accumulate, with two large sinuses.
- The two layers are separated by a small amount of fluid (~15–50mL), mainly comprising plasma ultra-filtrate.
- The transverse sinus lies above the heart between the ascending aorta and main pulmonary artery anteriorly, and between the SVC, left atrium, and pulmonary veins posteriorly.
- The oblique sinus lies between the left atrium and the fibrous pericardium behind.

Pericardial appearances on cardiac CT

The normal *pericardial surfaces* are seen as a thin grey line of soft-tissue density, delineated between the pericardial and epicardial fat layer.

- The thickness of normal pericardium is <2mm (Fig. 22.1).
- The pericardium is most evident on the anterior surface of the heart, in front of the right ventricle and right atrium, where the epicardial fat is most prominent and there is an area of ventral mediastinal fat.
- Several pericardial recesses may be visible which may contain fluid.
- It is important to recognize these normal variants as they may be misinterpreted as significant pathology.
- The *superior pericardial recess* is a crescentic structure to the right of the ascending aorta (Fig. 22.2a); it may be mistaken for aortic dissection, a mediastinal mass, lymph nodes, or the thymus gland.
- The *transverse pericardial sinus* (Fig. 22.2b), dorsal to the aorta, may also be mistaken for aortic dissection or lymphadenopathy.
- The *oblique pericardial fissure* (Fig. 22.2c) may be misinterpreted as a bronchogenic cyst or oesophageal pathology.

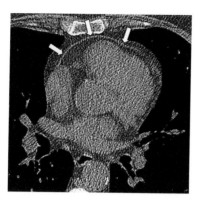

Fig. 22.1 Unenhanced CT demonstrating the normal pericardium (arrows) with a pericardial thickness of approximately 1–2mm.

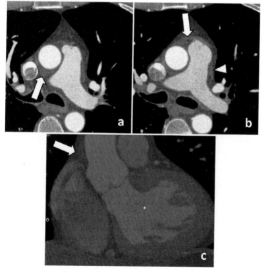

ig. 22.2 (a) Posterior superior pericardial recess, posterior to the ascending ᴐrta (arrow). (b) The pericardium extends around the lateral aspect of the aorta ᴐ form the anterior superior pericardial recess (arrow). The inferior aspect of the ᴇft pulmonary artery pericardial recess can also be seen (arrowhead). (c) Lateral ᴜperior aortic recess.

Pericardial imaging

Pericardial imaging is usually based on a staged, multimodality approach. The combination of echocardiography, CCT and CMR provide sufficient spatial resolution to visualize the pericardium, a wide FOV to look for associated pathology within the chest, a high temporal resolution to provide detailed information on myocardial function (and acute changes in function), and a means to differentiate tissue characteristics, such as calcium, blood, tumour, and fibrosis.

Echocardiography is usually the dominant modality used in the management of pericardial disease, with CCT and CMR reserved for patients in whom either there is a need to investigate possible underlying diagnoses, such as malignancy or there is concern about very localized effusions. Alternatively, assessment by CCT or CMR may be carried out as part of image acquisition for broader cardiac pathology with pericardial disease (particularly effusions) being noted incidentally.

Pericardial imaging with cardiac CT

CCT allows detailed imaging of pericardial pathology.
- CCT may be particularly useful in the assessment of loculated, haemorrhagic or localized effusions, or pneumopericardium, constrictive pericarditis, or pericardial masses.
- CCT may be indicated to investigate underlying causes of pericardial pathology such as malignancy.
- Pericardial effusions may be identified as an incidental finding during thoracic CT performed for investigation of symptoms such as shortness of breath.
- Strengths of CCT are:
  - Identification of calcification (including microcalcifications)
  - Inherent soft tissue contrast with tissue characterization, including fluid assessment based on attenuation
  - Wide FOV to identify associated chest pathology.
- CCT enables motion-free imaging of the pericardium, improving spatial resolution.
- MPR (see 📖 Multiplanar reformatting, p. 142) and multiphase reconstruction (see 📖 Multisegment reconstruction, p. 30) aid the assessment of associated changes in cardiac function.
- Gating (see 📖 ECG gating, p. 32) is required for accurate pericardial assessment: ungated studies are affected by motion artefact, which makes measurements inaccurate and hinders differentiation of thickened pericardium from fluid.
- The major limitations of CCT are the requirement for ionizing radiation and the use of iodinated contrast agents.

Pericardial effusion

Pericardial effusions occur following obstruction of venous or lymphatic drainage from the heart; many aetiologies can cause this obstruction. The key roles of cardiovascular imaging are to identify the size and location of the effusion, its likely cause, its haemodynamic effects, and the best approach to remove the effusion (pericardiocentesis).

Common causes

- Heart failure.
- Myocardial infarction.
- Renal insufficiency.
- Infection (bacterial, viral, tuberculous).
- Neoplasia (particularly lymphoma, lung and breast carcinoma).
- Trauma (including chylo-pericardium).
- Post-surgical.

Appearances on cardiac CT

Pericardial fluid usually has a CT number (see 📖 CT numbers and windowing, p. 138) similar to water and is seen as a thin line between the pericardial surfaces and the heart. Attenuation characteristics may ∴ allow characterization of the nature of an effusion.

- *Transudative effusions* usually have a similar CT number to water (Fig. 22.3).
- *Exudative effusions* (e.g. haemo-pericardium, purulent exudates, malignant effusions, chylous effusions) have higher protein content and hence higher CT numbers.
- The CT numbers of a haemo-pericardium vary with its age, with a gradual reduction over time and the emergence of heterogeneity due to the presence of thrombus.
- Inflammatory effusions may show ↑ contrast uptake by the pericardium.

CCT is particularly useful for detailed assessment of pericardial pathology associated with the effusion, in particular pericardial thickness, calcification, and the size, extent, and functional effects of pericardial masses (see 📖 Pericardial tumours and masses, p. 328). As the entire heart is captured in the standard CCT FOV, loculated or localized effusions and those around the anterior heart can be imaged within a standard protocol. The wide FOV should also be assessed for related pathology in the lungs and to define the extent of any masses associated with the pericardium. CCT is of limited value in the differentiation of a small effusion from pericardial thickening or when the effusion and pericardium have similar CT numbers.

Cardiac tamponade

Cardiac tamponade should have been identified clinically and on echocardiography prior to CCT. However, multidetector CT allows visualization of the entire cardiac cycle and may identify diastolic chamber collapse or changes in cardiac chamber size. If these findings are noted to be present during CT examination, immediate referral for treatment is warranted.

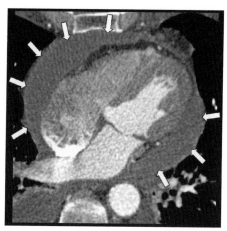

Fig. 22.3 Large pericardial effusion (arrows).

Constrictive pericarditis

Constrictive pericarditis usually presents with signs and symptoms of biventricular heart failure, with dyspnoea, orthopnoea, peripheral oedema, hepatomegaly, and, in severe cases, ascites. Diagnosis is important as pericardectomy may be beneficial.

Clinically, constrictive pericarditis may be difficult to distinguish from restrictive cardiomyopathy. Constrictive pericarditis is far more common and is more likely when there is a history of previous pericarditis, cardiac surgery/trauma, radiotherapy, or connective tissue disease.

Diagnosis is usually made by echocardiography, although the features of constriction and restriction occasionally overlap. Features suggesting constriction include septal motion towards the LV during inspiration, equalization of diastolic pressures in all four cardiac chambers, and peak systolic RV and LV pressures that are out of phase. Marked atrial enlargement and mitral/tricuspid regurgitation are more suggestive of restriction.

Common causes of constrictive pericarditis

- Mediastinal irradiation during radiotherapy.
- Post-surgical pericardiotomy.
- Post myocardial infarction (Dressler's syndrome).
- Infection (viral, bacterial, tuberculous, fungal, or parasitic).
- Systemic inflammatory disorders (rheumatoid arthritis, systemic lupus erythematosis).
- Neoplasia (particularly lymphoma, leukaemia, lung or breast carcinoma, mesothelioma).
- Post uraemic.
- Idiopathic.

Common causes of pericardial thickening

- Acute pericarditis.
- Uraemia.
- Rheumatic heart disease.
- Rheumatoid arthritis.
- Sarcoidosis.
- Mediastinal irradiation during radiotherapy.

Appearances on cardiac CT

- Pericardial thickness of >4mm on CCT is abnormal (Fig. 22.4) and, when accompanied by symptoms of heart failure, is highly suggestive of constrictive pericarditis.
- Pericardial calcification is also associated with constrictive pericarditis and is readily identified on CCT (Fig. 22.5).
- The right ventricle may be small, narrow, and tubular in structure.
- A sigmoid or 'D'-shaped septum may be observed.
- IVC and hepatic vein dilatation may be seen on review of wide field of view images.
- Ascites may be present in severe cases.

⚠ In the absence of appropriate symptoms and signs, neither pericardial thickening nor pericardial calcification are diagnostic of constrictive pericarditis.

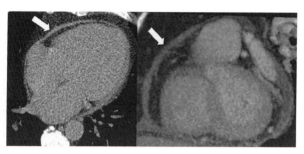

Fig. 22.4 Pericardial thickening (arrows).

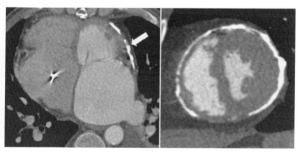

Fig. 22.5 Pericardial calcification (left, arrow), which may occasionally be concentric (right).

Pericardial tumours and masses

Pericardial tumours and masses include pericardial cysts, haematomas, and neoplasms.

Pseudotumours

Pericardial cysts are the most common pericardial masses and are formed when a portion of pericardium pinches off in development. They are most often diagnosed in middle age.

- Thin-walled with a non-enhancing rim and a central, fluid-filled portion; CT numbers similar to water (0–40HU) (Fig. 22.6).
- Often seen at the right costophrenic angle, but may be present anywhere in mediastinum.
- Rarely communicate with the pericardial cavity.
- May change in size and shape with respiration or body position.
- May be indistinguishable from a bronchogenic or thymic cyst.

Haematomas may also be seen within the pericardium. These may be acute, sub-acute, or chronic. In contrast to CMR, CCT is unable to distinguish reliably between acute and sub-acute haematomas, although calcification within a chronic haematoma may be seen readily.

Pericardial tumours

Pericardial tumours may be *1° or 2° to metastatic disease*, with the former much less common. Biopsy and histology are usually required to achieve a definitive diagnosis.

2° metastatic disease of the pericardium

Pericardial metastases are found in ~10% of all patients with a malignancy, although most are only recognized at post-mortem. They usually seed to the pericardium via the lymphatic or blood circulation. Pericardial metastases are most commonly due to carcinomas of the breast and lung, followed by lymphoma and melanoma. The pericardium usually has a thickened, nodular appearance; pericardial effusion is common.

Benign 1° pericardial tumours

Benign 1° pericardial tumours include:

- Lipomas (tissue density similar to fat)
- Fibromas (usually soft tissue density with poor or faint enhancement)
- Haemangiomas
- Teratomas.

Teratomas affect mainly infants and children, are mostly right-sided, and typically connect to the aorta or pulmonary artery via a pedicle through which it receives its blood supply.

- They are usually intra-pericardial (rarely intra-myocardial).
- They may be very large and associated with a pericardial effusion, with tamponade and/or respiratory distress.
- They are rarely malignant.
- CCT demonstrates a complex multicystic mass, with various tissue elements that may include calcified structures such as bone and teeth.

Malignant 1° pericardial tumours

Mesothelioma is the most common 1° pericardial malignancy, and affects both adults and children. It often presents with chest pain, shortness of breath, cough, and palpitation, and may mimic pericarditis. Widespread metastases may be present at diagnosis. CCT appearances include nodular or diffuse pericardial thickening, and occasionally pericardial effusion. Malignant pleural mesothelioma may invade the pericardium directly.

Lymphoma, *sarcoma* and *liposarcoma* may all affect the pericardium. They usually appear as large heterogeneous masses on CCT, often with large pericardial effusions.

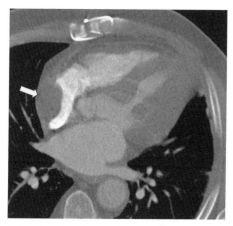

Fig. 22.6 Pericardial cyst (arrow) causing compression of the right atrium.

Congenital absence of pericardium

Congenital absence of the pericardium is rare but may be diagnosed definitively with CCT. Patients with pericardial defects are often asymptomatic. However, they may present with entrapment or herniation of cardiac chambers (especially the left atrial appendage) and become symptomatic, potentially requiring either surgical closure or enlargement of the pericardial defect to alleviate the herniation.

Congenital absence of the pericardium is often associated with one or more congenital heart defects, including:

- Atrial septal defects (see 📖 Atrial septal defects, p. 346)
- Patent ductus arteriosus (see 📖 Patent ductus arteriosus, p. 352)
- Mitral valve stenosis (see 📖 Mitral stenosis, p. 298)
- tetralogy of Fallot (see 📖 Tetralogy of Fallot, p. 364).

The aorto-pulmonary window is covered by pericardium and contains adipose tissue, so on CCT this region has fat-density CT numbers. Left-sided absence of the pericardium allows interposition of lung tissue between the aorta and pulmonary artery: CT numbers are ∴ closer to air. Occasionally, bulging of the left atrial appendage can be seen through the defect and may cause herniation and thrombus formation within the left atrial appendage. The heart is normally rotated to the left with left-sided absence of the pericardium.

Congenital heart disease

Introduction

CHD is the most common inborn defect affecting around 1% of new-borns. Over the last 30 years, advances in paediatric cardiology and cardiac surgery have revolutionized patient management, and as a result the majority of these patients now survive into adulthood.

Many undergo palliative or reparative surgery. However, few treatments are truly curative and subsequent close and often lifelong follow up is required to ensure optimum quality of life is maintained. These patients are at equal or ↑ risk of common cardiac conditions such as atherosclerosis and CAD and the need for imaging studies to provide comprehensive, non-invasive assessment is increasing.

Although CMR and TTE remain the techniques of choice for the routine assessment and follow-up of patients with ACHD, advances in CCT have led to its emergence as both a complementary technique and an alternative to CMR and TTE where these are unavailable or contraindicated.

Role of cardiac CT

CCT gives virtually isotropic images (see 📖 Detector terminology, p. 16) Intrathoracic structures may ∴ be viewed in any plane, a feature important in ACHD patients. Many have had previous cardiothoracic surgery, making alternative imaging such as echocardiography difficult due to poor ultrasound windows. The short acquisition time and superior spatial resolution of contrast-enhanced CT is advantageous, particularly for imaging the epicardial coronary arteries and other narrow structures. CCT also shows conduit calcification and stent location clearly. Retrospectively gated MPR allows measurements of biventricular size and function (see 📖 ECG gating, p. 34), providing an alternative to CMR in patients with a pacemaker or implantable cardiac defibrillator (ICD).

Given the complexity of many congenital cases, congenital CCT should ideally be undertaken by experienced congenital cardiovascular imaging specialists who have close and long-term collaboration with the cardiologists and cardiothoracic surgeons managing ACHD patients in their local tertiary referral centre.

Sequential segmental analysis

Knowledge of anatomy is crucial to accurate assessment of congenital CCT studies. In complex CHD the use of 'sequential segmental analysis' is advised.

- Analysis commences with description of, in turn, the atrial, ventricular, and arterial segments. The AV connections are described as concordant (normal) or discordant, as are the ventriculoarterial (VA) connections.
- A useful way of distinguishing which ventricle is morphologically the right ventricle is to compare the two surfaces of the interventricular septum. The LV surface is relatively smooth, with few trabeculations arising from it, whilst the RV side gives rise to the moderator band and multiple trabeculations in the apical region.
- Additionally, the position of the cardiac apex and situs of the atria should be described (Table 23.1).
- The normal heart is described as having AV and VA concordance, that is the right atrium connects to the right ventricle, the left atrium connects to the left ventricle, the right ventricle supports the pulmonary circulation and the left ventricle supports the systemic circulation. The right AV valve is a tricuspid valve and the left AV valve is a mitral valve.
- Having described the AV and VA connections, associated abnormalities such as septal defects or patent ductus arteriosus are described.
- The inlet and outlet valves should be fully described. For example, in tricuspid atresia, there is an absent right AV connection. In other cases both AV valves may connect predominantly to one ventricle, creating a double inlet-ventricle.
- It is important to be specific when describing anatomy in CHD, as conditions are tightly defined according to morphological appearance. For example, an over-riding aorta (as in tetralogy of Fallot, p. 364) is defined as an aortic valve that over-rides the interventricular septum by <50%. If the valve over-rides by >50%, it defines a double-outlet right ventricle.

Table 23.1 Atrial arrangement

	Atrial situs solitus: Normal	Atrial situs inversus	Right isomerism	Left isomerism
Atrial morphology	R-sided morphologic RA, L-sided morphologic LA	Mirror image: R-sided morphologic LA, L-sided morphologic RA	Bilateral morphological RA	Bilateral morphological LA
Atrial appendages	Broad based RA appendage, long narrow LA appendage	Mirror image	Bilateral RA appendages	Bilateral LA appendages
Sinus node	Single, R-sided	Single, L-sided	Bilateral	Absent
Pulmonary morphology	R lung trilobed, L lung bilobed	R lung bilobed, L lung trilobed	Bilateral trilobed lungs	Bilateral Bilobed lungs
Bronchial morphology*	Short R-sided main bronchus, Long L- sided main bronchus:	Mirror image	Bilateral short morphological R bronchi	Bilateral long morphological L bronchi
Abdominal arrangement** Aorta & IVC	Aorta to L of spine, IVC to R of spine	Normal or mirror image	Aorta and IVC on same side IVC anterior to aorta	Aorta and azygos on same side Azygos posterior to aorta
Stomach	L-sided	Normal or mirror image	Usually L sided	Usually R sided
Liver	R-sided		Midline	Midline
Spleen	R-sided		Usually absent	Often polysplenia.

IVC, inferior vena cava; L, left; LA, left atrium; R, right; RA, right atrium; SVC, superior vena cava

*Since bronchopulmonary situs nearly always follows atrial situs, atrial situs can be inferred from the chest radiograph

**Echocardiography shows the intra-abdominal relations of the great vessels.

Reproduced with permission from Thorne S and Clift P (2009). *Adult Congenital Heart Disease*. Oxford University Press.

Technical considerations in congenital cardiac CT

Contrast protocols

Standard retrospectively gated CT coronary angiography usually gives clear information about both LV function and coronary lumenography. However, certain considerations should be taken into account when timing contrast administration for patients with ACHD.

- A test bolus technique (see 📖 Optimizing scan timing, p. 102) tracked to determine the time to peak concentration at the aortic root is recommended in patients with CHD due to the variable transit time and venous haemodynamics; this also allows early identification of other late-filling structures.
- Care is required in those with presumed or likely pulmonary arterial hypertension, where transit times may be especially challenging.
- In ACHD, RV function is often of interest; reduced pulmonary transit time is likely to lead to better RV enhancement, but may be detrimental to analysis of the left ventricle; the scan timing or CT protocol can be adjusted to optimize RV opacification, but this may limit LV opacification and coronary artery assessment.
- Using specific intravenous contrast protocols, it is possible to combine CTPA with CT coronary angiography within a single scan protocol (see 📖 CT coronary angiography, p. 108) to allow comprehensive assessment of the pulmonary and coronary arteries, biventricular function and valvular anatomy without fundamentally altering the region of interest or the basic scan protocol.

Gating

In patients with ACHD, retrospective gating is most commonly used as the incidence of arrhythmia is higher and the functional information provided is helpful.

Anomalous coronary arteries (1)

The usual arrangement of the coronary arteries is described elsewhere in this book (📖 The coronary arteries and cardiac veins, p. 178). Autopsy data suggest that, in around 1% of individuals, this arrangement is altered, particularly in those with underlying abnormalities of cardiac morphology. Many referrals for CTA follow inability to fully visualize coronary anatomy on invasive angiography. CTA allows accurate assessment of the origin and course of anomalous coronary arteries.

Anatomical description

- The description of an anomalous coronary artery should begin with definition of the sinus from which it arises, according to the Leiden convention (see 📖 The coronary ostia and left coronary artery, p. 180).
- The following aspects of the coronary ostium should be described:
  - Angle of take-off: normal coronary arteries arise at ~90° to the coronary sinus; this angle is often much reduced ('acute take-off') in coronary anomalies.
  - Shape of the orifice: the usual shape of a coronary ostium is approximately circular; coronary anomalies typically demonstrate oval, tear-drop, or 'slit-like' orifices.
- The course of the artery should be described according to whether it passes:
  - Behind the aorta (retroaortic course, Fig. 23.1a and c)
  - Between the aorta and pulmonary trunk (inter-arterial or pre-aortic course (Fig. 23.1b) or
  - In front of the pulmonary trunk (pre-pulmonary course).
- A retroaortic course is common, particularly where the left circumflex artery arises from the RCA or sinus.
- An interarterial course is common when the RCA arises from the left coronary artery/ostium and vice versa.
- A pre-pulmonary course may be seen particularly in those with tetralogy of Fallot (TOF), where an anomalous LAD may arise from the right coronary sinus and pass in front of the right ventricular outflow tract (RVOT) to enter the AIVG. Damage may occur during surgery on the RVOT.

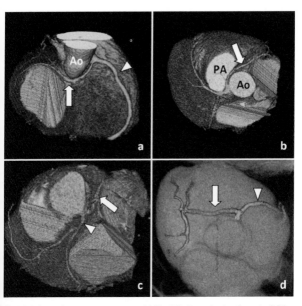

Fig. 23.1 Anomalous coronary arteries. (a) The LCx (arrow) arises from the RCA (arrowhead) close to its sinus and takes a retro-aortic course. (b) The RCA (arrow) arises from the left coronary sinus and passes between the pulmonary artery (PA) and aorta (Ao) to reach the RAVG. This pre-aortic course is said to carry an adverse prognosis. (c) The RCA (arrow) arises from the left coronary sinus (LMS, arrowhead) and follows a retro-aortic course. (d) LMS atresia. The left coronary artery (arrow) arises from the RCA (arrowhead) and takes a pre-aortic course to arrive in the AIVG, whereupon it bifurcates. A retrograde branch passes up the AIVG to give a left circumflex branch into the LAVG. (📖 Plate 7 for colour version).

Anomalous coronary arteries (2)

'Benign' and 'malignant' courses

- The course of the anomalous coronary artery is thought to determine prognosis, with the poorest associated with an interarterial course.
- A suggested mechanism is that compression occurs during systolic expansion of the great arteries, limiting coronary blood flow.
- Systolic pressures within the main pulmonary artery are relatively low, even during exertion; furthermore, coronary blood flow reaches a maximum during diastole, so compression alone may not offer the complete answer.
- Alternative adverse features include acute take-off from the aortic root, a slit-like orifice, and intramural course, all of which are more common for arteries taking an interarterial course.
- An acute take-off and slit-like orifice alter the shape of the coronary ostium and may plausibly affect coronary blood flow.
- An intramural course describes passage of the proximal coronary artery through the wall of the aorta. This is likely to increase coronary arterial wall tension (particularly during exertion), again with potentially negative consequences for coronary blood flow.
- These features offer more biologically plausible markers of adverse prognosis, rather than the interarterial course *per se*.

⚠ Most clinical data have come from autopsies of the young suffering sudden cardiac death (e.g. athletes, military recruits). Although there is no doubt that the interarterial phenotype is more common in this situation, extrapolation of this data to different groups, such as the elderly (who have lived with this undiscovered anomaly for their entire lives!), is confounded by studying only those who have died as a result of their condition. Prospective monitoring, probably at a national level, offers the highest likelihood of understanding the clinical relevance of these conditions.

Treatment

Surgical treatment is usually reserved for those with documented myocardial ischaemia. Reimplantation of the affected coronary artery may be considered, although excision of the roof of the intramural portion (*unroofing*) to create a single large ostial orifice has shown promising results.

Myocardial bridging

Coronary arteries are usually surrounded entirely by epicardial fat. Occasionally, a coronary artery will burrow into the myocardium for a variable distance before emerging distally as an epicardial vessel (Fig. 23.2). The artery may be completely or only partly surrounded by muscle. Autopsy data suggests some element of coronary artery muscle bridging in ~50% of hearts.

Assessment by cardiac CT

This should include:
- The artery and segment affected
- The approximate length of the bridge
- The diameter of the bridged segment in systole and diastole (and thus the approximate percentage compression during systole).

⚠ The functional significance of muscle bridging, and in particular its correlation with clinical symptoms, is uncertain. Although bridging leads to coronary artery compression during systole, coronary blood flow occurs predominantly during diastole when compression is at a minimum. There is further evidence that bridged coronary artery segments are spared from atherosclerosis.

If bridging is seen on CCT, referral for functional assessment, preferably using dynamic exercise, is probably appropriate if the patient is symptomatic.

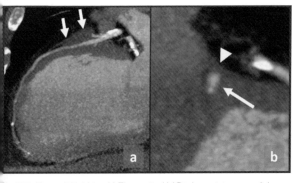

Fig. 23.2 Myocardial bridging. (a) The proximal LAD takes an intramyocardial course (arrows) before emerging to run epicardially in the mid and distal segments. (b) Viewing the proximal LAD in cross-section, it can be seen to lie entirely within the myocardium in the AIVG (arrow), with the overlying myocardium clearly visible (arrowhead).

Coronary assessment in adult congenital heart disease

Ischaemic heart disease
- High incidence of abnormal resting ECGs in patients with ACHD.
- Stress electrocardiography often unhelpful for the diagnosis of CAD.
- Abnormal ventricular anatomy may lead to difficulties in interpretation of myocardial perfusion scans.
- High incidence of investigation by ICA, although this may in itself be complicated by the presence of aortic root dilatation, variation in the site of the coronary ostia, and unusual coronary anatomy.
- Most ACHD patients presenting with chest pain do not have obstructive CAD.
- CTA offers excellent NPV for the exclusion of CAD and is a powerful alternative to ICA in this setting.
- CTA may be especially relevant outside tertiary congenital centres where the operator experience required for ICA in ACHD may be limited.

Kawasaki's disease
- Also known as mucocutaneous lymph node syndrome.
- Incidence ~10–30/100,000; ~80% <5 years of age; M>F 3:2.
- Leading cause of acquired heart disease in children.
- Systemic vasculitis with common features including fever ≥5 days, rash, lymphadenopathy, swollen hands and feet, and inflammation of the conjunctiva and mucous membranes.
- Cardiac features (~25%) include coronary artery aneurysms as well as myocarditis, pericarditis, and dysrhythmias.
- Intravenous immunoglobulin may limit the development of coronary artery aneurysms if given within 7 days of onset of fever.
- CTA allows measurement of the site, size, and number of coronary artery aneurysms, as well as the extent of calcification, thrombus, and contrast enhancement within any aneurysms seen (Fig. 23.3).

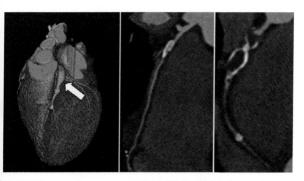

Fig. 23.3 Coronary artery aneurysms in Kawasaki's disease. Left: these are seen easily on volume-rendered imaging, although cMPR is required to assess patency. Middle: patent calcified aneurysm in the LAD with good distal run-off. Right: thrombosed and calcified aneurysm in the RCA with poor opacification (and a further small aneurysm) distally.

Other congenital coronary anomalies

Coronary fistulae

- Prevalence may be as high as 0.5%.
- Usually represent a connection between a coronary artery and either a cardiac chamber (right ventricle [40%] or atrium [25%]) or pulmonary artery (15%). Connections with the left heart, vena cavae, or pulmonary veins occur rarely.
- The abnormal connection is usually to a lower pressure system; blood flows preferentially into this 'sink' ('steal' phenomenon), potentially leading to myocardial ischaemia and dysfunction.
- Fistulae vary in size from small, direct connections to large, tortuous, and aneurysmal structures.
- CCT is a well-established technique for identifying and fully delineating coronary fistulae and may be useful in guiding intervention.

Anomalous left coronary artery from main pulmonary artery

- Acronym: ALCAPA; incidence 1 in 300,000 live births; M:F 2.3:1.
- Usually presents within the first few months of life as pulmonary vascular resistance falls.
- Usually presents with LV dysfunction ± shock as a result of delivery of deoxygenated blood to the left ventricle, although this depends on collateralization.
- Those with well-developed collateralization may present later with mitral regurgitation, cardiomegaly, and heart failure (~10–15%).
- CTA may provide the first diagnosis in patients with ALCAPA on the rare occasions that presentation occurs late (Fig. 23.4).

Single coronary artery and left main stem atresia

- Rarely, the left-sided coronary circulation is supplied entirely by branches from the RCA.
- This may be either as a continuation of the RCA around the left margin of the heart or by one or more aberrant branches, which usually follow either an anomalous interarterial or pre-pulmonary course.
- When an aberrant branch reaches the AIVG, classification is defined according to whether blood flows in an entirely anterograde (basal to apical) direction or partly retrograde (apical to basal) direction.
- If, on reaching the AIVG, the artery sends a branch down to the apex and another up the AIVG towards the aortic root, it defines the condition known as *LMS atresia* (Fig. 23.1d).
- If flow is anterograde only, it is classified a *single coronary artery*.
- Most cases of LMS atresia are probably in fact severe hypoplasia, with a string-like LMS in the usual position.
- Referral for ICA is probably appropriate for those with LMS atresia, with surgical correction the ultimate goal.

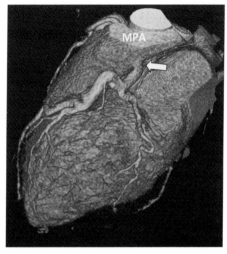

Fig. 23.4 Anomalous left coronary artery from pulmonary artery (arrow) arising from the proximal main pulmonary artery (MPA).

Atrial septal defects

Atrial septal defects (ASDs) account for ~10% of all CHD.

Secundum atrial septal defects

- Defect of the oval fossa.
- Interatrial shunting of blood (40% of L→R shunts in those >40 years).
- May present late if small.
- ASD causing RV dilatation and/or >1cm should be closed unless there is significant pulmonary vascular disease.
- Percutaneous closure preferred if <4cm and there is a sufficient rim of tissue on which to anchor the device (4–5mm away from AV valves and openings of the pulmonary/systemic veins).

Patent foramen ovale

- Common (30% of general population) and usually asymptomatic.
- Failure of oval foramen flap valve to close after birth.
- Flap valve allows only R→L shunting (provided right atrial > left atrial pressure).
- Associations include paradoxical embolism and migraine with aura.
- Contrast echocardiography ('bubble study') investigation of choice.
- Percutaneous closure as for secundum ASD.

Primum atrial septal defect

- Atrial component of atrioventricular septal defect (AVSD) (see 🕮 Atrio-ventricular septal defects, p. 350) due to defect of primum septum.

Sinus venosus atrial septal defect

- Atrial wall defect in the region of either the SVC (superior sinus venosus ASD) or IVC (inferior sinus venosus ASD, rarer) openings.
- Not a true defect of the atrial septum.
- The affected vena cava supplies both atria.
- Associated with partial anomalous right pulmonary venous drainage.
- Surgical closure; stenosis at the cavo-atrial junction may occur.

Coronary sinus defect

- Defect of atrial wall adjacent to mouth of coronary sinus, which empties into both atria.
- The defect may be small; in its severest form, the entire roof of the coronary sinus is absent ('unroofed' coronary sinus), with significant shunting of blood into the left atrium.
- Persistent left SVC is commonly seen with unroofed coronary sinus, exacerbating shunting.

Role of cardiac CT

- TTE remains the technique of choice for the detection of most ASDs.
- The high spatial resolution and 3D capabilities of CCT allow straightforward characterization of the location and size of the defect(s), especially in areas poorly visualized on TTE (Fig. 23.5).

- Additionally, biventricular size and function may be assessed (see 📖 Evaluation of ventricular and atrial function, p. 229), along with any associated anomalies such as anomalous pulmonary venous drainage.
- CCT may be used as a follow-up investigation after surgical or percutaneous ASD closure, either to evaluate RV function or to assess the state of a septal occlusion device (Fig. 23.6).
- CCT can also provide detailed anatomic information about the size and morphologic features of a patent foramen ovale (PFO). The presence of a short PFO tunnel length and atrial septal aneurysms on CCT correlates well with the presence of shunting on colour Doppler TTE.
- CCT is less effective at determining the presence of small defects and a TTE or TOE bubble study is recommended.

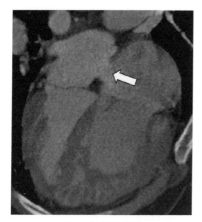

Fig. 23.5 Secundum atrial septal defect (arrow).

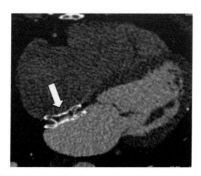

Fig. 23.6 ASD closed using an Amplatzer occlusion device (arrow).

Ventricular septal defects

Anatomy of the ventricular septum

- The ventricular septum has four components:
  - Inlet septum—separates RV inlet from LV outlet
  - Muscular septum—bounded by the attachments of tricuspid valve leaflets, apex, and supraventricular crest
  - Outlet septum—smooth-walled portion that extends from the supraventricular crest upwards to the pulmonary valve
  - Membranous septum—fibrous portion below aortic valve.
- A defect in any of these will result in a ventricular septal defect (VSD).

Classification

- Perimembranous (80%)—any VSD that has fibrous tissue or membranous septum as part of its border.
- Muscular (5–20%)—any VSD entirely surrounded by muscle.
- Subarterial (~5%)—any VSD bordered in part or over-ridden by aortic valve/pulmonary valve leaflets; AR may be a feature of these defects.
- As a group, VSDs are common (1.5–3.5 in 1000 live births) and account for ~20% of all CHD.
- May be associated with other congenital abnormalities, e.g. tetralogy of Fallot.

Physiology

- The degree of shunting across a VSD depends on defect size and systemic and pulmonary vascular resistance (PVR).
- Small VSDs (<$\frac{1}{3}$ size of the aortic root) have *restrictive* physiology, with a large pressure gradient between left and right ventricles and a variable degree of L→R shunting. RV/PA pressures are normal.
- At ~½ the size of the aortic root, VSDs become *moderately restrictive*, and show moderate to severe L→R shunting and raised RV pressures. PVR may be raised; left atrial/LV dilatation may result from volume overload.
- *Large non-restrictive* VSDs allow equalization of LV and RV pressures; uncorrected, irreversible increase in PVR occurs within 1–2 years, with progression to Eisenmenger's physiology (R→L shunt) by the end of the second decade.

Management

- Closure indicated if:
  - Symptomatic and >2:1 L→R shunting
  - Ventricular dysfunction and RV pressure/LV volume overload
  - Previous endocarditis
  - AR.
- Closure may be achieved via surgical or transcatheter approaches—see specialist texts for details.

Role of cardiac CT

- TTE remains the technique of choice for evaluation of VSDs.

- Straightforward characterization of the location and size of the defect(s), especially in areas poorly visualized on TTE (Fig. 23.7).
- Additionally, biventricular size and function may be assessed (see ⬚ Evaluation of ventricular and atrial function, p. 229), along with any associated anomalies.
- CCT may be used as a follow-up investigation after surgical or transcatheter closure, either to evaluate biventricular function or to assess the state of repair.
- Shunting cannot be evaluated by CCT.
- As for ASDs, small VSDs may be seen poorly on CCT; echocardiography is recommended.

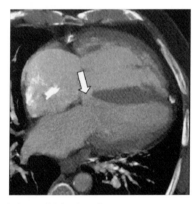

Fig. 23.7 Ventricular septal defect (arrow).

Atrio-ventricular septal defects

Anatomy and classification
- Failure of fusion of the junction between the atria and ventricles.
- There is a common AV junction guarded by a common AV valve.
- The common valve has five leaflets, which straddle the septum in the same plane: *superior* and *inferior bridging* leaflets which over-ride the septum and have attachments to both ventricles, a *left mural* leaflet, and *right inferior* and *antero-superior* leaflets.

⚠ The common AV valve may be described according to its 'left' and 'right' sided components but it is never correct to refer to the left or right AV valves as 'mitral' or 'trucuspid' as the anatomy is different.

- Atrioventricular septal defects (AVSDs) may be classified as:
  - Complete—there is both an ASD (primum ASD) and VSD, with 'floating' bridging leaflets; shunting occurs at both interatrial and interventricular levels
  - Partial—the bridging leaflets are adherent to the crest of the ventricular septum, dividing the common AV valve into two effective orifices; there is ∴ a primum ASD only and only interatrial shunting occurs.
- Occasionally, a partial AVSD occurs where the bridging leaflets adhere to the atrial septum; in this case, there is a VSD and interventricular shunting only.
- >75% of complete AVSDs but <10% of partial AVSDs occur in patients with trisomy 21.

Management
- Surgical closure indicated unless severe irreversible pulmonary vascular disease.
- Partial AVSDs are usually closed by pericardial patch, with concomitant repair of the left AV valve.
- Complete AVSDs require closure of the primum ASD and VSD and reconstruction of the AV valves.

Role of cardiac CT
- Anatomical characterization of AVSD, including assessment of bridging leaflets (Fig. 23.8).
- Evaluation of biventricular size and function (see 📖 Evaluation of ventricular and atrial function, p. 231), along with any associated anomalies.
- Follow-up investigation after surgery, either to evaluate biventricular function or to assess the state of repair.

⚠ CCT cannot evaluate shunting.

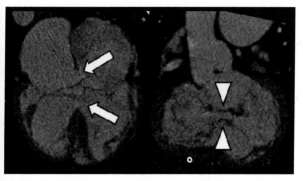

Fig. 23.8 Complete ASD (left, arrows) with a common AV valve. In the short-axis plane during diastole, the bridging leaflets of the common valve may be seen (right, arrowheads).

Patent ductus arteriosus

Background

- Persistent foetal connection between the aortic arch and proximal left pulmonary artery.
- May be associated with other malformations.
- May be required for survival in children with pulmonary atresia or hypoplastic left heart syndrome ('duct-dependent circulation').
- Usually isolated in adults.
- Prognosis depends on size, with large patent ductus arteriosus (PDA) prone to pulmonary hypertension and Eisenmenger's syndrome.
- Closure, by either trans-catheter or open surgical approaches, is recommended unless the PDA is small and clinically undetectable or if there is severe, irreversible pulmonary vascular disease.

Role of cardiac CT

- Occasionally found incidentally on CT acquisitions, particularly during investigation of pulmonary arterial hypertension (PAH).
- CCT can accurately determine the presence and size of a PDA and, with the use of 3D reconstruction techniques, provides accurate images prior to surgical correction where necessary (Fig. 23.9).
- CCT is also able to quantify calcification within the duct. Heavy PDA calcification is associated with a higher surgical risk; trans-catheter closure is preferable.

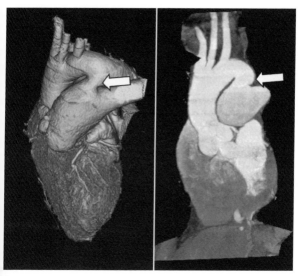

Fig. 23.9 Volume-rendered (left) and maximum-intensity projection (right) images of PDA (arrows).

Other congenital aortic abnormalities

Common arterial trunk

- A single arterial vessel arises form the heart, giving rise to the aorta, pulmonary, and coronary arteries.
- There is a common 'truncal' valve, which most commonly has three leaflets (~70%) but may have four (~20%), two (~10%), or, rarely, >4.
- Several classifications exist, including the Collett–Edwards classification.
  - Type 1 (~50–70%)—short main pulmonary artery (PA) arising from the common arterial trunk (CAT), giving rise to the right and left PAs.
  - Type 2 (30–50%)—no main PA; left and right PAs arise close together but separately from the CAT.
  - Type 3 (5–10%)—no PAs; lungs supplied by MAPCAs (see 📖 Major aorto-pulmonary collateral arteries, p. 362).
- Often straddles a large VSD, forming its superior roof.
- An interrupted aortic arch or coarctation may be present in 10–20%.
- Surgical repair is the 1° form of treatment:
  - Closure of VSD
  - Division of PA from CAT and creation of a valved conduit between the right ventricle and PA.

Role of cardiac CT

- Assessment of truncal anatomy (Fig. 23.10).
- Identification of pulmonary artery branches and collaterals, where present.
- In those who have undergone surgical repair, CCT is able to accurately assess conduit patency.

Aortopulmonary window

- Direct communication between the proximal aorta and pulmonary trunk due to incomplete division of the common arterial trunk during embryonic development.
- May be difficult to distinguish from PDA (see 📖 Patent ductus arteriosus, p. 352).
- The presence of separate aortic and pulmonary valves distinguishes this condition from CAT.
- Commonly associated with other abnormalities such as VSD, tetralogy of Fallot, ASD, and PDA.
- Symptoms include those of LV failure or pulmonary hypertension depending on direction of shunt and development of Eisenmenger's physiology.

Role of cardiac CT

- Assessment of location and size of the aortopulmonary (AP) window (Fig. 23.11).
- This may be useful if planning percutaneous closure as the superior and inferior rims of the defect may be assessed for adequacy to support an occlusion device.
- Associated lesions such as atrial and ventricular septal defects may be also evaluated from the same acquisition.

Coarctation of the aorta (see 📖 **Coarctation of the aorta,** p. 406)

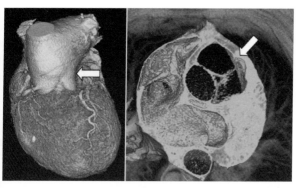

Fig. 23.10 Truncus arteriosus (left, arrow) and truncal valve (arrow, right).

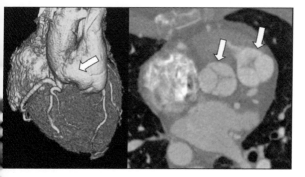

Fig. 23.11 Aortopulmonary window (left, arrow). Note the presence of separate aortic and pulmonary valves (arrows) that distinguishes this condition from truncus arteriosus.

Transposition of the great arteries

Complete transposition of the great arteries (TGA) accounts for ~5% of all CHD (~80% male). There is AV concordance but VA discordance, such that the morphological right and left ventricles support systemic and pulmonary circulations in closed circuits rather than in series.

Treatment is directed at returning blood to the correct sides of the circulation. Historically, patients were corrected surgically using interatrial approaches known eponymously as the Mustard and Senning repairs. Although rarely performed now, many survive into adulthood. The current surgical technique of choice is the arterial switch operation (also known as the Jatene procedure).

Interatrial repair

Atrial blood is 'baffled' via an AV channel to the contralateral ventricle such that the morphological left and right ventricles receive systemic and pulmonary venous blood, respectively, and return it to the physiologically correct destinations (i.e. the lungs and body, respectively). As VA discordance is maintained, the right ventricle continues to support the systemic circulation and is ∴ susceptible to failure.

The Mustard and Senning repairs are similar except that the former uses pericardium or prosthetic material to create the AV channel whilst the latter uses the septum and atrial wall.

Arterial switch

VA discordance is corrected by removing the aorta and pulmonary arteries and reattaching them to the (anatomically correct) contralateral ventricles. The coronary arteries are also removed and reimplanted into the neo-aorta. This operation is advantageous as it results in support of the systemic circulation by the left ventricle. Common complications involve stenosis or regurgitation at the sites of anastomosis, with the former particularly important in the case of reimplanted coronary arteries. There is also risk of early atherosclerosis.

Rastelli procedure

For patients with TGA, a large subaortic VSD, and pulmonary stenosis physiological correction of blood flow may be achieved by closing the VSD to redirect LV blood to the aorta, ligating the pulmonary artery and creating a conduit between the right ventricle and the PA. Again, the LV supports the systemic circulation. Conduit stenosis/regurgitation is common.

Role of cardiac CT

- Untreated, death occurs after closure of the ductus arteriosus and formen ovale, ∴ patients with TGA are usually evaluated after operative repair (Figs 23.12a and 23.13).
- CCT can help to assess the patency of intra-atrial baffles (Mustard and Senning procedures), VA conduits (Rastelli procedure), or the neo-aorta and neo-pulmonary arteries (arterial switch).

- Following arterial switching, the ostia of re-implanted coronary arteries may be readily assessed. Evidence of early atherosclerosis may also be detected.
- Precise knowledge of coronary anatomy is required prior to surgery and CCT is ideally suited to their non-invasive assessment.

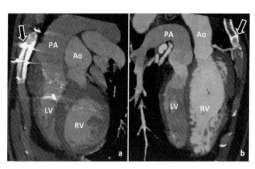

Fig. 23.12 (a) TGA. The morphological right ventricle (RV) is in the systemic postion and supplies the aorta (Ao). The morpholocial left ventricle (LV) is subpulmonary (PA). There is ∴ VA discordance. (b) Congenitally corrected transposition of the great arteries (ccTGA). Note the absence of sternal wires in this patient (outline arrows, a and b) implying ccTGA: all patients without congenital correction require operative repair.

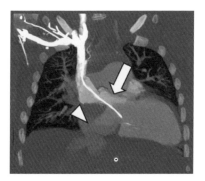

Fig. 23.13 Mustard repair for TGA. Flow from the superior (arrow) and inferior (arrowhead) venae cavae is directed to the sub-pulmonary ventricle. Note the pacemaker lead traversing the SVC channel which precludes CMR.

Congenitally corrected transposition of the great arteries

Background
- Rare—<1% of all CHD.
- Discordant AV and VA connections.
- The morphological left and right ventricles support the pulmonary and systemic circulations, respectively.
- Although this allows a 'physiologically correct' circulation, it leaves the morphological right ventricle to support the systemic circulation.
- Systemic RV failure is ∴ common, as is tricuspid incompetence.
- Dysrhythmia is also a common complication, particularly in older patients.
- Ninety-five per cent have associated abnormalities (VSD, Ebstein's anomaly (see ☐ Congenital heart disease, p. 331), aortic stenosis, AVSD, coarctation).

Surgical repair
- Usually performed using the 'double switch' operation—a combination of atrial and arterial switching (i.e. arterial switch plus interatrial repair).
- Associated abnormalities may also be repaired (e.g. VSD patch).

Role of cardiac CT
CCT can be useful in confirming AV and VA discordance (Fig. 23.12b) as well as evaluating the state of any anatomic repair and biventricular size and function.

Anomalous pulmonary venous connection

Background

- In the normal heart, four pulmonary veins (PVs) enter the back of the left atrium (NB: normal variants occur, see 📖 Left atrium and pulmonary veins, p. 276).
- ≥1 PVs connecting to the right-sided circulation (usually either right atrium or vena cavae) defines anomalous pulmonary venous connection.
- *Total anomalous pulmonary venous connection* (TAPVC)—all PVs drain into the right-sided circulation.
- *Partial anomalous pulmonary venous connection* (PAPVC)—≥1 PV drains into the LA, others drain into the right-sided circulation.

Total anomalous pulmonary venous connection

- 1 in 17,000 live births.
- Anomalous connections usually form a confluence before connecting into the right-sided circulation. The connection may be:
  - *Supracardiac*—PVs drain into the SVC, azygous, or innominate veins
  - *Cardiac*—PVs drain into the right atrium, coronary sinus, or persistent left superior vena cava (LSVC)
  - *Infracardiac*—PVs drain into the IVC or portal vein.
- As all PVs drain into the right heart, survival is only possible where a R→L shunt exists (usually at the atrial level through an ASD).
- Most present in infancy and are corrected surgically.
- Obstruction of re-implanted PVs may occur, leading to chest infections and ↑ pulmonary vascular resistance.

Partial anomalous pulmonary venous connection

- Commonly associated with ASD (10–15%) and is seen particularly in sinus venosus defects (80–90%) (see 📖 Atrial septal defects, p. 346).
- Wide anatomical variation; the most common are:
  - Right upper lobe (RUL) and right middle lobe (RML) PV to SVC or right atrium
  - Right PVs to IVC
  - Right lower PV to IVC (+ anomalous arterial supply to right lower lobe + hypoplasia of right lung = Scimitar syndrome)
  - Left upper PV to innominate vein (via an ascending vertical vein) or SVC (Fig. 23.14)
  - Left upper or lower PV to coronary sinus.
- Isolated PAPVC often asymptomatic, may be managed conservatively.
- >1 anomalous PV—symptoms are usually similar to ASD and depend on the degree of L→R shunt; pulmonary hypertension may develop.
- Surgical repair confers excellent prognosis.
- Obstruction of re-implanted PVs and, rarely, systemic veins may occur.

Role of cardiac CT

- Anatomical evaluation of course and patency of anomalous PVs, in addition to associated defects.

- Evaluation of biventricular size and function.
- After surgical repair, evaluation of PV anastomoses, systemic veins, and lung fields.

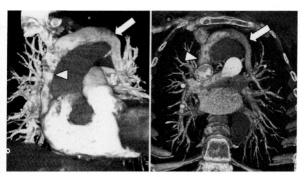

Fig. 23.14 Partial anomalous pulmonary venous connection. Maximum-intensity projection (left) and volume-rendered (right) images showing anomalous connection between the left upper pulmonary vein (arrow) with the SVC (arrowhead). (📖 Plate 8 for colour version).

Major aorto-pulmonary collateral arteries

MAPCAs develop in conditions such as pulmonary atresia when blood fails to reach the lungs via the pulmonary arteries.

- The anatomy of these collateral arteries varies widely, and accurate delineation is crucial to clinical management (Figs 23.15 and 23.16).
- The high spatial resolution and 3D nature of CCT lends itself well to accurate anatomical localization.
- CCT compares well with measurements made by ICA and can ∴ guide interventional or surgical management.

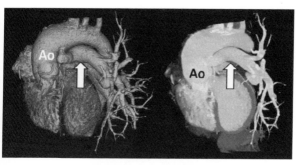

Fig. 23.15 Left pulmonary artery (arrow) arising directly from the aorta (Ao).

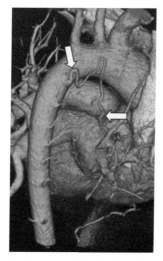

Fig. 23.16 Major aortopulmonary collateral artery in a patient with pulmonary atresia.

Tetralogy of Fallot

Tetralogy of Fallot accounts for around 10% of all CHD. Fifteen per cent have chromosome 22q11 deletion. The condition arises as a result of:

- Anterocephalad deviation of the outlet septum (the muscular structure separating the sub aortic and subpulmonary outlets).
- Hypertrophy of the septoparietal trabeculae (muscular bands in the infundibulum of the RVOT).

The former leads to a VSD and aortic over-ride, whilst both lead to pulmonary stenosis and 2° RV hypertrophy. These four features together constitute the tetralogy (Fig. 23.17).

Wide variation exists in the severity of the lesions, from mild pulmonary stenosis to pulmonary atresia. The degree of aortic over-ride may vary from 5% to 95%. Over-ride of >50% defines a double outlet right ventricle, which may thus coexist with tetralogy of Fallot. The distinction is important as it has implications for surgical repair.

Associated cardiovascular anomalies

- Right-sided aortic arch.
- Persistent left SVC (which usually drains into the coronary sinus).
- Patent foramen ovale.
- Secundum ASD.
- Concomitant muscular VSD or atrioventricular septal defect (AVSD).
- Pre-pulmonary anomalous LAD from right coronary sinus.

Role of cardiac CT

- As effective as TTE for the diagnosis of tetralogy of Fallot. However, CMR remains the modality of choice for the assessment and follow up of adults with repaired tetralogy of Fallot.
- If CMR is unavailable or contraindicated, CCT becomes the assessment of choice for ventricular morphology and function. ⚠ Flow and shunts cannot be assessed.
- Assessment of the coronary and pulmonary arteries, with information on anomalous courses in the former and stenoses in the latter. This is relevant when planning operative repair.
- Measurements of global and regional RV and LV function, RVOT obstruction, conduit, or pulmonary artery stenoses and aortic root size—all contribute to decisions on management, particularly for the timing of pulmonary valve replacement in the presence of PR.
- In patients who have undergone surgical repair, patency, size, and potential stenoses within shunts and valved conduits (Fig. 23.18) is required.
- In those with stenotic or regurgitant valved conduits referred for percutaneous pulmonary valve replacement, assessment of the conduit and its spatial relationship to other structures, particularly anomalous coronary arteries between the conduit and adjacent epicardium is required. Expansion of a stented pulmonary valve within the conduit could lead to compression of an underlying anomalous coronary artery resulting in myocardial ischaemia and, if uncorrected, infarction.

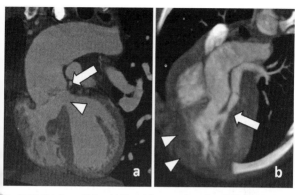

Fig. 23.17 Tetralogy of Fallot. (a) Over-riding aorta (arrow) and VSD (arrowhead). In this projection, the aorta over-rides the septum by >50%, thus defining a double-outlet right ventricle. This may coexist as part of the spectrum of Tetralogy of Fallot. (b) Severe stenosis of the RVOT (arrow) and RV hypertrophy (arrowheads).

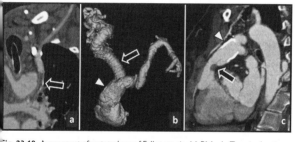

Fig. 23.18 Assessment after tetralogy of Fallot repair. (a) Blalock–Taussig shunt with distal thrombosis (arrow). (b) Calcified RVOT homograft (arrowhead) and conduit to the right pulmonary artery (arrow). (c) MPR image of the same patient as in (b) showing the calcified homograft (arrowhead) and sub-pulmonary stenosis (arrow).

The functionally univentricular heart

- Describes a heart in which there is only one functional ventricle and in which anatomical repair is impossible.
- True single ventricle morphology is rare; obstructions of either systemic or pulmonary outflows with shunting away from the obstructed side, usually at the atrial level, are more common (Fig. 23.19).
- The functional ventricle may have either a morphological LV or RV phenotype and is usually accompanied by a rudimentary non-functional ventricle.
- Common causes include tricuspid or pulmonary atresia, double inlet left ventricle, and hypoplastic left heart syndrome.
- The anatomy of inflow/outflow obstructions and the associated systemic and pulmonary circulations are critical in deciding management.
- CCT is able to identify virtually all causes of both systemic and pulmonary outflow tract obstructions, listed under separate headings here, in addition to allowing evaluation of biventricular function.
- Treatment involves surgical correction by creation of a Fontan-type circulation. CCT may be used to assess the patency of these connections in patients unsuitable for CMR.

Fontan circulation

There are many variations of Fontan circulation. In all forms, the single ventricle supports the systemic circulation whilst systemic venous blood is returned to the pulmonary arteries directly. Pulmonary blood flow relies on:

- High systemic venous pressure
- Low pulmonary vascular resistance.

Frequently, a Fontan-type circulation is created using a staged approach, with the SVC connected to the right pulmonary artery first (Glenn anastomosis, Fig. 23.20a), followed by connection of the IVC at a later date (creating a total cavopulmonary connection, Fig. 23.20b). The classical Fontan operation involves creation of an atriopulmonary connection (e.g. right atrium to PA). However, total cavopulmonary connection, bypassing the right atrium altogether, is now the procedure of choice for palliation of functionally univentricular hearts.

Role of cardiac CT

- Patency of the associated connections and low pulmonary artery pressures are crucial to maintain pulmonary blood flow.
- Connections are readily assessed by CCT, which is especially useful at delineating the complex vascular anatomy using 3D reconstruction techniques.
- From this data, abnormal vessel dimensions, stenoses and post-stenotic dilatation, mural damage (such as dissection or calcification), and *in situ* thrombosis may all be identified.
- Right atrial size and pulmonary venous return may also be readily assessed.

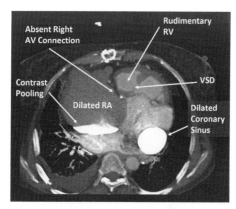

Fig. 23.19 Functionally univentricular heart in a patient with tricuspid atresia. AV, atrioventricular; RV, right ventricle; RA, right atrium; VSD, ventricular septal defect.

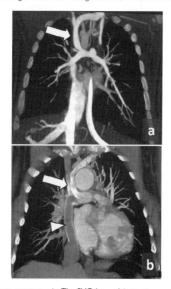

Fig. 23.20 (a) Glenn anastomosis. The SVC (arrow) is anastomosed to the right pulmonary artery. (b) Total cavopulmonary connection. There is direct anastamosis of the SVC with the right pulmonary artery (arrow) whilst the IVC is connected using a conduit (arrowhead). Note that the IVC conduit is unenhanced due to injection of contrast medium via an antecubital vein. To evaluate both limbs of the Fontan circulation, contrast must be injected simultaneously via the upper and lower limbs. Alternatively, imaging may be delayed until contrast has equilibrated throughout the blood pool.

Congenital valve pathology

Aortic valve (see ☐☐ Valve imaging, p. 283)

- CCT accurately identifies bicuspid aortic valve morphology (Fig. 23.21) when compared with TOE, and is potentially more accurate than TTE.
- Aortic valve calcification may be assessed, with moderate to severe calcification correlating well with TTE measurement of stenosis severity (Fig. 23.21).
- Aortic valve area may be measured using planimetry, although, as with coronary assessment, dense calcification may lead to underestimation of valve area.

Mitral valve (see ☐☐ Mitral stenosis, p. 298)

- The mitral valve leaflets may be assessed for thickening and calcification, the latter also being seen in the annulus; these features correlate with the presence of mitral stenosis on TTE.
- Assessment of congenital mitral valve anomalies, such as the parachute-like mitral valve, may also be possible, but data are limited to case reports at present.
- Mitral valve planimetry by CCT correlates well with TTE.
- Retrospective gating (see ☐ ECG gating, p. 34) allows assessment of valve leaflet mobility and coaptation throughout the cardiac cycle.

Right-sided valves (see ☐☐ Tricuspid regurgitation, p. 304)

- Right-sided valve assessment is often more difficult in the normal heart because of poor contrast density in the right heart.
- In patients with ACHD, such as in those with ASD, VSD, or pulmonary hypertension, assessment is more straightforward, as RV contrast is improved as a result of either impaired RV outflow or an abnormal communication between the left and right sides of the circulation.

Ebstein's malformation (see ☐☐ Chapter 21, p. 306)

- Assessment of right atrial and ventricular anatomy allows identification of Ebstein's malformation (Fig. 23.22), along with any coexistent ASD.
- Tricuspid valve displacement and malfunction may be assessed, as may RV function.
- ~50% of adults with Ebstein's malformation have an associated ASD, usually due to distension and gaping of a PFO.
- Functional imaging may show diastolic compression of the left ventricle by the dilated right heart, impairing LV filling and limiting the cardiac output.

Pulmonary valve (see ☐☐ Pulmonary regurgitation, p. 310)

- Free PR, with little or no effective valve function, is common after repair of tetralogy of Fallot (see ☐ Tetralogy of Fallot, p. 364); it may be tolerated without symptoms for decades, but may also lead to RV dysfunction, arrhythmia, and premature death.

Post valve surgery

- Stenosis or regurgitation of replaced valves is common, especially in the case of the RV-PA homograft conduit used in tetralogy of Fallot (see 📖 Tetralogy of Fallot, p. 364) or the Ross procedure (see 📖 Prosthetic valves, p. 315).
- Stenosis may be due to shrinkage of the homograft tube or a suture line, or to stiffening of the valve leaflets.
- After the Ross procedure, autograft valves in the aortic position should be assessed for possible dilatation and regurgitation, particularly beyond 10 years after operation.
- After aortic root replacement and coronary re-implantation, CTA may be indicated to evaluate ostial anastomoses.

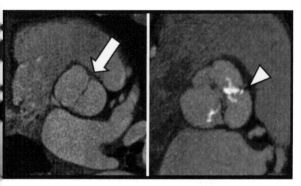

Fig. 23.21 Left: bicuspid aortic valve. Right: calcified bicuspid aortic valve. The left and right coronary cusps are fused and calcified (arrow). Calcium is also seen in the non-coronary cusp.

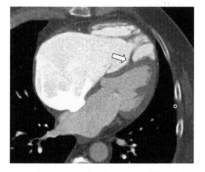

Fig. 23.22 Ebstein's malformation of the tricuspid valve. There is incomplete delamination of the septal leaflet of the tricuspid valve such that its hinge point occurs in the mid septum (arrow).

Non-cardiac findings on cardiac CT

Introduction

In addition to imaging the heart and coronary arteries, most centres use a wide FOV that incorporates a variety of other non-cardiac structures such as the lung parenchyma, mediastinum, upper abdominal structures, pleura, and chest wall. Each of these systems has numerous potential pathologies, some of critical clinical importance and others that require no follow-up.

Most studies suggest incidental non-cardiac findings are present in between 8 and 70% of all cardiac CT studies. Of these, between 5 and 20% are clinically important. Incidental non-cardiac findings include:

- Malignancy (lung, breast, thyroid, liver)
- Lung nodules
- Pleural thickening/calcification
- Mediastinal lymphadenopathy.

The type of cardiac study performed determines the prevalence of non-cardiac pathology detected. This is in part technical and in part due to the population studied with each type of protocol in clinical practice.

- Non-contrast studies (i.e. coronary calcium scoring) have a low detection rate for incidental pathology, partly due to its use as a screening tool in a low-risk population and partly because no contrast is used.
- Standard CT coronary angiography protocols (see 📖 CT coronary angiography, p. 108) aim to maximize contrast in the left coronary circulation and ∴ often result in suboptimal opacification of the pulmonary system and aortic arch. This reduces the likelihood of diagnostic quality images of these areas and caution should be used in coming to firm diagnoses in these areas.
- A triple rule-out protocol (see 📖 The triple rule-out, p. 430) allows assessment of the pulmonary, coronary, and aortic vasculature but comes at the cost of higher doses of both ionizing radiation and iodinated contrast.

The spectrum of potential extracardiac pathology highlights the importance of collaboration between cardiologists and radiologists in this field for both quality and clinical governance purposes.

Lung parenchyma

Lung window settings

CT produces images with a wide dynamic range of contrast definition
In the case of the chest, CT images are viewed three times, with window
settings specific for lung detail (Fig. 24.1), as well as standard soft tissue
mediastinal detail, illustrated in images in the previous chapters. Bone detai
is also important for delineation of the structures that form the thoracic
wall (Fig. 24.2).

Lung anatomy

Lobes

The right lung is divided into upper, middle, and lower lobes whilst the left
lung is divided into upper and lower lobes.

Bronchopulmonary segments

Each lobe is subdivided as follows:

- *Right upper lobe*—apical, anterior, and posterior segments
- *Right middle lobe*—lateral and medial segments
- *Right lower lobe*—superior, anterior basal, medial basal, posterior basal,
  and lateral basal segments
- *Left upper lobe*—apicoposterior and anterior segments; the lingula is
  divided into superior and inferior segments, and is really considered
  part of the left upper lobe
- *Left lower lobe*—superior, anterior basal, posterior basal, and lateral
  basal segments.

Fissures

- Consist of a double layer of enfolded visceral pleura.
- In the right lung there is an oblique fissure and horizontal fissure.
- The major/oblique fissure separates the middle and lower lobes on the
  right and runs from the level of the T3 vertebra posteriorly to the 6th
  costochondral junction anteriorly.
- The minor/horizontal fissure runs forward and laterally in a horizontal
  direction from the right hilum and separates the anterior segment of
  the right upper lobe from right middle lobe.
- In the left lung, there is an oblique fissure only, which separates the
  upper and lower lobes.

Lung parenchyma

The 2° pulmonary lobule (SPL) is the smallest radiologically visible uni
of the lung and is the basis for the morphological framework of the lung
The borders consist of interlobular septa. Centrally, it consists of a lobula
bronchiole and its accompanying pulmonary artery. Lymphatics cours
along the interlobular septa, the central bronchovascular bundle, and i
the pleura.

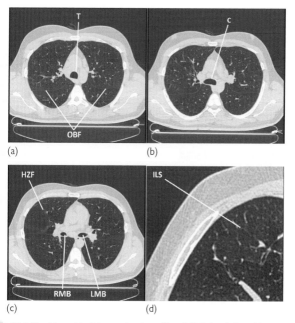

Fig 24.1 Caudal-cranial axial reconstructions of lung field (using dedicated lung window settings). T, trachea ; OBF, oblique fissures ; C, carina ; HZF, horizontal fissure ; RMB, right main bronchus; LMB, left main bronchus; ILS, inter-lobular septum.

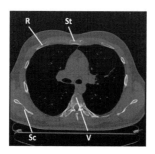

Fig. 24.2 Caudal-cranial axial reconstruction of skeletal structures (bone windows). St, sternum; R, rib; Sc, scapula; V, vertebral body.

Lung nodules

Non-calcified pulmonary nodules are the most common non-cardiac finding on CCT. Two critical components are required when assessing pulmonary nodules; the nodule appearance and the patient risk factors.

Nodule appearance

Assess size

- Increasing malignancy risk with increasing size.
- Almost all lesions >3cm are malignant whereas almost all <5mm are benign.

Assess density

- There are several patterns of density and calcification that increase the likelihood that a mass is benign.
- Lesions can be classified as *solid*, *part-solid*, or *ground glass*:
  - *Solid* nodules completely obscure underlying tissue.
  - *Part solid* nodules contain both solid and ground glass components.
  - *Ground glass* describes hazy, ↑ opacification; nodules diplaying this appearance are more likely to be malignant (i.e. adenocarcinoma or broncheoalveolar cell carcinoma (BAC)).
- If a lesion is of predominantly fat density (<−50HU), it is most likely to be a hamartoma.
- Calcification is usually associated with benign lesions, and patterns that confer a greater likelihood of benign character include lamellar, central (likely calcified granulomas, usually from old TB) or popcorn calcification (hamartoma).
- Be suspicious of eccentric calcification, which can occur in 1° lung carcinomas.
- Cavitating lesions are more likely to be benign if <5mm but more likely to be malignant if >15mm.

Assess location

- There are several well recognized locations for certain types of lesion.
- 6–9mm triangular or ovoid nodules abutting the pleura usually represent intrapulmonary lymph nodes.
- Multiple clustered nodules (>7) increase the likelihood of an infective aetiology.
- 1° lung carcinomas are more prevalent in the upper lobes.
- Pulmonary metastases are usually multiple, of various sizes, and most common in the lung bases.

Assess border

- Most 1° lung malignancies have spiculated or irregular borders.
- Pulmonary metastases are usually smooth edged.
- Small smooth nodules usually require no follow-up.

Management of lung nodules

Fleischner Society guidelines[1] on appropriate investigation and follow-up of incidental lung nodules are shown in Table 24.1.

Table 24.1 Fleischner Society guidelines for the management of incidental lung nodules in patients >35 years of age.[1] Nodule size is determined by the average of length and width. Patients are high risk if they have a history of smoking or other risk factors for bronchial carcinoma such family history in a first-degree relative or exposure to asbestos.

Nodule size	Low-risk patient	High-risk patient
≤4mm	No follow-up	Follow-up at 12 months If no change no further follow up
4–6mm	Follow-up at 12 months If no change no further follow-up	Follow-up at 6–12 months Then 18–24 months if no change
>6–8mm	Follow-up at 6–12 months Then 18–24 months if no change	Follow-up at 3 and 9 months Then 18–24 months if no change
>8mm	Follow-up at 3, 9, and 24 months Consider PET, biopsy, or both	Follow-up at 3, 9, and 24 months Consider PET, biopsy, or both

Further reading

1 MacMahon H, Austin JHM, Gamsu G, et al. (2005) Guidelines for Management of Small Pulmonary Nodules Detected on CT Scans: A Statement from the Fleischner Society. *Radiology* **237**, 395–400.

Parenchymal lung disease

Many aetiologies underlie parenchymal lung disease.
- The most common is multifocal pneumonia, which is usually caused by *Streptococcus pneumoniae*, *Haemophilus influenzae* and *Mycoplasma pneumoniae*.
- Pulmonary oedema and pulmonary haemorrhage can also cause diffuse consolidation.

Idiopathic pulmonary fibrosis is the most common cause of fibrotic lung disease and is often associated with progressively worsening dyspnoea.
- Fibrotic lung disease is characterized by ground-glass attenuation (hazy ↑ attenuation without obscuration of the underlying bronchial or vascular strutures), linear and reticular opacities, and smooth thickening of interlobular septae.
- Irregular peribronchial and perivascular interstitial thickening may be seen in pulmonary fibrosis.
- Other causes of similar CT patters include sarcoidosis (usually with smooth peribronchial interstial thickening and egg shell calcification of mediatinal lymph nodes), collagen vascular diseases, and fibrosing alveolitis.

Emphysema is a common incidental finding on CCT studies (~10%).
- Centrilobular emphysema is the most common subtype and is associated with cigarette smoking.
- It usually affects the apical and posterior upper lobes and superior segments of the lower lobes.
- There is marked loss of lung parenchyma (Fig. 24.3) in the centre of the 2° pulmonary lobule surrounding the bronchovascular bundle.
- Panacinar emphysema affects the lower lobes predominantly and is associated with α-1 anti-trypsin deficiency.
- Patients with coexistent pulmonary nodules have a higher malignancy risk than those without emphysema.

Bronchiectasis is irreversible localized or diffuse bronchial dilatation usually as a result of chronic or recurrent infection, proximal airway obstruction, or congenital bronchial malformation.
- It is diagnosed on CCT when the bronchial lumen diameter exceeds the accompanying pulmonary artery diameter (signet-ring sign) (Fig. 24.4).
- Additional features on CT include bronchi within 1cm of the pleura and uniformity of distal caliber bronchi (i.e. no bronchial tapering).

Other important pathologies in patients presenting with chest pain are pulmonary embolus (see 📖 Pulmonary artery imaging, p. 420) and aortic dissection (see 📖 Aortic dissection, p. 402).

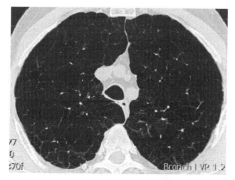

Fig. 24.3 Widespread loss of lung parenchyma characteristic of emphysema.

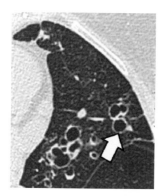

Fig. 24.4 Bronchiectasis. The peripheral airway diameter exceeds that of the accompanying arterial vessel (arrow).

Mediastinal anatomy

- The mediastinum is the space in the thorax that lies between the pleural cavities and is arbitrarily divided into superior and inferior compartments by a line extending from the manubriosternal joint to the lower border of the T4 vertebrae trachea (Fig. 24.5).
- This plane passes through the tracheal bifurcation, just above the main pulmonary artery bifurcation and just under the aortic arch.
- Superior mediastinum contains the aortic arch and adjacent structures.
- Inferior mediastinum—divided into anterior, middle, and posterior compartments by the fibrous pericardium. Anterior and posterior compartments are anatomically continuous with the superior mediastinum.
- The major components of the inferior mediastinum are:
  - Anterior—thymus, lymph nodes, and internal thoracic vessels
  - Middle—heart, pericardium, adjoining great vessels, lung roots, and lymph nodes
  - Posterior—oesophagus, descending aorta, azygous vein, thoracic duct, and lymph nodes.

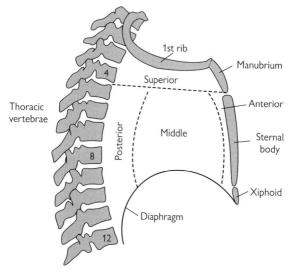

Fig. 24.5 Divisions of the mediastinum.

Mediastinal pathology

Introduction

- Incidental mediastinal pathologies include diseases such as aortic aneurysms (see 📖 Aortic aneurysms and dilatation, p. 400), penetrating ulcers, and intramural haematomas (see 📖 Aortic intramural haematoma, p. 404).
- Soft tissue mediastinal masses are usually due to nodal enlargement or thymic, thyroid, or germ cell tumours.
- Cardiac and pericardial pathology will usually be encountered in patients who have been found to have an abnormality on echocardiography.

Approach to interpretation and tissue characterization

The 1° aim is to determine whether a mass is benign or malignant, 1° or 2°. Correct diagnosis is based on presentation, anatomical localisation, morphology, and probability.

Presentation

- Age—differential diagnoses vary between adults and children.
- An incidental asymptomatic lesion is likely benign.
- Symptomatic disease suggests a more aggressive/malignant nature.
- Those with a known 1° malignancy or multiple lesions in different locations have a high chance of metastatic disease.

Anatomical location

- Location within a particular mediastinal compartment allows narrowing of the differential diagnosis (see 📖 Differential diagnosis of mediastinal tumours and masses, p. 384).

Morphology

- The CT number (see 📖 Reconstruction of the CT image, p. 136) may be helpful in distinguishing different tissue types (Table 24.2).
- For example, a mass in the inferior portion of the anterior mediastinum that has a density similar to fat is most likely to represent a pericardial fat pad.

Probability

- Seventy per cent of 1° cardiac tumours are benign. Of these myxomas (adults) or rhabdomyomas (paediatric) are the most likely.
- Most anterior mediastinal masses in children are due to Hodgkin's disease.
- 15% of patients with myasthenia gravis have thymoma.

Table 24.2 Attenuation values of different tissue types

Tissue	HU
Fat	<−50
Pure water	0
Unenhanced soft tissue	+40 to 60
Contrast	>+100
Calcium	>+100

Differential diagnosis of mediastinal tumours and masses

Anterior mediastinal masses

Superior portion
- Retrosternal goitre—confluent with thyroid (Fig. 24.6).
- Tortuous brachiocephalic artery,
- Lymphadenopathy (see 📖 Patterns of mediastinal lymphadenopathy, p. 388).
- Thymic tumours (Fig. 24.7):
  - Normal thymus—usually small and arrowhead in shape; fatty involution after age 30 years
  - Lobulation/focal distortion of contour suggests pathological
  - Thymoma may contain calcium (Fig. 24.7)
  - Thymolipoma—often large
  - Thymic carcinoma—spreads along pleura, although effusion uncommon.
  - Other tumours include thymic carcinoid and thymic lymphoma
- Ascending aortic aneurysm.

Mid-portion
- Germ cell tumours:
  - Most are teratomas and most are benign
  - Contain multiple cell lines—calcium, fat, cyst, soft tissue
  - Others—seminoma, embryonal cell carcinoma, choriocarcinoma.
- Thymic tumours.
- Metastases—lung, breast are common.

Inferior portion
- Pericardial fat pad.
- Morgagni hernia.
- Pericardial cyst.

Other causes in children
- Normal thymus.
- Cystic hygroma.
- Morgagni hernia.
- Tumours:
  - Hodgkin's and non-Hodgkins lymphoma, leukaemia
  - Germ cell tumours—as above
  - Thymic tumours.

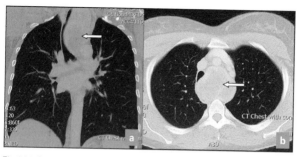

Fig. 24.6 Superior mediastinal mass. (a) Large retrosternal thyroid goitre (white arrow) that is compressing the trachea and causing tracheal deviation to the right. (b) Inferior extent of the goitre behind the ascending aorta.

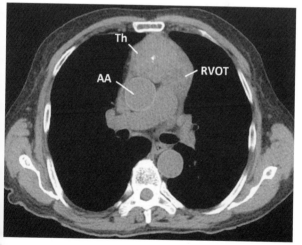

Fig. 24.7 Anterior mediastinal mass. A thymoma (Th) with central calcification anterior to the ascending aorta (AA) and adjacent to the right ventricular outflow tract (RVOT).

- Lymphadenopathy.

Middle mediastinal masses

- Masses arising from the heart and pericardium are listed elsewhere.
- Lymphadenopathy.
- Bronchial carcinoma.
- Aortic aneurysm.
- Bronchogenic cyst.

Other causes in children

- Any anterior mediastinal tumour may extend into the middle mediastinum.
- Foregut duplication cysts (Fig. 24.8).
- Cystic hygroma.
- Hiatus hernia.
- Oesophageal dilatation.

Posterior mediastinal masses

If associated with the spine

- Metastases, myeloma, lymphoma—there are often bony abnormalities but with preservation of the discs.
- Extramedullary haemopoiesis—haemolytic anaemias.
- Paravertebral abscess—bone and disc space destruction.
- Ganglioneuroma.

Otherwise

- Oesophageal dilatation.
- Aortic aneurysm.
- Hiatus hernia.

Other causes in children

- Bochdalek hernia—usually presents neonatally with respiratory distress.
- Ganglion cell tumours:
  - Neuroblastoma—most malignant, age <5 years
  - Ganglioneuroblastoma—age 5–10 years
  - Ganglioneuroma—benign, usually >10 years
  - All have similar imaging appearances
  - 90% calcify
  - Look for extradural extension.

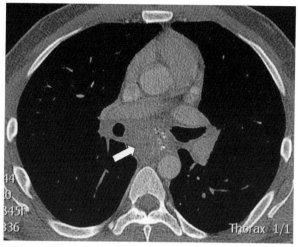

Fig. 24.8 Posterior mediastinal mass. A foregut duplication cyst in the azygo-oesophageal recess (arrow).

Patterns of mediastinal lymphadenopathy

Introduction

- Normal lymph nodes (LN) are smooth and either ovoid or triangular in shape.
- The normal size of a LN is variable and dependent on its location. However, a LN >10mm in its shortest dimension is likely to be abnormal.
- Attention should be paid to both the internal mammary and diaphragmatic LN, which drain the breast and chest wall, respectively, as these are often overlooked.
- Pericardial recesses (see 🔲 The pericardium, p. 320) should be distinguished from LNs.

Unilateral hilar lymphadenoapthy

- Should be considered to be due to bronchial carcinoma until proven otherwise.
- Other causes are rare:
  - Infective (TB, mycoplasma)
  - Lymphoma and sarcoidosis occasionally cause unilateral hilar lymphadenoapthy; bilateral involvement is much more common.

Bilateral hilar lymphadenoapthy

- Sarcoidosis and lymphoma are the most common causes.
- Viral infection may lead to reactive lymphadenopathy; nodes are usually low volume and return to normal after resolution of infection.
- Other causes include TB (rarely bilateral), histoplasmosis, fungal infection, and silicosis.

Patterns of attenuation

- Low attenuation LN should be taken seriously as they may be malignant and represent central necrosis.
- Causes of low attenuation LN include local malignancy (if necrotic, may be aggressive), lymphoma, TB, fungi, or metastases from renal, thyroid, melanoma, small cell carcinomas.
- Calcified lymph nodes (Fig. 24.9) are commonly caused by silicosis, sarcoidosis, and as a delayed effect of radiotherapy for lymphoma.

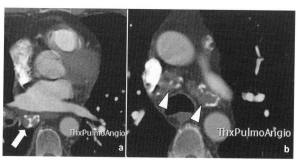

Fig. 24.9 (a) Enlarged azygo-oesophageal lymph node with central calcification consistent with previous tuberculosis. (b) Two middle mediastinal lymph nodes with eccentric (or egg-shell) calcification in a patient with sarcoidosis.

Chest wall and pleural pathology

Breast tissue is often included in cardiac CT studies and is often overlooked during reporting.

- ~1% of CCT will show an abnormality of breast tissue.
- Up to 50% of these abnormalities may be malignant.
- CT cannot detect microcalcification; soft tissue lesions with irregular shape and border and rim enhancement should raise the suspicion of breast malignancy.
- All patients with breast pathology should be referred for a specialist opinion and further investigation.

Pleural effusions are the most common pleural pathology identified on CCT studies.

- The most common cause is left heart failure and they are transudative effusions.
- Pleural effusions usually have a low attenuation (0–20HU).
- It is necessary to distinguish pleural effusions from ascites.

Solid pleural pathology includes pleural plaques following asbestos exposure, mesothelioma, or metastatic disease from adenocarcinoma or lymphoma.

Upper abdominal pathology

Abdominal viscera included in the CCT study include the upper liver, oesophagus, and descending thoracic and upper abdominal aorta.

The most common incidental liver lesions seen are *simple liver cysts* (Fig. 24.10).

- Present in ~5% of the general population.
- CCT appearances: well-defined, homogeneous low-density lesions that do not communicate with the biliary tree.
- Asymptomatic unless extremely large.
- Rarer causes include hydatid disease, polycystic liver or kidney disease, or cystic tumours (these usually have thicker walls and are often more heterogenous in nature).
- Ultrasound may be recommended to confirm a cystic nature with smaller or atypical lesions.

Haemangiomas are also a common incidental finding, classically showing nodular filling in at the periphery during the venous portal phase of imaging. Ultrasound may be recommended for confirmation of typical appearances.

Liver metastases

- The liver is the second most common site for metastases after the lungs.
- Common primaries include lung, breast, colon, pancreas, and stomach.
- Liver metastases on CCT are usually low soft tissue density and require the usual work-up employed for incidental solid liver lesions.

Hiatus hernias (Fig. 24.11) are also a common finding on CCT studies and are present in 10% of the population.

- Incidence increases with age.
- May be an alternative cause of epigastric and retrosternal chest pain in patients with no flow-limiting coronary disease.
- No follow-up is required for hiatus hernia.

Conclusions

Extracardiac structures within the standard CCT FOV should be scrutinized as a matter of routine. There are both medico-legal and moral obligations to ensure that the whole FOV is interpreted to the highest standards. The prevalence of pathology is determined by both the scan protocol and patient population under investigation.

Analysis of extracardiac structures should be systematic and may allow diagnosis of alternative causes for symptoms or important co-morbidities.

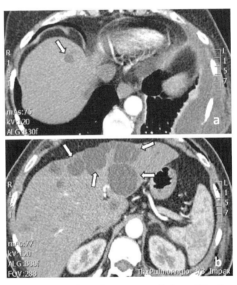

Fig. 24.10 Simple liver cysts (arrows) are a common finding on CT and may be (a) single or (b) multiple.

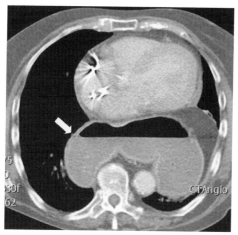

Fig. 24.11 A very large hiatus hernia (arrow) with fluid level within the stomach.

Thoracic aortic imaging

Normal anatomy of the thoracic aorta

The type of imaging performed on the thoracic aorta is usually dependent on the clinical presentation, local clinical practice, and availability of imaging techniques. Cardiovascular CT remains the gold standard for aortic assessment, but increasingly cardiac MRI angiography is used, particularly in patients who are young and require serial follow-up. Other standard cardiac imaging procedures are also used in the assessment of aortic pathology, including the PA chest radiograph, TTE, and TOE. Invasive aortography is occasionally also used.

Normal anatomy (Fig. 25.1)

- *Ascending aorta*—extends from the aortic valve to the first branch of the arch, the innominate (brachiocephalic) artery.
- *Aortic root*—proximal portion of the aorta.
- *Aortic arch*—commences at the innominate artery and ends at the ligamentum arteriosum; the most distal aspect of the arch is often slightly narrowed.
- *Descending thoracic aorta*—commences at the ligamentum arteriosum and extends to the diaphragmatic hiatus.

In the majority (70%) of individuals, three major arterial branches arise from the superior surface of the arch of the aorta:
- Innominate (brachiocephalic) artery
- Left common carotid artery
- Left subclavian artery.

The right subclavian artery and right common carotid arteries arise as terminal branches of the right innominate artery. The left and right vertebral arteries arise from the respective subclavian arteries.

The next most common variation of branching is a combined origin of the innominate artery and left common carotid artery. A number of additional variations are also quite commonly encountered.

The usual diameter of the ascending aorta internally is 35mm in females and 38mm in males. There is a linear association of increasing diameter with increasing age. The aorta tapers distally and the descending aorta, in a normal individual, is always smaller in calibre than the ascending aorta. The abdominal aorta is considered normal if less than 20mm in diameter.

Development of the aorta

To recognize normal variant anatomy and the pathology of the aorta, it is useful to understand basic aortic embryology according to a hypothetical double arch system.
- In utero, there is both a right- and left-sided aortic arch, each with a potential ductus arteriosus.
- Normal anatomy results from disruption of the hypothetical right arch distal to the right subclavian artery.
- The right subclavian and carotid artery fuse to form the right brachiocephalic artery.
- The proximal portion of the hypothetical right arch is incorporated into the left arch.
- This results in the normal left-sided aortic arch.

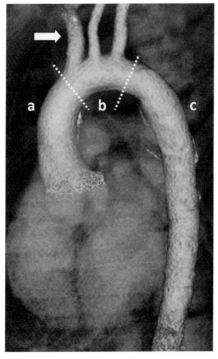

Fig. 25.1 Volume-rendered image of the normal ascending aorta (a), arch (b), and descending aorta (c). The main head and neck vessels (arrow) are, from left to right, the brachiocephalic, left common carotid, and left subclavian arteries.

CT angiography
- Aortic imaging is ideally performed on MSCT scanners, with ECG gating and dose modulation.
- The scan should be extended to include femoral arteries if aortic pathology extends below the diaphragm or there is suspicion of intra-abdominal pathology (e.g. trauma).
- Initial scanning will be in the arterial phase, with delayed phases in certain clinical scenarios.
- Aortography may be performed as part of a double or triple rule-out protocol (see 📖 The triple rule-out, p. 430).

Indications for aortic CT imaging
- Co•genital pathology, e.g. coarctation, interupted aortic arch, right-sided or double arch.
- Acute chest pain—often as part of triple rule-out of CAD, aortic dissection, and pulmonary embolism.
- Chronic pathology, including follow-up.
- Trauma.
- Pre operative—to access anatomy and plan operative approach.
- Assessment prior to percutaneous procedures, e.g. percutaneous aorta vale replacement.

Aortic aneurysms and dilatation

An aortic aneurysm is defined as an irreversible dilatation of the aorta to at least twice normal size. In the dilated segment, all layers of the aortic wall must be affected. Aortic size is age-related and age should be taken into account when assessing aortic dimensions.

Causes of aortic dilatation

- Degenerative disease.
- Connective tissue disease (Marfans syndrome, Ehlers-Danlos).
- Trauma.
- Aortitis (infective, i.e. syphilitic or bacterial, and inflammatory).
- Post surgical.
- Post stenotic (i.e. aortic stenosis).
- False or pseudo-aneurysms represent saccular dilatation that does not include the intimal layer, and are usually associated with previous surgery, infection, trauma, or, less commonly, penetrating ulcers.

Features on contrast-enhanced CCT (Fig. 25.2)

- Site of dilatation, diameter, and length.
- Perianeurysmal thickening and haemorrhage.
- Intraluminal thrombus.
- Displacement or erosion of adjacent structures.
- Involvement of the major branches.
- Extent of mural calcification and thrombus (important in surgical clamping).

The morphological appearance of aneurysms of the ascending aorta and arch are usually predictable based on the underlying aetiology.

- Cystic medial necrosis (such as is seen in Marfan's syndrome) results in aneurysmal involvement of the sinuses of Valsalva, with smooth tapering into a normal arch; these aneurysms result in a classically tulip- (or pear-) shaped aorta.
- Atherosclerotic aneurysms or post-stenotic dilatation in longstanding aortic valve disease usually spare the sinuses but extend into the transverse arch.

Treatment and follow-up

- The most serious complication is rupture, which is almost invariably fatal.
- Absolute size as well as speed of dilatation and aetiology are all important determinants of risk of rupture; serial CT allows prompt surgical decision-making in cases of rapid enlargement.
- Most centres treat aggressively with β-blockers at 4.5–5.0cm, and repair ascending aortic aneurysms at 5.0–5.5cm.
- Descending thoracic aortic aneurysms may be treated conservatively until 6.0–6.5cm; patients with significant co-morbidity are increasingly treated with percutanous stents.

CT can be used to follow the evolution of aneurysms, although careful consideration is required with regard to repeated exposure to ionizing radiation and intravenous contrast agents.

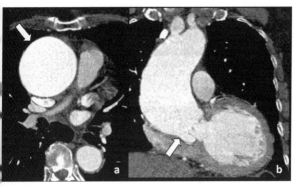

Fig. 25.2 Massive dilatation of ascending aorta (a, arrow) with effacement of the sinotubular junction (b, arrow).

Aortic dissection

Introduction

Aortic dissection has a high mortality rate and clinically may be difficult to distinguish from acute myocardial infarction or pulmonary embolism if presenting acutely. However, aortic dissection may also present insidiously and may be picked up incidentally as a widened mediastinum on plain PA chest radiography.

Aortic dissection involves a separation (dissection) of the aortic media by infiltrating blood, associated with an intimal tear. The tracking of blood between the medial layers distinguishes it from an aortic intramural haematoma. The false lumen may extend proximally or distally and potentially may re-enter the true lumen distal to the intial intimal tear.

Several conditions predispose to aortic dissection:
- Hypertension
- Those that predispose to dilatation and aneurysm formation (see 📖 Aortic aneurysms and dilatation, p. 400)
- Atherosclerotic disease causing a penetrating ulcer
- Iatrogenic causes, including aortic cross-clamping in cardiothoracic surgery, coronary catheterization, and IABP placement.

Classification of aortic dissection

Acute vs chronic dissection
- Acute (<2 weeks old) has a much higher mortality (75% vs 25%).
- Prognostically useful classification.

Anatomical extent of thoracic aortic involvement. (Fig. 25.3)
- Debakey classification.
- Stanford classification.

Acute proximal dissections (Stanford Type A, Debakey Type I and II) are most common (75% of all cases) and have a high mortality rate.
- May extend into the coronary arteries or aortic root (causing severe aortic regurgitation).
- Rupture into the pericardium causes effusion and tamponade, or haemothorax if into the pleural space.
- Usually diagnosed on TOE at the bedside, although this may not always be available.

Chronic proximal dissections usually result from cystic medial necrosis. Both acute and chronic proximal dissections should be surgically repaired as soon as possible.

Distal aortic dissections (Stanford Type B, Debakey Type III) originate, by definition, distal to the left subclavian artery.
- Acutely, these are treated medically with aggressive blood pressure control (aiming for <100mmHg systolic if tolerated),
- Surgical intervention may be indicated in cases of rupture, end-organ ischaemia, progression of dissection, or severe pain,
- Chronic dissections may require surgery if symptomatic or if associated with aneurysmal dilatation ≥5cm or >1cm increase in any one year.

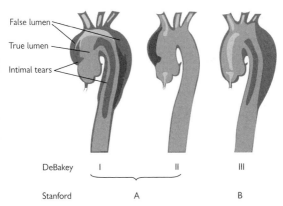

False lumen

True lumen

Intimal tears

DeBakey   I   II   III

Stanford   A   B

Fig. 25.3 Classifications of aortic dissection.

CCT imaging of aortic dissection

CCT is a robust and reliable way of confirming or excluding aortic dissection. Caution should be used when evaluating the aortic root as motion artefact may mimic aortic dissection. Gated studies may be more accurate when root assessment is required.

- Unenhanced scans are useful for detecting blood in the aortic wall (dissection or intramural haematoma [IMH]).
- Displaced intimal calcification may also be seen, but does not distingish between acute and chronic aetiology.
- Contrast enhancement allows diagnosis of dissection by identification of two separate lumens separated by an intimal flap (Fig. 25.4).
- Supporting findings include:
  - Differential flow between lumens
  - Compression or irregularity of the true lumen
  - Aortic dilatation
  - Pericardial effusion.
- The most specific marker of a false lumen is strands of media giving the appearance of 'cobwebs'.
- The false lumen is often larger, although this marker is less specific.

Full assessment of dissection involves:
- Assessment of the type
- Distinguishing between the true and false lumens
- Identification of the intimal tear and entry point
- Identification of an exit point if present
- Measurement and description of aortic dilatation
- Identification of involvement of major branches.

Aortic intramural haematoma

Aortic IMH may be thought of as a subset of aortic dissection, accounting for ~25% of cases. It is caused by localized haemorrhage into the aortic medial layer, probably as a result of rupture of the vasa vasorum. In pure IMH there is no intimal flap, although progression to full dissection may occur.

- Similar risk factors and clinical presentation to aortic dissection.
- Poorly defined aetiology.
- Significant imaging overlap between IMH and aortic dissection.
- Non-contrast studies demonstrate a low attenuation crescentic defect within the aortic wall, with higher attenuation than blood.
- The haematoma does not enhance following administration of contrast unless progression to dissection has occurred.

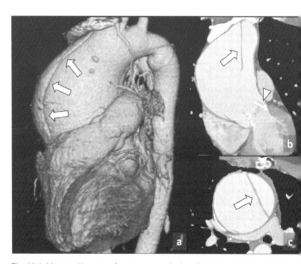

Fig. 25.4 Massive dilatation of aortic root with clear dissection (a and b, arrows) in a patient with previous aortic valve and root repair (b, arrowhead). Cross-sectional imaging clearly demonstrates the dissection flap and double lumen (c, arrow); differentiation between the true and false lumen may be difficult.

Coarctation of the aorta

Background
- Localized narrowing of an aortic segment due to medial and intimal thickening.
- Uncertain aetiology.
- ~8% of all CHD; M:F 3:1.
- Most commonly affects the aorta in the vicinity of the ductus arteriosus (juxta-ductal).
- May be defined in relation to the duct:
  - Proximal to duct (pre-ductal)
  - At the level of the duct (ductal)
  - Distal to duct (post-ductal)
- May present rarely in the distal thoracic or abdominal aorta.
- ~80% have bicuspid aortic valve.
- Other associated anomalies—patent ductus arteriosus (see 📖 Patent ductus arteriosus, p. 352), ventricular septal defect (see 📖 Ventricular septal defects, p. 348), mitral valve abnormalities.
- Unoperated outlook is poor—most die by 50 years of age due to premature CAD, stroke, or aortic dissection.

Role of cardiac CT
- CCT allows accurate determination of the location and extent of aortic coarctation as well as evaluation of post-stenotic dilatation and collateralization.
- Compares well with assessment by TTE.
- Although CMR offers information about flow through the coarctation, the aorta in such patients may be tortuous and it can be difficult to ensure that the correct imaging planes are selected.
- The isotropic nature of voxels acquired using CCT allows the selection of any desired imaging plane after acquisition has been completed.
- In this regard CCT may be particularly useful in isthmic coarctation.
- CCT is superior to both CMR and TTE in the assessment of stent patency after percutaneous treatment, and can be a valuable tool in both the diagnosis and follow-up of these patients.

If detected in an adult, assessment of aortic coarctation should include:
- Degree of stenosis
- Associated findings, e.g. bicuspid aortic valve
- Collateral circulation (Fig. 25.5)
- LV hypertrophy.

Follow up of treated coarctation is required to look for evidence of rest enosis. Whilst this is probably best performed by CMR, CCT may have role in patients with previous stents (Fig. 25.6) or other metallic device that preclude CMR.

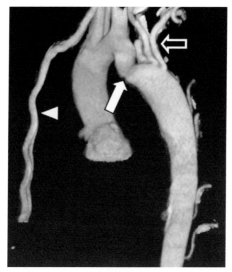

Fig. 25.5 Unrepaired coarctation of the aorta (white arrow). Note the dilated collateral arteries (outline arrow), including the internal mammary arteries (arrowhead).

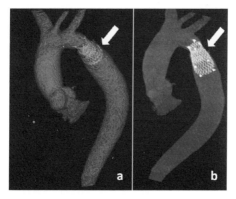

Fig. 25.6 (a) Volume-rendered image of a stented coarctation. (b) Thick MIP images allow assessment of stent deployment; the aortic lumen may be assessed using curved MPR images. (□ Plate 9 for colour version).

Other congenital aortic abnormalities

Double aortic arch
- Persistence of both aortic arches can form a vascular ring compressing the trachea and causing respiratory symptoms (Fig. 25.7).
- Right arch usually dominant, with the left dominant in around 25% and codominance in 5%.
- Patients with symptoms require surgical correction.

Left-sided aortic arch anomalies
- Most commonly associated with aberrant right subclavian artery (0.5% studies) and dilatation at right subclavian artery origin (Kommerell diverticulum).
- True right subclavian artery dilatation requires surgical intervention.

Right-sided aortic arch anomalies
- Associated with aberrant left subclavian artery.

Right aortic arch with mirror image branching
- Associated with concomitant CHD.

Interrupted aortic arch
- Usually occurs at one of three sites:
  - Distal to origin of left subclavian artery
  - Between left common carotid and left subclavian artery
  - Between innominate and left common carotid artery.
- Often associated with a large patent arterial duct supplying the descending aorta.

Aortitis

Takayasus's vascultis is the most common cause of aortitis and usually affects young Asian females.

- It may affect the aortic arch and accompanying vessels, the thoraco-abdominal aorta and its branches, and the pulmonary arteries.
- Mural thickening usually affects the tunica media and adventitia layers.
- Aortitis can cause stenoses, occlusion, dilatation, and aneuysm formation, which commonly coexist in the same patient.
- Classically, patients lose their peripheral pulses, but this is usually preceded by an acute 'flu-like' illness with rigors, myalgia, arthralgia, normocytic anaemia, and a raised erythrocyte sedimentation rate (ESR).

On non-contrast CCT, aortitis is seen as high attenuation within the inflamed area, often with associated mural or intimal calcification. Mural enhancement is seen in both patients with clinically active disease and those with disease in remission (healed lesions often contain fibrous and connective tissue that may undergo dystrophic calcification).

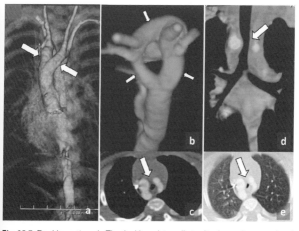

Fig. 25.7 Double aortic arch. The double arch is well visualized on volume-rendered imaging (a, arrows), particularly for the definition of the resulting vascular ring (b, arrows). The patency of the trachea within the vascular ring may be evaluated on the transaxial images (c and e, arrows), with the classical indentation of the trachea seen best on MIP images (d, arrow). (🕮 Plate 10 for colour version).

Pre- and post-surgical assessment

CT is increasingly used to assess the aorta and coronary vessels prior to coronary artery bypass grafting, aortic valve or ascending aortic surgery, and in the planning of percutaneous procedures such as transcatheter aortic valve implantation (TAVI). In the latter, CT allows accurate measurement of the aortic root and assessment of the most appropriate vascular access.

Post surgery, CT may be particularly useful for delineation of pseudoaneurysms following aortic valve replacement, CABG, or any other procedure performed under cardiopulmonary bypass.

Assessment prior to transcatheter aortic valve implantation (TAVI) (1)

Introduction

Patients with severe symptomatic aortic stenosis are traditionally referred for surgical replacement of the aortic valve. However, some patients are turned down for conventional surgery on the grounds of excessive surgical risk. TAVI now offers a realistic alternative to open-chest surgery in such patients. However, the procedure is complex and requires careful planning. Two considerations are paramount:

1 sizing and placement of the valve
2 vascular access.

Assessment of the aortic valve and root

The most crucial aspects of implantation of a stented valve (see Fig. 25.8) in the aortic position are appropriate sizing of the valve and accurate positioning within the aortic outflow. For example, an undersized or inappropriately expanded valve can lead to paravalvular regurgitation, reduced valve lifespan, or, at worst, device embolization. Conversely, overexpansion of the valve may lead to aortic root rupture.

Prior to the use of CCT, conventional angiography and echocardiography were used to measure aortic dimensions. Initial data comparing CCT with these techniques showed small discrepancies in the measurements of the aortic annulus. However, the isotropic nature of CCT allows a true 3D assessment of the aortic valve and root. Both CCT and CMR series have demonstrated that the aortic annulus is oval in shape (and thus not annular!), which may account for this variability. There appears to be no correlation between the shape of the aortic annulus and the likelihood of post-procedure paravalvular regurgitation, although routine oversizing of valves may account for this.

Required aortic measurements

- Sub-aortic inflow diameter (Fig. 25.9a).
- Annular diameter (Fig. 25.9b).
- Coronal and sagittal diameters typically differ by 3–4mm, with little difference between systole and diastole.
- Sino-tubular junction diameter (Fig. 25.9c).
- Ascending aortic diameter (Fig. 25.9d).
- Aortic sinus to commissure distances (Fig. 25.9e).
- Distance from the valve annulus to the coronary artery ostia (Fig. 25.10).
  - Typically in the range 14–17mm.

The burden of aortic wall calcification should also be reported. Comment should also be made about the transverse arch, the tortuosity and calibre of the innominate and subclavian arteries, and the general state of the thoracic aorta, abdominal aorta, and the pelvic side wall vessels.

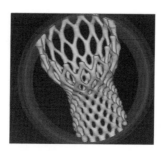

Fig. 25.8 An expanded TAVI stent.

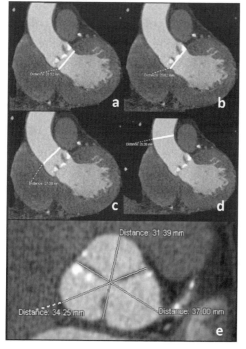

Fig. 25.9 Standard aortic dimensions required prior to TAVI include the
(a) subaortic left ventricular outflow tract, (b) aortic annulus, (c) sinotubular
junction, (d) ascending aorta, and (e) aortic sinus to commisure measurements.

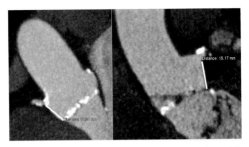

Fig. 25.10 Measurement of the distance between the aortic annulus and the ostia of the coronary arteries (white lines).

Assessment prior to transcatheter aortic valve implantation (TAVI) (2)

Assessment of vascular access

It is necessary to establish the state of the thoracic and abdominal aorta, as well as of the major branches, as part of the work up for TAVI. Arteries should be assessed for:

- Discrete or diffuse luminal narrowing
- Aneurysm formation
- Ectasia (Fig. 25.11)
- Irregular atheromatous plaque formation (Fig. 25.12a).

In particular, the diameter of the ilio-femoral arteries (usually at the level of the common femoral artery) should be measured on both sides (Fig. 25.12b). Current device delivery systems require minimal internal luminal dimensions of 7mm for a transfemoral approach. If there is concentric calcification, particularly in association with ectasia, alternative routes of access should be considered. Furthermore, the presence of discrete stenoses and circumferential calcification, which would not allow arterial expansion, with or without ectasia, would prompt consideration of an alternative strategy such as a transapical procedure or conventional open surgery.

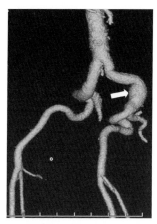

Fig. 25.11 Ectasia of the left common iliac artery (arrow) in a patient undergoing assessment prior to TAVI.

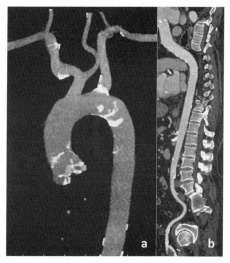

Fig. 25.12 (a) Volume-rendered CT aortogram demonstrating severely calcified aortic valve with calcification of the aortic root, aortic arch, and great vessels. (b) Imaging should include the iliofemorals to evaluate the suitability of vascular access.

Pulmonary artery imaging

Introduction

Indications for pulmonary artery imaging may be divided into acute pulmonary thromboembolic disease and assessment of chronic pulmonary artery hypertension. These will be discussed separately. Although recurrent acute thromboembolic disease may eventually evolve into pulmonary hypertension, the two are essentially separate indications for CT scanning.

Acute pulmonary embolus

Pulmonary emboli most commonly arise in patients in whom there are predisposing factors such as recent surgery, medical illness, or residential care. Risk factors are identified in approximately 75% of patients. The clinical presentation of acute thromboembolic disease has been well characterized. Features such as dyspnoea, tachypnoea, and pleuritic chest pain are present in the majority of patients. Unfortunately these symptoms are frequently present in patients who do not turn out to have acute thromboembolic disease.

- Near-patient testing, such as pulse oximetry, is helpful but not sufficient to distinguish patients with and without PE.
- Similarly, blood testing for D-dimers, the subject of much research over the last 10 years, has a useful NPV but is frequently positive in patients who do not have PE.
- Many current modelling approaches suggest that a negative D-dimer test in a patient with a low or intermediate clinical probability of PE should prompt alternative diagnoses to be pursued in the first instance: this would significantly reduce the number of unwarranted imaging studies.

CT pulmonary angiography

CTPA is now the imaging method of choice in patients where there is clinical suspicion of acute PE disease.

- Initial studies from 1992 demonstrated the accuracy of CT in the diagnosis of acute PE.
- There was initial concern over the degree of accuracy for emboli confined to the sub-segmental vessels, but the increasing detail available from modern multichannel CT systems has allayed these concerns.
- Initially CT was compared to the gold standard of conventional invasive pulmonary angiography, but it seems likely that modern 64-slice CT systems are actually more accurate.
- Of particular interest are the very high levels of inter- and intraobserver agreement, and the small number of non-diagnostic CT studies.
- Furthermore, when a patient presents with acute chest symptoms, a CT scan may reveal an alternative cause for the presentation, including pneumonia, malignancy, pleural disease, or oesophageal, pericardial, or aortic pathology.
- A number of studies have demonstrated that spiral CT provides an alternative explanation for a patient's symptoms in between 25 and 50% of cases.

CT pulmonary angiography acquisition

Modern CT scanners can achieve a volumetric dataset of the entire thorax at submillimetre collimation with consistent optimal opacification of the pulmonary arterial tree.

- It is common practice to scan the thorax in a caudal-cranial direction so that breathing artefact, usually more pronounced later on in the study, has less influence on the quality of images.
- As in other forms of CT angiography, optimal bolus timing can be achieved by bolus-tracking software or by using a fixed scan delay which may be calculated using a test bolus technique.
- The amount of contrast administered will depend on the duration of the acquisition, which itself is a function of the particular CT scanner.
- The aim is to achieve a density of at least 250HU in the pulmonary arteries.

CT pulmonary angiography interpretation

Images are reviewed on a computer workstation, which allows scrolling through the large numbers of slices in the data stack and also facilitates manipulation of the window and level settings to demonstrate filling defects optimally within the contrast column in the arterial tree.

- The interpretation of CTPA is entirely analogous to the interpretation of a conventional pulmonary angiogram, the key diagnostic finding being the presence of filling defects within the contrast column (Fig. 26.1).
- In the majority of patients with a positive scan there will be multiple emboli.

- Most of the filling defects will be within the central or lobar vessels, with the segmental vessel being the site of the largest embolus in approximately 25% of patients and isolated sub-segmental emboli occurring in approximately 20% of patients.
- Most emboli are non-occluding and ∴ may be outlined by contrast around the majority of the circumference.
- Emboli are slightly more common in the lower lobes than the upper lobes.
- Most emboli originate in the deep veins of the extremities and are ∴ often long and narrow in configuration and may straddle the divisions of the pulmonary artery braches; this configuration is sometimes described as a saddle embolus.
- Most emboli can be detected on several contiguous images, and apparent emboli that are confined to a single slice should be viewed with considerable suspicion.
- The exact appearance of an embolus within an opacified artery branch will depend on the orientation of the vessel relative to the plane of the scan.
- Multiplanar reformats may allow more convincing demonstration of thrombo-emboli.

Severity assessment

The great majority of emboli are not of sufficient size to cause acute RV compromise or reduced cardiac output. However, signs of RV dilatation and strain may be apparent on non-gated CT scanning with paradoxical movement off the septum into the LV cavity. Reflux of contrast into the IVC and the azygos vein may also be observed.

A number of programs have been developed and designed to assess clot burden and so predict outcome.

Pitfalls in CT pulmonary angiography interpretation

- Motion—Severe respiratory motion artefact can severely degrade image quality to the extent that the study is non-diagnostic, ∴ each study should be acquired during the shortest possible breath hold.
- Image noise—Larger patients may also degrade the quality of images due to overall image noise.
- Contrast density—There may be difficulties with adequate contrast opacification. In some patients there is clearly adequate contrast in the SVC and the right heart as well as in the left-sided chambers and aorta, but the pulmonary arteries are not adequately pacified. There is effectively a bolus of non-opacified blood within the pulmonary arterial tree dividing two adequately opacified contrast columns. This artefact is usually associated with a deep inspiratory effort which encourages non-opacified blood from the abdomen, via the IVC, to interrupt the contrast bolus.
- An alternative cause for failure of opacification is the result of a Valsalva maneouver which temporarily opens a right to left right shunt through a patent foramen ovale.

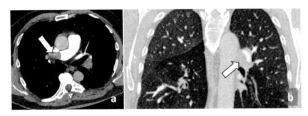

Fig. 26.1 CT pulmonary angiogram demonstrating a large filling in the right (a, arrow) and left (b, arrow) pulmonary arteries.

Peripheral venous imaging

A number of authors have proposed assessment of the deep venous system of the pelvis and lower limbs in combination with the CT pulmonary angiogram. This is an attractive diagnostic approach since both deep vein thrombosis and PE are manifestations of the same disorder, and both require anticoagulation.

- Generally compression ultrasound of the legs is undertaken as the first procedure whenever there are symptoms or signs to suggest deep vein thrombosis.
- Ultrasound is usually more readily available, has no associated radiation burden, and is of low cost.
- CT venography may be substituted for ultrasound in certain clinical situations.
- CT can image pelvic sidewall vessels and the IVC, two areas that provide technical challenges to ultrasound.
- The usual technique is to undertake a CT pulmonary angiogram then, after a delay of 2–3min, to examine the IVC, pelvic veins, and leg veins to down to the mid-calf.
- Signs of acute deep venous thrombosis include:
  - Venous distension
  - Venous wall enhancement
  - Intraluminal filling defects (Fig. 26.2)
  - Peri-venous soft tissue oedema.

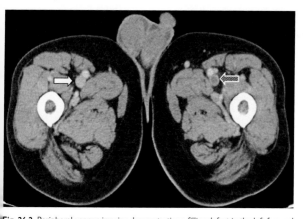

Fig. 26.2 Peripheral venous imaging demonstrating a filling defect in the left femoral vein (hatched arrow). The right femoral vein (white arrow) shows normal contrast opacification for comparison.

Chronic pulmonary hypertension

There are a number of causes of chronic pulmonary hypertension. The disease may be idiopathic, formerly known as 1° pulmonary hypertension. The disease classification is now usually divided into:

Pre-capillary hypertension, including:
- Small vessel disease
- Pulmonary artery obstruction due to chronic thromboembolic disease (Fig. 26.3) or non-thrombotic emboli
- CHD, causing shunting
- Chronic pulmonary disease
- Alveolar hyperventilation

Post-capillary hypertension:
- Pulmonary veno-occlusive disease
- Capillary haemangiomatosis
- Left-sided heart failure
- Mitral valve disease
- Pulmonary venous stenosis or anomalous connections.

The diagnosis of pulmonary hypertension can be difficult: the onset is usually insidious and non-specific. Exercise tolerance usually deteriorates steadily and exertional chest pain or syncope may develop.

- CCT is an important step in the assessment of patients with suspected pulmonary hypertension, particularly since high-resolution images of the lungs can be obtained at the same investigation.
- When the study is ECG-gated, an assessment of cardiac chamber size, degree of TR (see 📖 Tricuspid regurgitation, p. 304), and evaluation of right-sided ventricular function can also be combined in a single investigation (see 📖 Combined CT coronary and pulmonary angiography, p 432),
- Dilatation of the central pulmonary arteries is the cardinal sign in the CT assessment of pulmonary hypertension.
  - Absolute measurements of pulmonary artery diameter or size relative to the aorta have both been validated.
  - When the pulmonary artery diameter is larger than the thoracic aorta, pulmonary hypertension is highly likely with a PPV of over 90%.
- Other features include:
  - Peripheral arterial pruning
  - Right atrium and right ventricle may become dilated and encroach on the left-sided chambers
  - Paradoxical movement of the septum, best appreciated on gated images.

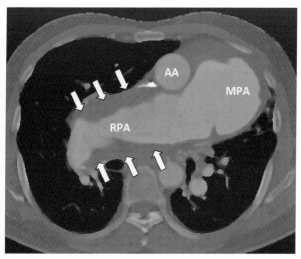

Fig. 26.3 Chronic pulmonary thromboembolic disease. A large main pulmonary artery (MPA) and right pulmonary artery (RPA) with *in situ* thrombus (arrows) and mural calcification. A ratio of pulmonary artery to ascending aorta (AA) diameter of >1 suggests pulmonary hypertension.

Combined multivessel angiography

The triple rule-out

These protocols have become increasingly popular in the setting of acute chest pain for the simultaneous identification or exclusion of CAD, aortic dissection, and pulmonary embolism. The concept of 'triple rule-out' is appealing as it offers the potential to exclude life-threatening conditions quickly using only a single test.

Particular concerns about the triple rule-out are high radiation exposure and the use of the protocol as a substitute for clinical judgment. The vast majority of cases of acute chest pain can be settled by thorough history, clinical examination (e.g. blood pressure in both arms), and routine investigations such as blood tests (e.g. D-dimer, cardiac enzymes), ECG, and arterial blood gases. Only where these fail to differentiate between or exclude these three conditions should a triple rule-out protocol be considered.

CT findings (Fig. 27.1)

- CAD (see 📖 Imaging atherosclerotic plaque, p. 191) ± myocardial infarction (see 📖 Evaluation of myocardial scarring and perfusion, p. 259).
- Aortic dissection (see 📖 Aortic dissection, p. 402).
- Pulmonary embolus (see 📖 Pulmonary artery imaging, p. 419).

Specific issues

Contrast administration

- Contrast enhancement of the pulmonary arteries precedes that of the aorta and coronary arteries.
- The difference between pulmonary and coronary artery enhancement is typically 10–15s, although this may be reduced in those with poor LV function.
- Bolus-tracking or test bolus protocols (see 📖 Optimizing scan timing, p. 102) may be used to optimize enhancement; no clear benefit has been demonstrated for either.
- A test-bolus protocol results in higher contrast delivery but improves the likelihood of simultaneous opacification of all three vessels as scan delay can be calculated and subsequently applied to the main scan.
- Bolus tracking requires no additional contrast administration but requires the operator to initiate the scan when simultaneous enhancement is seen, potentially introducing uncertainty.
- Biphasic (see 📖 CT coronary angiography, p. 108) or triphasic (see 📖 Gated CT pulmonary angiogram, p. 110) contrast protocols provide adequate opacification of the aorta, coronary, and pulmonary arteries.

Radiation

- Triple rule-out requires a scanning FOV that encompasses the whole chest. The associated radiation exposure is ∴ higher than for either CTPA or CTA alone.
- Reported exposures vary between 17–19mSv for retrospectively-gated acquisitions without ECG tube current modulation (see 📖 ECG gating, p. 34) and 8–9mSv with tube current modulation applied.

- Heart rate is a crucial determinant of diagnostic quality of CTA; those with heart rates >70bpm probably benefit from wide temporal padding (e.g. 30–80% R–R interval, see 📖 ECG gating, p. 34).

Other issues

- β-blockade may be inappropriate if haemodynamically compromised; high heart rate may ∴ lead to a significant reduction in diagnostic quality.

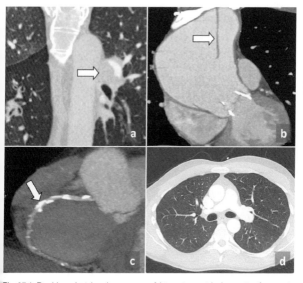

Fig. 27.1 Double and triple rule-out are useful in patients with chest pain of uncertain aetiology and can confirm or exclude pulmonary embolism (a, arrow), aortic dissection (b, arrow), and CAD (c, arrow). These protocols allow assessment of the aorta, pulmonary arteries, and coronary arteries in addition to the lung fields (d).

Combined CT coronary and pulmonary angiography

A combined, retrospectively-gated, contrast-enhanced CTPA and CT coronary angiography protocol provides a comprehensive non-invasive assessment of the pulmonary and coronary vasculature. In addition, biventricular functional assessment can be performed.

- This study can be performed in a single breath hold of around 10–20s, depending on the type of scanner.
- It is particularly useful in patients with PAH (see 📖 Pulmonary artery imaging, p. 419) where it provides a comprehensive non-invasive assessment of the aetiology and cardiopulmonary consequences of raised pulmonary arterial pressure.
- Additionally, underlying cardiac morphology can be accurately assessed, and complex congenital heart malformations (see 📖 Congenital heart disease, p. 331) do not compromise the assessment of relevant cardiac and extracardiac parameters.

Protocol

For assessment of both pulmonary and coronary anatomy, iodinated contrast is required in both the pulmonary and coronary arteries.

- A long contrast bolus is required to attenuate these structures in addition to the RV and LV blood pool.
- RV opacification may present problems when interpreting CT coronary angiography as streak artefact may affect the proximal RCA (see 📖 Beam hardening, p. 152), ∴ a protocol is required which achieves sufficient PA and RV attenuation without hindering proximal RCA interpretation.

As with standard CT coronary angiography an initial test bolus is often used to determine the time to peak concentration in the aortic root, and to identify late filling structures. After the tracking acquisition, we recommend a triphasic venous injection using a dual-headed power injector:

- 70mL contrast at 5mL/s, followed by
- 60mL saline/contrast (30:70 mix) at 5mL/s, with a final
- 40mL saline/contrast (50:50 mix) at 5mL/s.

This protocol allows sufficient attenuation of the RV blood pool but does not lead to streak artefact affecting the proximal RCA.

Peripheral arterial imaging

Introduction

Accurate mapping and assessment of the upper limb, abdominal, and pelvic arterial tree has become a standard CT request (Fig. 28.1) and is now a pre-requisite for appropriate planning of interventional procedures in the thorax. In particular, the delivery systems of interventional devices (such as transcatheter aortic valve implantation, see 📖 Assessment prior to transcatheter aortic valve implantation, p. 412) have a minimum require-ment for vessel calibre. Marked tortuosity of the vessels that comprise the access route to cardiac or thoracic vascular structures will also influence the choice of procedure undertaken. Access difficulties from the groin may convert a femoral approach into an axillary approach, or require conventional thoracotomy or a minimally invasive transapical technique. Further information may also be required on other important structures such as the mesenteric and renal vessels. This chapter will not deal with peripheral vascular disease below the inguinal ligaments.

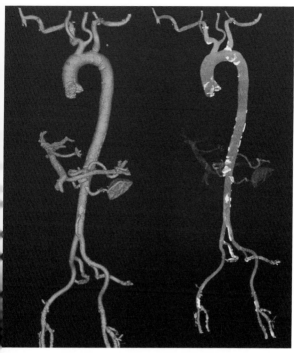

Fig. 28.1 Volume-rendered (left) and MIP (right) images of the whole aorta and terminal branches. (□ Plate 11 for colour version).

CT technique

There are a number of common principles that apply to all multidetector CT studies. However, the success of vascular acquisition depends on multiple variables, including the CT scanner, the patient's individual contrast medium transit time, injector flow rate, duration of injection, duration of acquisition, and contrast concentration. There is no single or series of protocols that is likely to be universally successful.

Contrast delivery

In order to maximize contrast enhancement, it is usual to administer at least 100mL of contrast, typically of strength 350mgI/mL (see 📖 Adverse contrast reactions, p 92), aiming for enhancement in the descending aorta of at least 250HU. Injection rate should be between 3 and 5mL/s. On a typical 64-slice CT scanner, tube voltage and current should be 120kV and 600–800mA, respectively. Tube voltage should be reduced in slim patients (see 📖 X-ray tube voltageCT, p. 23).

Contrast timing

Since acquisition times vary according to the gantry rotation time (see 📖 Gantry, p. 10) and the z-axis dimension of the detector array (see 📖 Detectors, p. 15), a standard delay from initiation of contrast delivery to start of acquisition cannot be prescribed. It is possible, with very short acquisition times, to completely miss the bolus of contrast if the delay is not correctly calculated. The appropriate delay may be as little as 2s for faster scanners or, if it is necessary to cover a large area of anatomy in optimum detail, as long as 40s, depending on scanner and patient-related factors.

In all cases, either a test bolus or test tracking technique should be used. If the study is acquired as part of a CT coronary angiogram protocol, then scan timing should be calculated as described earlier (see 📖 CT coronary angiography, p. 108). If the vascular tree is to be analysed in isolation, either technique may be employed but with the ROI placed in the abdominal aorta. For the test bolus technique, the time to peak enhancement of the abdominal aorta should be used to calculate the scan delay for the main scan. For bolus tracking, serial low-dose scans should be performed through the abdominal aortic ROI and the main scan initiated automatically when attenuation in the ROI reaches 100HU.

Saline flush

It is normal practise to flush the venous system with saline, using a dual-headed injector (see 📖 Adverse contrast reactions, p. 92). This 'tightens' the contrast bolus, thereby improving arterial enhancement and reducing venous streak artefacts as dense contrast is washed out from the brachiocephalic veins and SVC.

Image reconstrcution and post processing

Images are acquired during suspended respiration. A contiguous dataset through the area examined is then reconstructed at thin collimation with 50% overlap. Axial data is analysed using appropriate software.

Abdominal aorta and branches

Anatomy

From the level of the diaphragm, the abdominal aorta extends to the fourth lumbar vertebra, where it bifurcates into the *common iliac arteries*. In order, the major branches of the abdominal aorta below the diaphragm (Fig. 28.2) are:

- *Coeliac artery* or trunk, supplying the liver, spleen, and upper abdominal viscera
- *Superior mesenteric artery*, supplying the majority of the small intestine and proximal large intestine up to the transverse colon
- *Renal arteries*
- *Inferior mesenteric artery*, supplying the distal large intestine, including the descending and sigmoid colons and upper rectum.

A number of additional paired arteries are present:

- Inferior phrenic arteries
- Supra-renal arteries
- Gonadal arteries

They are additionally numerous pairs of lumbar arteries.

Below the aortic bifurcation, the common iliac artery divides into the *internal* and *external iliac arteries*. The external iliac arteries lie against the pelvic sidewalls and extend to the *common femoral arteries* at the level of the femoral heads, which in turn divide into the *superficial femoral* and *profunda femoris arteries*. Most vascular punctures, for access purposes, are made into the common femoral arteries.

Indications for cardiac CT

- TAVI (see 📖 Assessment prior to transcatheter aortic valve implantation, p. 412).
- Aortic pathology (see 📖 Thoracic aortic imaging, p. 412).

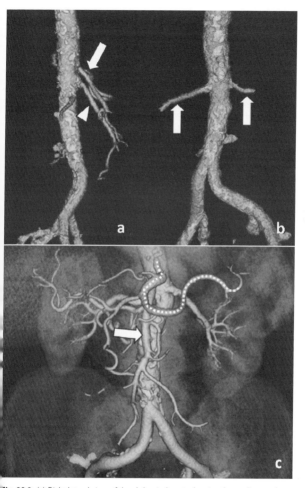

Fig. 28.2 (a) Right lateral view of the abdominal aorta showing the coeliac trunk (arrow) and superior mesenteric artery (arrowhead). (b) Anteroposterior view showing the renal arteries (arrows). (c) The coeliac trunk sends branches to the spleen (dotted line) and liver, whilst the superior mesenteric artery (arrow) passes downwards to supply the bowel. (📖 Plate 12 colour version).

Renal artery imaging

CT angiography is ideally suited to the assessment of small stationary vessels such as the renal arteries, which may be evaluated as part of wider assessment of the arterial tree or as a more targeted investigation (Fig. 28.3). Much like coronary artery imaging, the presence of calcified atherosclerotic plaque within the renal arteries may hinder accurate evaluation.

Indications
- Suspected renal vascular hypertension.
- Preoperative assessment of renal transplant candidates.
- Repeat evaluation after renal artery stenting.

Normal CT angiography of the renal arteries virtually excludes renal artery stenosis. CT may also be used to evaluate variant renal arterial and venous anatomy as well as the renal parenchyma.

It is important to achieve adequate coverage to include all possible branches to the renal arteries. When renal artery assessment is required in a patient with renal impairment, alternative techniques should be considered. If CCT is to be performed, the Royal College of Radiology guidelines on administration of contrast agents should be followed (see Adminstration of intravenous contrast, p. 88).

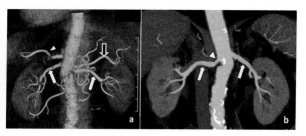

Fig. 28.3 (a) Postero-anterior view of the aorta showing the renal arteries. The splenic (arrowhead) and hepatic (outline arrow) branches of the coeliac trunk are also visible. (b) MIP of the renal arteries (arrows) showing mild stenosis at the ostium of the right renal artery (arrowhead).

Carotid artery imaging

The assessment of the carotid arteries prior to coronary artery bypass grafting or other major vascular or valvular intervention is now routine. Although Doppler ultrasound is the initial screening test of choice, CT is frequently used as a second non-invasive imaging modality to confirm ultrasound findings. Magnetic resonance is an equally well-validated non-invasive technique, but access to this modality is often more restricted than access to multislice CT.

CT angiography of the carotids is a well-validated and robust technique that allows excellent visualization of the vessel lumen from origin to skull base, and can be extended to include the circle of Willis. In the context of acute stroke, the study can be combined with functional imaging of cerebral perfusion.

Stenosis severity and plaque burden may be readily assessed by CT (Fig. 28.4). A number of large clinical trials have clarified the indications for surgical or percutaneous intervention for carotid artery stenosis in symptomatic and asymptomatic populations, with conventional angiography as the gold standard for assessment. The ability of non-invasive techniques to determine the need for definitive treatment can obviate conventional invasive angiography, which is not without risk.

Variant carotid anatomy may also be assessed by CT, particularly if surgical procedures are planned (Fig. 28.5).

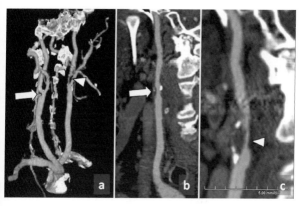

Fig. 28.4 Assessment of the carotid arteries. (a) Volume-rendered image showing narrowing proximal to the right carotid bifurcation (arrow) and in the proximal left internal carotid artery (arrowhead). (b) The stenosis on the right side is eccentric and not causing significant luminal narrowing (arrow). (c) However, the stenois of the proximal left internal carotid artery is significant (arrowhead).

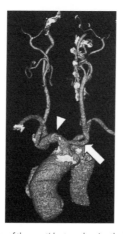

Fig. 28.5 Variant anatomy of the carotid artery showing the left carotid artery (arrow) arising from the innominate artery (arrowhead) rather than the aortic arch. Such a pattern is often referred to as a 'bovine arch', although it bears no relation to the true bovine branching pattern.

Systemic veins

Introduction

Most contrast-enhanced scanning protocols of the thorax are designed to provide optimal visualization of the lungs, pulmonary arteries, heart or aorta and its branches. Nevertheless, the systemic venous system is routinely imaged during CT examinations, but is often regarded as of 2° importance to the main indication for the scan.

However, there are many clinical situations where the visualization of the systemic veins is of prime interest. These include:

• Assessment of SVC obstruction
• Assessment of IVC involvement by renal and other intra-abdominal neoplasms (Fig. 29.1)
• Assessment of potential access routes for central venous line or pacing wire placement
• Pre-operative assessment of venous anatomy prior to surgery for complex CHD
• Post-operative assessment of shunts and anastomoses in complex CHD, e.g Glenn shunt, total cavopulmonary connection, intra-atrial baffles (Mustard, Senning) (Fig. 29.2)
• Delayed scanning of the thighs, pelvis, and abdomen may also be performed as an adjunct to CTPA to identify the source of pulmonary emboli.

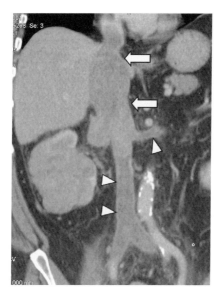

Fig. 29.1 The IVC above the level of the renal veins (arrows) is expanded and occluded by tumour extending from a right renal cell carcinoma. Thrombus can be seen in the IVC and internal iliac veins peripheral to the intraluminal tumour and also in the left renal vein (arrowheads).

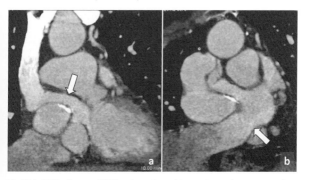

Fig. 29.2 (a) Unobstructed SVC pathway (arrow) in a patient with an intra-atrial baffle for transposition of the great arteries. (b) Alteration of the imaging plane shows that the IVC channel is also unobstructed (arrow).

Systemic venous anatomy

Normal anatomy of the systemic veins is somewhat variable. For descriptive purposes they can be regarded as either superficial or deep (Table 29.1). In health the superficial veins drain the chest wall and spine, and the deep veins drain the head and neck, infra-diaphragmatic structures, and the superficial veins of the thorax. In clinical practice the superficial veins are most obviously visualized in pathological situations (such as SVC obstruction) when abnormal venous pathways cause them to dilate and abnormal flow may cause them to opacify on scans.

- The SVC (Figs 29.3 and 29.4) is formed by the confluence of the right and left brachiocephalic veins. It is situated in the right side of the middle mediastinum and drains directly into the right atrium.
- In 0.3–0.5% of the normal population and more frequently in association with CHD (c. 4–12%) there is a *persistent left* SVC. This receives flow from the left subclavian and left jugular veins and usually drains into the coronary sinus (Fig. 29.5).
- Many individuals with a left SVC also have a right SVC, and in such cases a bridging vein often passes between them.
- The *subclavian veins* commence at the outer edge of the first ribs as a continuation of the *axillary veins*. The *jugular veins* join the subclavian veins posterior to the sterno-clavicular joints to form the *brachiocephalic* (or innominate) *veins*. The right brachiocephalic vein passes more-or-less caudally to reach the SVC, whereas the left brachiocephalic vein passes across the mid-line anterior to the aorta to reach the SVC.
- The *internal mammary veins* draining to the brachiocephalic veins and the *lateral thoracic veins* draining to the subclavian veins receive flow from the anterior intercostal veins.

Table 29.1 Systemic veins of the thorax

Deep veins
SVC and IVC
Innominate, jugular, and subclavian veins
Thymic, inferior thyroid, and interbrachiocephalic veins
Pericardiophrenic and cardiac veins and coronary sinus
Superficial veins
Azygos and hemi-azygos veins
Internal mammary and lateral thoracic veins
Intercostal and chest wall veins

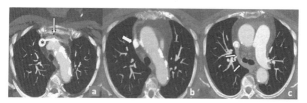

Fig. 29.3 (a) Transaxial scan at the level of top of transverse aortic arch shows the left brachiocephalic vein (straight arrow) passing anterior to the aorta to enter the SVC (asterisk). A pacing wire is in the brachiocephalic vein. (b) Transaxial scan at level of mid aortic arch shows right internal mammary vein entering SVC (arrow). (c) Transaxial scan at level main pulmonary artery shows the azygos vein entering SVC (arrows).

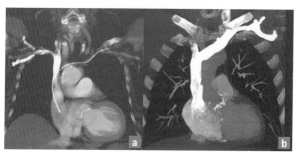

Fig. 29.4 (a) Thick MIP shows right subclavian and jugular veins forming right brachiocephalic vein and draining into SVC. A pacing wire is present in the left brachiocephalic vein. (b) Thick MIP shows left subclavian and jugular veins forming left brachiocephalic vein and joining right brachiocephalic vein to form SVC.

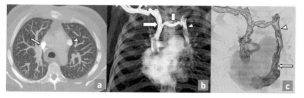

Fig. 29.5 (a) Transaxial MIP shows persistent left SVC (arrowhead) in addition to right SVC (straight arrow). (b) Coronal MIP shows a right SVC (horizontal arrow), bridging vein (vertical arrow), and persistent left SVC (arrowhead). (c) Volume-rendered reformat shows bridging vein and left SVC (arrowhead) draining to coronary sinus (straight arrow). (☐ Plate 13 for colour version).

- The *azygos vein* is formed by the junction of the ascending right lumbar vein and the right subcostal vein at about the level of the diaphragm. It passes cephalad in close relation to the right side of the spine (Fig. 29.6a), oesophagus, and thoracic duct, and then arches over the right hilum to drain into the SVC (Fig. 29.6b). In about 1% of people the azygos arch is associated with invagination of the pleura producing an azygos fissure. The azygos vein receives flow from the right intercostal veins, the hemi-azygos veins, and oesophageal, bronchial, and other mediastinal veins.
- The *hemi-azygos vein* is formed by confluence of the left ascending lumbar and sub-costal veins (Fig. 29.6b). It passes cephalad to the left of the spine and usually receives flow from above from the *accessory hemi-azygos vein*, although this vein may drain across the mid-line to the azygos vein.
- The hemi-azygos veins receive flow from left intercostal veins and bronchial and other mediastinal veins.
- The IVC is formed by the confluence of the iliac veins and passes cephalad traversing the central tendon of the diaphragm to drain into the right atrium (Fig. 29.7). Its largest tributaries are the renal and hepatic veins.
- Occasionally there is congenital absence of the infrahepatic part of the IVC.
- This anomaly is usually associated with CHD; most of the systemic venous return from the abdomen is then to the azygos system (so-called *azygos continuation of the IVC*) and the hepatic veins usually drain directly to the right atrium.

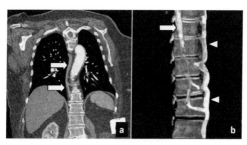

Fig. 29.6 (a) Azygos vein (arrows) ascending in the right para-spinal position. (b) Hemi-azygos and accessory hemi-azygos veins (arrowheads) in left para-spinal position. The connecting veins to the azygos vein (arrow) pass anterior to the spine.

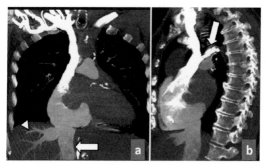

Fig. 29.7 (a) Coronal MIP shows reflux of contrast medium (due to tricuspid incompetence) into IVC (arrow) and hepatic veins (arrowhead). (b) Sagittal MIP showing contrast reflux into azygos arch (arrow).

Imaging the systemic veins

Scan protocols

For assessment of the thoracic veins a non-contrast enhanced scan is rarely required. During contrast-enhanced scans of the thorax for most indications there will be opacification of the thoracic veins to a lesser or greater degree.

- For specific examination of the thoracic systemic veins injection of 100–120mL of non-ionic contrast medium containing 350mg/mL of iodine at 3mL/s via an 18–20 gauge cannula in an antecubital vein and scanning with a 25–30-s delay will usually provide adequate data.
- If imaging of the IVC and pelvic veins is required a delay of about 2min is recommended before scanning these areas.

Artefacts and pitfalls

Two commonly seen artefacts in the SVC may lead to misinterpretation of scans:

- Dense (undiluted) contrast medium in the SVC often causes *streak artefacts*, which may obscure the lumen of the SVC and adjacent structures (see 🕮 Beam hardening, p. 152). A similar problem may also be caused by pacing leads traversing the SVC.
- *Flow-related artefacts* due to inhomogeneous mixing of contrast medium and blood or due to non-opacified blood entering the SVC from the brachio-cephalic, jugular, or azygos veins may mimic intraluminal filling defects (Fig, 29.8). Similar flow-related artefacts are often seen in the IVC from non-opacified renal venous blood.

Post processing

Venous anatomy and pathology can often be adequately assessed using axial and multiplanar reconstructions. However, thoracic veins and collaterals are often tortuous and do not conveniently fit into single planes. Moreover, venous opacification may not be particularly dense, making MIP images less satisfactory than for arterial imaging. Venous anatomy is ∴ often best demonstrated using volume rendering.

Superior vena caval obstruction

Most cases of SVC obstruction are due to malignant disease (Fig. 29.1), usually lung cancer, but also metastatic disease and lymphoma. Benign causes include fibrosing mediastinitis (Fig. 29.9a) and a complication of central venous line placement. CT can usually define the cause and level of obstruction, and can be used to assess the structures adjacent to the SVC and to plan therapeutic intervention. SVC obstrcution usually causes diversion of systemic venous return to the more superficial thoracic veins, which is well-demonstrated by CT (Fig. 29.9b).

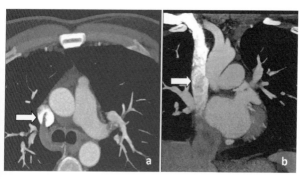

Fig. 29.8 (a) 'Filling defect' in the SVC (arrow) is caused by mixing with non-opacified blood from the azygos vein. (b) Coronal MIP showing poor mixing of contrast medium and non-opacified blood in the SVC (arrow).

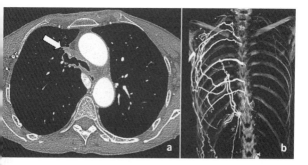

Fig. 29.9 (a) SVC obstruction caused by fibrosing mediastinitis. The SVC is constricted to almost a pinhole (arrow) by fibrotic tissue in the mediastinum which is also distorting the airways. (b) Volume-rendered reformat shows numerous large collateral chest wall veins 2° to SVC obstruction.

Guidelines, accreditation, and certification

Cardiovascular CT guidelines

Cardiac imaging is a rapidly expanding field. The increasing availability of CCT as an alternative non-invasive cardiac imaging modality has led to widespread use. CCT offers complementary information to echocardiography, cardiac radionuclide imaging, conventional invasive catheter angiography, and CMR in the management of CAD and cardiac disease as a whole.

The most appropriate test for a given patient depends on:
- The specific clinical requirements of the referrer, e.g.:
  - Exclusion of CAD of any severity
  - Exclusion of functionally significant CAD
  - Investigation of LV dysfunction
  - Evaluation of cardiothoracic anatomy
- The PTL of disease
- Locally available expertise.

General considerations

Renal dysfunction

CCT should be used with caution in patients with borderline or compromised renal function (see 📖 Adverse contrast reactions, p. 92), especially if the likelihood of requiring additional contrast from ICA is high.

Radiation exposure

With increasing use of dual-source and >64-detector row CT scanners, as well as prospective gating techniques, radiation burden from CTA is now well within the domain of other cardiovascular imaging techniques that involve exposure to ionizing radiation (e.g. diagnostic ICA, ^{99m}Tc SPECT MPS). When clinically justified, there should be no higher concern about the exposure from CTA than for other techniques and all reasonable dose-sparing techniques should be employed. However, the need for repeat exposure over time should be considered when embarking on a diagnostic investigation strategy and, if possible, a non-ionizing technique sought when the patient is young or likely to require serial imaging.

Prognostic data

It is important to emphasise the high NPV that CT coronary angiography affords and the more accepted clinical utility of accurately excluding CAD. Although there are increasing data regarding the prognostic value of CT coronary angiography, there is a need for long-term prospective studies investigating hard end points or future clinical events, particularly in those who have had a previously 'negative' CT coronary angiogram.

Further reading

Waugh N, Black C, Walker S, McIntyre L, Cummins E, and Hillis G (2006) The effectiveness and cost-effectiveness of computed tomography screening for coronary artery disease: systematic review. *Health Technol Assess* **10**(39), iii–iv, ix–x, 1–41.

Appropriate use criteria for cardiac CT

Appropriate use criteria for CCT were released in 2006 by the American College of Cardiology Foundation (ACCF) Task Force on Clinical Expert Consensus Documents, in association with other related US societies. These criteria were broadly endorsed by the European Society of Cardiology in 2008. The ACCF have recently released revised criteria reflecting progress over the intervening 4 years. In particular, the number of rated potential indications has ↑ nearly threefold.

2010 ACCF criteria

In patients without known CAD, appropriateness depends in part upon the PTL of CAD. Low, intermediate, and high PTL values are defined as <10%, 10–20%, and >20% 10-year absolute coronary heart disease risk, respectively. Indications are summarized below; there remain several where the use of CCT is considered uncertain.

Symptomatic patients without known coronary artery disease

CT coronary angiography (CTA) is considered appropriate in:
- Patients with stable chest pain and:
  - Intermediate PTL, whether or not the ECG is interpretable and exercise is possible
  - Low PTL and uninterpretable ECG or unable to exercise
- Patients with acute chest pain and:
  - Low or intermediate PTL and normal/equivocal ECG and cardiac biomarkers.

Patients with stable chest pain who have a low PTL, an interpretable ECG and who are able to exercise should not undergo CTA (although there is no stipulation that they should have coronary calcium scoring, as suggested in the UK NICE guidelines, see 📖 Guidelines, accreditation, and certification, p. 455). Patients with definite myocardial infarction should not be investigated using CTA.

Other permutations in this setting are considered uncertain indications for CTA, including the evaluation of other patients with high PTL of CAD and the use of the triple-rule-out (see 📖 The triple rule-out, p. 430).

Asymptomatic patients without known coronary artery disease

Coronary calcium scoring is considered:
- Appropriate in patients with low PTL and a family history of premature CAD
- Also appropriate in asymptomatic patients without known CAD and an intermediate PTL (this may be controversial)
- Inappropriate in low PTL patients; use in high PTL patients uncertain.

CTA is generally considered inappropriate in this patient group, although its role in patients with high PTL is deemed uncertain.

CT coronary angiography in the setting of prior test results

After coronary calcium scoring

- Appropriate provided CCS is <400.
- Inappropriate in the setting of any positive CCS >2 years prior.
- Uncertain appropriateness if CCS >400 or if zero CCS >5 years prior.

After exercise testing

- Appropriate in the setting of a normal exercise ECG test and continued symptoms or where the Duke Treadmill Score suggests intermediate cardiac risk.
- Inappropriate in the setting of a low or high Duke Treadmill Score.

After stress imaging

- Appropriate when stress imaging is equivocal or discrepant with exercise ECG testing.
- Also appropriate for the evaluation of new onset symptoms in the setting of a previously normal stress imaging test.
- Inappropriate if stress imaging shows moderate to severe ischaemia.
- Uncertain appropriateness in the setting of mild ischaemia.

CTA after revascularization

- Appropriate for the evaluation of bypass grafts in the symptomatic patient and LMS stents >3mm in the asymptomatic patient.
- Inappropriate in asymptomatic patients after bypass grafting and patients with stents <3mm regardless of symptoms.
- Uncertain appropriateness in patients with stents >3mm who remain asymptomatic after 2 years or who develop new symptoms.

Cardiac CT to evaluate cardiac structure and function

CCT is generally considered appropriate in all patients requiring evaluation of cardiac structure and function (coronary anomalies, CHD, prior to electrophysiological mapping, location of bypass grafts prior to repeat thoracotomy, etc.) except as an initial test of LV function and in those requiring investigation of cardiac masses.

Other clinical scenarios

CTA is considered appropriate in the following settings:

- Detection of CAD in patients with low or intermediate PTL and new-onset heart failure.
- Coronary evaluation in patients at intermediate PTL prior to non-coronary cardiac surgery.

Other indications considered inappropriate

- Evaluation of new onset atrial fibrillation.
- Repeat testing in asymptomatic patients with known CAD or in those with stable symptoms and previous stress imaging or ICA.
- Pre-operative risk assessment in patients without active cardiac conditions.

Cardiac CT in other clinical guidelines

Indications that CCT has become accepted across the international medical community have been provided by the publication of the recent UK NICE guidelines for stable chest pain.

2010 NICE guidelines for stable chest pain

The 2010 NICE guidelines for the diagnosis of stable chest pain (available at http://guidance.nice.org.uk/CG95) include specific recommendations for CCT in patients with low (10–29%) PTL of CAD.

Pre-test likelihood

- Evaluated using the supplied chart based on a modified Diamond and Forrester scoring system.
- Four characteristics require evaluation in each case: age, gender, cardiovascular risk factors, and category of chest pain.
- The latter may be decided according to whether the chest pain is:
  - Central
  - Brought on by exertion
  - Relieved by rest or GTN.
- If the answer is yes to the above three questions, the patient has angina by definition. Answering yes to two or one question(s) defines atypical and non-anginal pain, respectively.
- Patients with cardiovascular risk factors that include diabetes mellitus, smoking, and hyperlipidaemia are classified as high-risk; patients without any of these risk factors are classified as low-risk.

Guidelines

In brief, this guidance recommends coronary calcium scoring in the following patients, according to presenting symptoms and risk factors:

- *Angina, low risk*—women <45 years (and possibly men <35 years)
- *Atypical chest pain, low risk*—women aged 55–65 years and men <45 years
- *Non-anginal chest pain*—NICE expects that most people with non-anginal chest pain will be investigated for causes other than CAD. However, those with 10–29% pre-test probability include all women with risk factors and men without risk factors aged 45–55 years.

If the CCS is:
- Zero—no further imaging recommended
- 1–400—CTA suggested
- >400—ICA recommended provided it is clinically appropriate and acceptable to the person *and* coronary revascularization is being considered; otherwise offer functional testing.

If the CTA shows CAD of uncertain significance, functional testing (e.g. SPECT MPS see 📖 Myocardial perfusion single photon emission CT, p. 472 or stress echo, see 📖 Stress echocardiography, p. 486) is recommended.

⚠ These guidelines are controversial for several reasons:
- The reassuring prognostic value of a CCS of zero is derived mainly from asymptomatic cohorts, and may not be applicable to patients with chest pain.
- A CCS of zero does not exclude patients with non-calcified plaque and coronary remodelling, both of which may be markers for an ↑ risk of plaque rupture.
- CCS >400 does not necessarily indicate obstructive coronary lesions; automatic referral of these patients for ICA may lead to a dramatic increase in the number of normal diagnostic angiograms and the rare but significant complications that may occur.
- CTA has actually been shown to be most cost-effective in patients with *intermediate* PTL of CAD.

2006 ESC stable angina guidelines

With regards to CTA, these guidelines are now relatively old. Nonetheless, the guidance suggests that CTA is indicated for the investigation of patients with chest pain who have a low PTL of CAD and non-conclusive exercise ECG or stress imaging test.

Further reading

Bluemke DA, Achenbach S, Budoff M, *et al.* (2008) Noninvasive coronary artery imaging: magnetic resonance angiography and multidetector computed tomography angiography: a scientific statement from the American Heart Association Committee on Cardiovascular Imaging and Intervention, Council on Cardiovascular Radiology and Intervention, and Committee on Cardiac Imaging, Council on Clinical Cardiology. *Circulation* **118**(5), 586–606.

Budoff MJ, Achenbach S, Blumenthal RS, *et al.* (2006) Assessment of coronary artery disease by cardiac computed tomography: a scientific statement from the American Heart Association Committee on Cardiovascular Imaging and Intervention, Council on Cardiovascular Radiology and Intervention, and Committee on Cardiac Imaging, Council on Clinical Cardiology. *Circulation* **14**(16), 1761–1791.

Budoff MJ, Cohen MC, Garcia MJ, *et al.* (2005) ACC/AHA clinical competence statement on cardiac imaging with computed tomography and magnetic resonance: a report of the American College of Cardiology Foundation/American Heart Association/American College of Physicians Task Force on Clinical Competence (ACC/AHA Committee on CV Tomography). *J Am Coll Cardiol* **46**, 383–402.

Cooper A, Calvert N, Skinner J, *et al.* (2010) Chest pain of recent onset: Assessment and diagnosis of recent onset chest pain or discomfort of suspected cardiac origin. National Clinical Guideline Centre for Acute and Chronic Conditions, London.

International Commission on Radiological Protection (2007) Managing patient dose in multi-detector computed tomography (MDCT), Publication 102. *Annals of the ICRP* **37**, 1.

Jacobs JE, Boxt LM, Desjardins B, *et al.* (2006) ACR Practice Guidelines for the Performance and Interpretation of Cardiac Computed Tomography. *J Am Coll Radiol* **3**(9), 677–685.

Mark DB, Berman DS, Budoff M, *et al.* (2010) ACCF/ACR/AHA/NASCI /SAIP/SCAI/SCCT 2010 expert consensus document on coronary computed tomographic angiography. *J Am Coll Cardiol* **55**, 2663–2699.

Schroeder S, Achenbach S, Bengel F, *et al.* (2008) Cardiac computed tomography: indications, applications, limitations, and training requirements: report of a Writing Group deployed by the Working Group Nuclear Cardiology and Cardiac CT of the European Society of Cardiology and the European Council of Nuclear Cardiology. *Eur Heart J* **29**(4), 531–556.

Taylor AJ, Cerqueira M, Hodgson JM, *et al.* (2010) ACCF/SCCT/ACR/AHA /ASE/ASNC/SCAI/ SCMR 2010 Appropriate Use Criteria for Cardiac Computed Tomography. *Circulation* **122**(21), e525–555.

Accreditation in cardiac CT

Although radiologists and cardiologists receive core training in cardiovascular physiology and imaging, CCT remains an emerging technique and gaining sufficient experience in CCT during basic training in either specialty is unusual. Specific training ∴ is recommended prior to independently performing CCT.

To this end, international levels of clinical competency have been established in the USA by the Society of Cardiovascular CT (SCCT), which are widely accepted as being appropriate. In the UK, the British Society of Cardiovascular Imaging (BSCI) has endorsed the principle that high standards of clinical training and competency are vital to ensure the appropriate use of CCT at acceptable radiation dosage. Accordingly the BSCI have produced a document that sets out the standards required to support best practice in CCT.*

Based on this guidance, both the BSCI and SCCT offer accreditation for individual clinicians. Although there are many courses offered for both level 1 and level 2 accreditation, ongoing clinical experience is increasingly required for all but the most basic level of accreditation.

Competency levels

Both the SCCT and BSCI recognize three broadly comparable levels of training and competency in CCT.

Level 1

This is an introductory level that is likely, in time, to form the basis of core training for both cardiologists and radiologists. To obtain level 1 accreditation one must:

- Undertake core lectures in CCT covering technical and clinical aspects, normal cross-sectional anatomy and common pathology
- Have exposure to at least 50 CT coronary angiograms with the opportunity to perform supervised/mentored interpretation.

Level 2

This is the minimum recommended level for independent performance and interpretation of CCT. Whilst this level of training can be considered an extension of level 1 training, the applicant is required to have a regular and on-going commitment to the reporting of scans post-accreditation. To obtain level 2 accreditation one must:

- Undertake further lectures in CCT, including technical and clinical aspects and more detailed pathological findings
- Have exposure to at least 150 CT coronary angiograms, including both enhanced and unenhanced scans; cases should include coronary calcium scoring and graft and stent cases, with the opportunity to perform supervised/mentored interpretation; opportunity to compare with other cardiac modalities is important to appreciate the relative strengths and weaknesses of CCT
- Demonstrate an ongoing commitment to CCT reporting.

Level 3

Applicants should be able to demonstrate not only considerable expertise in performing and interpreting CCT, but also of running a successful academic or clinical CCT unit. These individuals would be expected to be directly responsible for quality assurance and training of radiographers and other physicians. The requirements to gain level 3 accreditation are more stringent than lower levels. One must:

• Undertake further lectures in CCT, including detailed technical and clinical aspects involving extensive pathological findings and evidence of attendance at clinical meetings
• Have exposure to at least 300 CT coronary angiograms, including both enhanced and unenhanced scans; cases should include coronary calcium scoring, graft and stent cases, with the opportunity to be involved in scan acquisition, post-processing and reporting; opportunity to compare with other cardiac modalities is important to appreciate the relative strengths and weaknesses of CCT
• Demonstrate ongoing teaching and/or research involvement, either as a lecturer on a faculty teaching accredited courses or via publication of peer-reviewed research articles.

Logbook

For all levels, and for those wishing to apply for the certification exams (see 📖 Guidelines, accreditation, and certification, p. 455), it is good practice to maintain a logbook of cases for presentation to the relevant bodies. This should comprise:

Numerical listing of cases, including date and an anonymous identifier
Scan indication
Scan procedure, including type and scope of CCT examination
(e.g. native coronaries, bypass grafts, congenital, etc.)
Radiation dose (DLP)
Key findings
Supervisor.

Further reading

Budoff MJ, Achenbach S, Blumenthal RS, et al. (2006) Assessment of coronary artery disease by cardiac computed tomography: a scientific statement from the American Heart Association Committee on Cardiovascular Imaging and Intervention, Council on Cardiovascular Radiology and Intervention, and Committee on Cardiac Imaging, Council on Clinical Cardiology. *Circulation* **114**, 1761–1791.

Recommended Standards in ECG Gated Cardiac CT Training: British Society of Cardiac Imaging (BSCI) available at: 🔗 http://www.bsci.org.uk/accreditation.

Certification in cardiac CT

Separate from the process of accreditation, certification exams in CCT are available. At present, these are only available through US institutions: the Certification Board of Cardiovascular CT ($\wp$ www.CBCCT.org) or the American College of Radiology (Cardiac CT—Certificate of Advanced Proficiency, $\wp$ www.acr.org). Both examinations cover similar material, broadly in line with the contents of this book. Certification through these pathways demonstrates attainment of a certain level of experience (through eligibility criteria), and theoretical and clinical understanding (through computer-based examination). Passing the examination confers no special rights or privileges, nor does it qualify the successful candidate to practise CCT. It does not confer any post-nominal qualification (although the editors have seen it used as such, despite explicit guidelines to the contrary). At present, neither examination is formally recognized in Europe. However, the ESC now recognizes the examination of the Certification Board of Nuclear Cardiology, with successful candidates receiving an accreditation letter from the ESC. It is anticipated that the CCT certification exams will follow a similar path.

Eligibility

The reader is directed to the above websites for full details as there are variations in eligibility criteria both between the two examinations and within them, depending on the $1°$ specialty of the candidate.

For both, candidates must hold an unrestricted licence to practise medicine in their country of origin. They must also be board-certified in cardiology, nuclear medicine, or radiology. For UK candidates, full membership of the Royal College of Physicians or Fellowship of the Royal College of Radiology is sufficient.

Required CCT experience varies according to specialty. Presentation of a logbook (see 📖 Accreditation in cardiovascular CT, p. 462) as evidence of experience is usually required, along with written confirmation of experience from course or programme directors. Generally, the candidate should have been present and involved in the acquisition and interpretation of 150–500 cases, of which 50–75 should have been reported personally. Evidence of continuing medical education in CT is also required.

Examination

CBCCT

One hundred and seventy best-of-four multiple choice questions answered at a computer terminal over 4½ hours.

ACR CCT CoAP

Sixty best-of-x multiple choice questions and 12 radiology cases. The latter are answered by selecting appropriate findings on a 'Case Finding' form, similar to a standard radiology report. Questions are answered at a computer terminal over 4 hours.

Comparison of multimodality imaging

Introduction

CCT is currently the only non-invasive imaging modality able to image coronary anatomy reliably and directly. However, other cardiac imaging has been used to provide physiological information about the coronary circulation for at least 35 years, beginning with exercise radionuclide ventriculography (now seldom performed).

Currently, myocardial perfusion SPECT and stress echocardiography (echo) are extensively used worldwide and are very well validated. Myocardial perfusion PET and stress cardiac MRI are increasingly available in expert centres, and their evidence-base is growing.

Functional information is commonly used to assess the likelihood of flow-limiting coronary stenoses in patients with suspected CAD. By convention, the different techniques have been compared with ICA as the gold standard. In such terms, the diagnostic performance of CCT is undoubtedly superior to that of any functional imaging technique. This is not surprising given that CCT is an angiographic technique, but in no way negates the independent value of physiological information. The presence or absence of stress-induced hypoperfusion or LV wall motion abnormalities provides important symptomatic and prognostic information, even in patients with documented coronary stenoses.

CCT is seen by some as being in competition with the functional techniques. However, there are already data to suggest that in many patients a combination of non-invasive angiographic and physiological information, such as that provided by SPECT-CT or PET-CT scanner as a single investigation, provides a better overall assessment than either type of information alone. Nevertheless, there is certainly an element of competition between advocates of the various functional modalities, all of which provide roughly equivalent clinical information. None of these has yet emerged as clearly superior to all the others in both practical and clinical terms, and, for the moment, local expertise tends to determine which is/are favoured in a given institution.

To understand the role, place, and timing of cardiovascular CT imaging in the assessment and management of cardiac patients, it is important to recognize the value and limitations of currently available techniques. This chapter summarizes these alternative techniques; for more in-depth information the reader is directed to the relevant dedicated *Oxford Specialist Handbook in Cardiology*.

Basis of functional imaging: coronary physiology and stress testing

Normal coronary anatomy and physiology

The coronary arterial system consists of two functional parts:
- Epicardial coronary arteries—range in diameter from several millimetres down to about 400μm; do not normally exert significant resistance to blood flow
- Microvasculature—arterioles and capillaries; modulate blood flow by varying their resistance over a five-fold range.

In contrast to most tissues, myocardial oxygen extraction is high (approximately 60%) at rest and cannot increase significantly when demand increases during exercise. The necessary increase in myocardial oxygen uptake can only be achieved by a virtually linear increase in myocardial perfusion (Fig. 31.1).

Coronary physiology in the presence of epicardial stenoses

In the presence of a significant epicardial coronary stenosis, the arterioles distal to the lesion vasodilate to compensate for the resistance it offers. Myocardial perfusion at rest remains normal until an epicardial stenosis is severe (80–85% by diameter, 60–80% by area).

The use of vasodilator reserve to maintain resting perfusion limits the maximal coronary flow that can be achieved during exercise, to a degree that depends on the severity of the stenosis. Thus stress perfusion becomes heterogeneous in the presence of significant coronary disease, with myocardium subtended by stenosed arteries achieving lower levels than myocardium subtended by unobstructed arteries.

The mismatch between increasing myocardial oxygen demand and limited vasodilator reserve leads to metabolic ischaemia, myocardial diastolic and systolic dysfunction, ischaemic ECG changes, and anginal symptoms: the so-called 'ischaemic cascade'.

Elements of the ischaemic cascade can be imaged using a number of imaging modalities:
- Inducible perfusion abnormalities: SPECT, PET, myocardial contrast echo, perfusion CMR
- Inducible myocardial wall motion abnormalities: echo, CMR.

Effects of pharmacological stress on coronary blood flow

When dynamic exercise is impractical for clinical or technical reasons, cardiac stress can be achieved pharmacologically using:
- 1° vasodilator (dipyridamole or adenosine)
- Inotrope (dobutamine)

Vasodilator drugs provoke a four- to fivefold increase in flow within a normal coronary territory, in the absence of any direct effect on myocardial oxygen demand. Such agents are most suitable in combination with modalities that image myocardial perfusion rather than wall motion, as they only rarely provoke metabolic ischaemia.

Dobutamine, like exercise, provokes coronary vasodilatation as a 2° effect of ↑ myocardial oxygen demand, and smaller increases in flow are achieved (two- to threefold). This drug is ∴ preferred in combination with modalities which depend on the induction of myocardial ischaemia and contractile dysfunction.

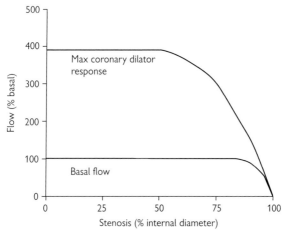

Fig. 31.1 Relationship between coronary stenosis severity and flow at rest and during maximal coronary vasodilatation.

Cardiac stress for functional imaging

Dynamic exercise

Exercise is the most physiological form of stress and provides important clinical information that may complement imaging findings.

- Treadmill exercise is most commonly performed according to the Bruce or modified Bruce protocols (Table 31.1).
- Bicycle ergometer exercise can be performed in upright, supine, or semisupine positions, with the patient typically pedalling at a constant 50rpm against increasing workload (e.g. starting at 25W and increasing by 25W every 2–3min).

Adequate stress is taken to be:

- Sustained achievement of target heart rate, i.e. 85% of maximum predicted heart rate (220 – age for males, 210 – age for females); or
- Limiting chest pain.

Otherwise pharmacological stress is preferable.

Vasodilator drugs

Dipyridamole and adenosine are $1°$ coronary arteriolar dilators. Adenosine acts directly via A_{2a}-receptors. Dipyridamole raises extracellular levels of endogenous adenosine by inhibiting reuptake into cells.

Adenosine is given as a continuous infusion at 140mcg/kg/min, typically for 6min, which produces maximal hyperaemia in 92% of subjects within 1–2min. Plasma half-life is very short (10s) due to avid uptake by red blood cells.

Dipyridamole is given as an injection at 0.56mg/kg over 4min. Maximal hyperaemia occurs 3–4min after injection. Plasma half-life is 20–30min, so its actions are more prolonged than with adenosine.

Important contraindications/complications of vasodilator drugs are:

- Proven asthma/risk of A3-mediated bronchoconstriction
- Unpaced second- or third-degree heart block/risk of A1-mediated AV-nodal blockade.

Dobutamine

Dobutamine is a positive chronotrope and inotrope via β-1- and α-1-adrenoceptor stimulation.

Dobutamine is given as a continuous infusion, typically commencing at 10mcg/kg/min and increasing by 10mcg/kg/min every 3min to a peak of 40mcg/kg/min. Lower doses (2.5 and 5mcg/kg/min) are used when looking for contractile reserve in suspected hibernating myocardium. Boluses of atropine may be given to achieve target heart rate. Dobutamine has a plasma half-life of approximately 2min due to rapid metabolism in the liver.

Contraindications to dobutamine are similar to exercise. Dobutamine is more dysrhythmogenic than other forms of stress, and caution is necessary in patients known to have severe LV impairment.

Table 31.1 Bruce and modified Bruce treadmill protocols

Stage	Time (min)	Speed (mph)	Slope (%)
0 (mod)	3	1.7	0
½ (mod)	3	1.7	5
1	3	1.7	10
2	3	2.5	12
3	3	3.4	14
4	3	4.2	16
5	3	5.0	18
6	3	5.5	20
7	3	6.0	22

Myocardial perfusion single photon emission CT (1)

Overview

A radiopharmaceutical perfusion tracer is injected during cardiac stress, and is taken up and retained by cardiac myocytes in relation to blood flow. Subsequent imaging is performed on an Anger gamma camera, and the distribution of radionuclide reflects myocardial viability and perfusion at the time of tracer injection, i.e. during stress. A separate imaging study is performed after injection of tracer at rest (technetium-99m-labelled tracers) or following redistribution of the stress injection (thallium-201). The resting distribution of radionuclide primarily reflects viability. An area of reduced stress uptake but normal resting uptake (inducible perfusion defect) indicates viable myocardium supplied through a flow-limiting coronary stenosis. An area of reduced stress *and* rest uptake (fixed perfusion defect) indicates scar following myocardial infarction.

Radiopharmaceutical perfusion tracers

A radiopharmaceutical has both chemical and physical properties, which determine its physiological and imaging characteristics, respectively. Three radiopharmaceuticals are in routine clinical use in myocardial perfusion SPECT:

- Thallium-201 (^{201}Tl) as thallous chloride
- Technetium-99m (^{99m}Tc) sestamibi
- Technetium-99m (^{99m}Tc) tetrofosmin.

The properties of these tracers are summarized in Table 31.2.

^{201}Tl has the best physiological characteristics, as its myocardial uptake is most linearly related to perfusion during stress, whilst its ability to redistribute at rest provides an assessment of viability that is independent of perfusion. The ^{99m}Tc tracers have superior physical characteristics, producing higher energy photons for optimal gamma camera imaging, with a relatively short half-life and hence a lower radiation exposure for a given administered activity.

The Anger gamma camera

Crystal

The key component of a gamma camera is a large flat circular or rectangular sodium iodide crystal, activated by non-radioactive thallium, NaI(Tl). The crystal is a 'scintillator', i.e. absorption of a gamma photon via the photoelectric effect yields a burst of photons of visible light within 1mm of the interaction.

Photomultiplier tubes

The side of the crystal away from the patient is viewed by a hexagonal array of up to 100 photomultiplier tubes (PMTs). These convert the weak signal carried by photons of visible light leaving the crystal into a detectable electrical pulse. The pattern of activation of PMTs signals the location of the originating scintillation event, with the largest electrical pulse being generated in the PMT closest to the event.

Collimators

The side of the crystal facing the patient is shielded by a parallel-hole collimator, a lead disc penetrated by thousands of uniform parallel channels separated by thin septa. Only photons travelling perpendicular to the collimator can penetrate the channels and enter the crystal, whilst the remainder are absorbed by the lead septa. Thus gamma-photons originating from a particular area of the heart can only enter a selected area of the NaI(Tl) crystal, maintaining spatial information.

Table 31.2 Comparison of available radiopharmaceuticals used in MPS

	^{201}Tl	^{99m}Tc-labelled tracers
Decay	Electron capture	Isomeric transition to ^{99}Tc
Main photon	X-ray 68–80keV	Gamma 140keV
Physical $t_{1/2}$	73h	6h
Effective dose equivalent (UK)	18mSv	8–10mSv
Production	Commercial cyclotron	Pharmaceutical labelled with ^{99m}Tc from generator
Chemical properties	Monovalent cation (K$^+$ analogue)	Lipophilic monovalent cation
	Enters myocytes down electrochemical gradient	Enters myocytes down electrochemical gradient
First-pass extraction fraction	0.85	Sestamibi 0.65
		Tetrofosmin 0.54
Myocardial retention	Redistributes at rest	Bound in mitochondria: no redistribution
Excretion	Renal	Hepatobiliary
Typical protocol (UK doses)	80MBq stress injection	Two-day: 400MBq stress and rest injections
	Immediate post-stress imaging	One-day stress-rest or rest-stress: 250MBq then 750MBq injections
	Redistribution imaging at 4h	Imaging 15–45min post injection
	(40MBq may be reinjected at rest to optimize viability assessment)	(Sublingual GTN may be given before rest injection to optimize viability assessment)

Myocardial perfusion single photon emission CT (2)

Single photon emission CT image acquisition and display

Acquisition and summation of scintillations by the head of a gamma camera for a few minutes yields a planar scan that represents the 3D distribution of radiopharmaceutical within a patient as a 2D image.

- SPECT imaging involves the acquisition of a series of planar projections at different angles as the head(s) of the gamma camera orbit(s) the patient.
- A dual-headed camera is preferred, with the heads positioned at 90° to one another to halve acquisition time.
- A typical acquisition might involve 64 projections (32 per head) acquired over a 180° orbit and take 16min.

Filtered back-projection or iterative reconstruction is used to produce a set of transaxial sections through the patient. The transaxial slices can then be reorientated to the axes of the heart to produce vertical long-axis, horizontal long-axis, and short-axis slices. The count density of each pixel within the reorientated slices is displayed relative to the pixel of maximal counts in the myocardium (0–100%) using a grey scale or colour spectrum. Stress slices are displayed above corresponding rest slices to facilitate comparison.

Gated single photon emission CT

SPECT acquisitions can be 'gated' to the electrocardiogram. The R–R interval is divided into 8 or 16 frames, and each planar projection is acquired as 8 or 16 corresponding images. Each frame is reconstructed and reorientated separately to produce SPECT slices that represent the left ventricle at a particular point in the cardiac cycle. Static slices to assess perfusion can be obtained from the same acquisition by summing the frames for each planar projection.

Gated slices can be viewed in a looped cine format to assess regional function in terms of wall excursion and thickening. Commercially available software is used to fit endocardial and epicardial boundaries and determine end-diastolic volume, end-systolic volume, and ejection fraction.

Attenuation correction

Gamma photons emitted from the heart are variably attenuated by soft tissue. This can produce spurious apparent perfusion abnormalities in the processed slices (attenuation artifacts). Many modern gamma cameras allow attenuation correction (AC). A *transmission* acquisition is performed using one or more scanning gadolinium sources or X-ray CT, and an attenuation map is reconstructed. This is used to correct the *emission* acquisition, which is acquired simultaneously (gadolinium approach) or separately (CT approach).

Myocardial perfusion single photon emission CT in clinical practice

MPS is a well-established technique for the assessment of CAD and the detection of myocardial ischaemia. MPS provides a functional rather than an anatomical evaluation of the significance of coronary stenosis, which guides clinical decision-making with regard to the need for coronary revascularization.

Clinical indications

- Detection and estimation of the extent and severity of obstructive CAD.
- Assessment of myocardial viability and hibernation.
- Assessment of the functional significance of non-atherosclerotic causes of myocardial ischaemia (e.g. anomalous coronary arteries, myocardial bridging).
- Initial assessment of patients with acute chest pain and non-specific ECG changes (popular in the USA, less so in the UK).

Diagnosis of coronary artery disease

- MPS is best performed in symptomatic patients with intermediate pre-test probability of angiographically significant disease according to Diamond and Forrester criteria.[1]
- Within this category, it is considered the first-line diagnostic test in patients unable to exercise, in women, and in patients with diabetes or conduction abnormalities on their resting ECG (NICE recommendations at http://guidance.nice.org.uk/TA73).
- MPS allows further stratification into low- or high-risk categories, and adds incremental prognostic value to clinical history, exercise ECG, and even coronary angiography.
- MPS may also be indicated in patients with low or high pre-test probability of disease and previous inconclusive tests or unexpected results.

Patients with known coronary artery disease

MPS may be performed to:
- Document the site, extent, and severity of inducible ischaemia in patients with recurrence or exacerbation of anginal symptoms.
- Assess the functional significance of angiographic disease, particularly in the presence of angiographically moderate coronary artery stenosis.
- Assess and risk-stratify patients after PCI or CABG, particularly those with diabetes, incomplete revascularization, proximal left anterior descending CAD, or other high-risk factors; the value of MPS in this setting relies on its ability to determine the site and severity of ischaemia, an important consideration for further management that cannot be assessed accurately by the exercise ECG.
- Determine the total ischaemic burden and hence the need for revascularization after an uncomplicated acute coronary syndrome.

Advantages of myocardial perfusion scintigraphy

- High sensitivity and specificity for the detection of CAD (83–91%, and 71–94%, respectively[2]).
- Powerful prognostic tool that helps distinguish patients at low risk for coronary events (<1%/year) from those at ↑ risk who may benefit from more aggressive medical therapy and/or intervention.
- Highly cost-effective strategy that directs ICA to patients more likely to benefit from revascularization.

Limitations of myocardial perfusion scintigraphy

- Image quality and interpretation can be affected by photon scatter, photon absorption, and patient motion during the acquisition; impact on the final images can be minimized by applying the appropriate reconstruction algorithms.
- Exposure to ionizing radiation: effective dose equivalent varies from 6 to 21mSv depending on patient characteristics, imaging protocol, and radionuclide used.
- At the doses currently administered in the UK, the individual risk of malignancy associated with radiation exposure during MPS is small.
- Preliminary studies using new-generation camera systems have shown that radiation exposure can be reduced significantly, with total exposures as low as 3–4mSv being achievable for a complete ECG-gated stress–rest myocardial perfusion study.

Further reading

1 Diamond GA and Forrester JS (1079) Analysis of probability as an aid in the clinical diagnosis of coronary-artery disease. *N Engl J Med* **300**, 1350–1358.

2 Underwood SR, Anagnostopoulos C, Cerqueira M, *et al.* (2004) Myocardial perfusion scintigraphy: the evidence. *Eur J Nucl Med Mol Imaging* **31**, 261–291.

Myocardial perfusion positron emission tomography (PET)

Overview

A PET perfusion tracer is injected at rest and is taken up and retained by cardiac myocytes in relation to blood flow. Immediate imaging is performed on a PET camera. A separate imaging study is performed immediately after injection of tracer during pharmacological stress. PET has many principles in common with SPECT, although different radiopharmaceuticals and imaging hardware are used.

Two important developments have generated particular interest in cardiac PET:
- Availability of rubidium-82 (^{82}Rb) generators, making perfusion imaging practical without an on-site cyclotron
- Availability of PET cameras and commercially produced 18F-fluorodeoxyglucose (^{18}F-FDG) to service oncological imaging.

Positron emission tomography tracers

Two PET perfusion tracers are in clinical use for perfusion imaging:
- ^{13}N-ammonia
- Rubidium-82 (^{82}Rb)

^{13}N-ammonia can only be used in a centre with an on-site cyclotron, which restricts its use in routine clinical imaging.

^{82}Rb is obtained from a commercially available generator with a working life of 4 weeks, giving it broader applicability. ^{82}Rb has a half-life of only 75s and is eluted from the generator and administered directly to the patient. The resting study is performed first, with stress 10–15min later.

^{18}F-fluorodeoxyglucose (^{18}F-FDG) is a metabolic tracer, the myocardial uptake of which demonstrates myocardial viability. The relatively long half-life of ^{18}F (110min) allows ^{18}F-FDG to be commercially produced and distributed, without the need for an on-site cyclotron.

Positron emission tomography camera

A PET camera consists of a series of circular or hexagonal arrays of scintillation detectors, each of which is paired via a coincidence circuit with a large number of detectors on the opposite side.

The radionuclides used in PET decay by positron ('anti-electron') emission. Within a short distance, positrons annihilate by combining with an electron, producing two 511keV gamma-photons travelling in opposite directions (180° apart). If each of a pair of detectors simultaneously registers a scintillation event (coincidence), positron annihilation is assumed to have occurred along a narrow corridor between the two detectors. Coincidence detection is ∴ able to localize the site of decay within the patient without collimation.

Attenuation is a bigger problem in PET than in SPECT, as both annihilation photons must reach a detector for a coincidence to be registered. Attenuation correction is ∴ essential in PET, and is achieved using a rotating line source (germanium-68 or cesium-137) or X-ray CT (Fig. 31.2).

Myocardial perfusion positron emission tomography in clinical practice

Cardiac PET remains the standard reference for quantitative assessment of myocardial perfusion and detection of viability. However, high costs and limited availability of dedicated scanners are major barriers to the widespread use of PET in clinical practice.

Hybrid devices that incorporate high-speed multi-detector CT along with SPECT or PET detector systems can provide a one-stop shop for the evaluation of patients with known or suspected CAD by allowing simultaneous anatomical and functional assessment. However, the application of such devices in routine practice remains to be elucidated.

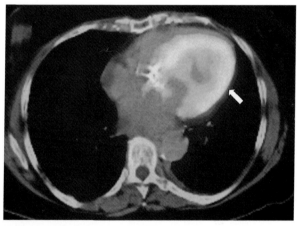

Fig. 31.2 Attenuation correction of myocardial perfusion PET. The PET image (arrow) is registered with the chest CT; attenuation values from the latter are used to correct the former. (📖 Plate 14 for colour version).

Radionuclide ventriculography

Radionuclide ventriculography (RNV) has largely been superseded by echocardiography and MRI for the assessment of cardiac function. However, it remains the preferred method in cases where accurate and reproducible measurements of LV function are essential for planning further management (e.g. monitoring cardiac effects of cardiotoxic drugs).

During RNV, radiolabelled erythrocytes are imaged during first-pass through the heart or after reaching equilibrium with the blood pool (Fig. 31.3). The latter is the most widely used technique, although the former is occasionally useful in the evaluation of intracardiac shunts. Equilibrium RNV may be used to assess LV function in response to increasing workload during dynamic exercise.

In the UK, radiation exposure during radionuclide ventriculography is ~6mSv for the recommended dose of 800MBq of 99mTc-pertechnetate.

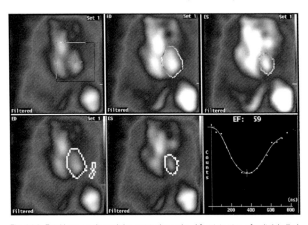

Fig. 31.3 Equilibrium radionuclide ventriculography. After injection of radiolabelled erythrocytes, a region of interest is selected around the left ventricle (top left) and the endocardial contour traced in end-diastole (top middle) and end-systole (top right). After correction for background counts, LVEF may be calculated by comparing counts within the left ventricle in end-diastole and end-systole (bottom row). (☐ Plate 15 for colour version).

Echocardiography

Echocardiography remains the most important non-invasive imaging modality in clinical cardiology. It is the test of first choice for the assessment of cardiac anatomy, ventricular function, and valve physiology. It has become the most widely used diagnostic technique because of its high accuracy, real-time capabilities, low costs, portability, and tolerability.

Echo machine

Ultrasound transducer

The key component of an ultrasound (echo) machine is the transducer or probe. This contains a piezoelectric crystal (lead zirconate-titanate) cut into thin slices, each wired individually. A piezoelectric material mechanically deforms when an electrical potential is applied, and generates an electrical potential when deformed. Application of a voltage causes the slices to vibrate at a frequency determined by their dimensions, typically 1.5–7MHz, with the production of ultrasound waves. The same slices vibrate in response to returning ultrasound waves of appropriate frequency, with generation of a voltage.

By comparing the frequency of transmitted sound waves with the returned wave frequency reflected off moving blood cells, Doppler imaging allows estimation of blood flow velocity, direction, and quality (laminar vs turbulent), and hence the assessment of valve disease, ventricular outflow tract obstruction, septal defects, and vascular stenosis (e.g. coarctation, pulmonary artery branch stenosis).

Image formation

The transducer generates a beam of 1–2µs ultrasound pulses, which are transmitted into the thorax through an aqueous gel. Pulses encounter a series of tissue interfaces, each of which reflects a proportion of the incident energy back to the transducer. The delays between emission of an ultrasound pulse and detection of its echoes allow the depths of the reflecting interfaces to be determined:

$$\text{depth} = \tfrac{1}{2} \times \text{propagation velocity} \times \text{echo delay}$$

In a phased array transducer, the small ultrasound wavelets from each crystal slice combine to form a compound wave. Varying the activation sequence of the crystal slices causes the compound wave to sweep rapidly backwards and forwards across a sector of the heart. A 2D real-time image can be constructed from the series of radial lines which comprise the sector, with depth and intensity information being provided by the delay and amplitude of the returning echoes.

Most examinations include single-dimension or M-mode (motion mode), 2D (cross-sectional), and Doppler imaging. Although 3D echocardiography may overcome some of the shortcomings of 2D imaging, it has yet to become part of the routine echocardiographic examination.

Progressive improvements in ultrasound processing have led to greatly improved image quality, which has made stress echo (see 📖 Comparison of multimodality imaging, p. 465) increasingly reliable. An important recent refinement has been harmonic imaging, where the image is formed from the second harmonic of the transmitted ultrasound frequency. This offers improved spatial resolution with no loss of penetration and reduces imaging artefacts.

Standard views

Ultrasound transmission is obstructed by the ribs and lungs. TTE is ∴ restricted to a limited number of acoustic 'windows' (most importantly at the lower left sternal edge and apex). Images are acquired as a series of standardized 2D digital cine loops, triggered by the electrocardiogram.

Transoesophageal echocardiography

Although the transthoracic method is more common, TOE may be indicated in cases of limited transthoracic access. Particular applications of TOE include diagnosis of prosthetic valve endocarditis, intracardiac thrombi or other source of systemic emboli, aortic dissection, and intra-operatively during valve surgery, especially during mitral valve repair.

Echocardiography in clinical practice

Indications

- Assessment of global and regional left ventricular function.
  - Visual assessment and quantification of LV volumes and function forms the basis for the majority of referrals.
  - Quantification of volumes and function relies on geometric assumptions and hence may result in inaccurate measurements, particularly in the presence of regional abnormalities of contractile function or significant distortion of normal ventricular morphology.
  - Suboptimal image quality can be improved by using contrast agents to enhance the LV endocardial border.
  - Other applications of contrast echocardiography include visual enhancement of regurgitant jets and assessment of myocardial perfusion.
- Evaluation of valve anatomy and function.
- Diagnosis of pericardial effusion and cardiac tamponade.
- Evaluation of constrictive and restrictive disorders of the heart.
- Assessment of cardiac morphology (e.g. congenital heart disease).
  - The site of origin and proximal course of the main coronary arteries can be visualized on standard echocardiography, although TOE may be required; echocardiography may ∴ be indicated in the assessment of suspected anomalous coronary arteries, although CTA may be preferred.
- Diagnosis of obstructive coronary artery disease (stress echo; see 🕮 Stress echocardiography, p. 486).

Advantages of echocardiography

- Rapid and reliable method for visual and quantitative assessment of cardiac morphology and function.
- Safe, well-tolerated technique that can be performed in almost every subject almost anywhere.
- No documented adverse effects from exposure to current ultrasound frequencies.

Limitations of echocardiography

- Diagnostic yield depends greatly on image quality.
- Non-diagnostic images are common in cases of poor tissue penetration or limited access; TOE or other imaging modalities may be considered.
- Artefacts and unusual anatomical arrangements may also interfere with interpretation and result in misdiagnosis.

Stress echocardiography

Overview

The combination of echocardiography with cardiac stress testing provides an accurate method for the diagnosis of obstructive CAD by detecting ischaemia-induced changes of regional myocardial contractile function. In patients with CAD and LV impairment, stress echocardiography is useful in the assessment of myocardial viability and hibernation.

Myocardial thickening and excursion are imaged using an echo machine at rest in standard transthoracic views. An echo contrast agent is frequently used to optimize endocardial border definition. Identical views are acquired at each stage of (ergometer exercise, dobutamine) or immediately after (treadmill) cardiac stress.

A resting regional wall motion abnormality suggests previous infarction, or occasionally stunned or hibernating myocardium. An inducible wall motion abnormality developing during stress suggests regional ischaemia. A resting wall motion abnormality that improves with low-dose dobutamine indicates the presence of viable myocardium; deterioration at higher doses ('biphasic response') suggests hibernating myocardium.

Standard views

Ultrasound transmission is obstructed by the ribs and lungs. TTE is ∴ restricted to a limited number of acoustic 'windows' (most importantly at the lower left sternal edge and apex). Images are acquired as a series of standardized 2D digital cine loops, triggered by the ECG.

Loops are obtained at rest and at each stage of, or immediately after, cardiac stress (Fig. 31.4). Some operators acquire parasternal long and short and apical four-chamber and two-chamber views. Others acquire apical four-chamber, two-chamber and three-chamber views, perhaps using the multiplane function of a 3D probe to minimize imaging time. In any event, it is important that identically orientated images are obtained throughout, and that all LV segments are imaged on at least one view. Modern software allows loops of each view to be saved in a predetermined order at each stage. Ideally the baseline loop of a given view is displayed alongside the live imaging to ensure equivalent positioning.

Transpulmonary echo contrast agents

Excellent image quality with clear delineation of the endocardial border of all myocardial segments is essential for reliable stress echo. Echo contrast agents allow this to be achieved even in patients with suboptimal imaging windows. These consist of a suspension of microbubbles, each composed of an inert fluorine-based gas bounded by an albumin or phospholipid shell. These bubbles are highly reflective of ultrasound, and being the size of red blood cells can traverse the pulmonary microvasculature. Thus they can opacify the LVr blood pool following intravenous injection, providing excellent contrast between the endocardium and the blood (Fig. 31.5).

Two echo contrast agents are currently available in the UK:
- Optison (GE Healthcare)
- SonoVue (Bracco).

The contrast agent is reconstituted in a vial and needs to be regularly agitated to avoid settling of the microbubbles. It is given as a series of boluses (typically 0.2–0.4mL with harmonic imaging) or as an infusion. Low-power imaging is used to reduce destruction of bubbles by the ultrasound beam.

In skilled hands, echo contrast agents can be used to image myocardial perfusion as well as wall motion. However, this is technically demanding and echo myocardial perfusion cannot yet be regarded as a routine investigation beyond a small number of expert centres.

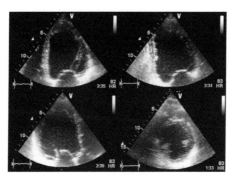

Fig. 31.4 Standard baseline images acquired in the (clockwise from top left) apical four-chamber, apical two-chamber, apical three-chamber and parasternal short-axis views.

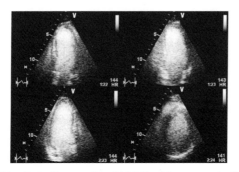

Fig. 31.5 In patients with poor endocardial definition, intravenous contrast bubbles are used to further delineate the endocardial border as in this example at peak stress.

Cardiovascular magnetic resonance imaging

CMR is a high-resolution, cross-sectional imaging technique that has been used increasingly in clinical cardiology over the last decade. It is a versatile diagnostic tool that can provide a comprehensive assessment of patients with suspected or known cardiovascular disease in a single examination.

Technical aspects

CMR is conceptually more complex than the other imaging modalities; a full understanding requires advanced knowledge of quantum mechanics.

Magnet

The patient lies within an electromagnet comprising a superconducting niobium-titanium wire bathed in liquid helium. This generates a powerful uniform magnetic field (1.5T for most current clinical scanners; 3T scanners are starting to be installed). The magnetic moments of the hydrogen nuclei (protons) within the patient align in the direction of the field.

Radiofrequency coils

The RF coils emit pulses of RF waves which are absorbed by the protons and cause them to change their alignment. The RF frequency required for this to occur is given by the equation

$$frequency = (magnetogyric\ ratio \times local\ field\ strength)/2\pi$$

As they return to equilibrium, the protons resonate and emit RF waves at a frequency determined by the field strength at the time of emission (e.g. 64MHz for a 1.5T scanner). These are detected by the RF coils.

Gradient coils

Spatial information in CMR is provided by varying the magnetic field strength across the patient in a graded manner, by turning gradient coils on and off. A magnetic gradient is applied along a given axis, so that each plane along that axis has a characteristic and different resonant frequency. A specific plane can ∴ be excited by a 90° RF pulse of appropriate frequency. Subsequent application of a magnetic gradient parallel to the plane causes the protons to resonate at decreasing frequency with reducing field strength across the plane. This codes spatial information.

Differences in intensity within the imaging plane depend on variations in the concentration of resonating nuclei, and also their magnetic relaxation times: T1 (longitudinal), T2 (transverse), and $T2^*$ ('effective T2'). A carefully chosen pattern of RF pulses can be used to emphasize differences in these relaxation times within the body, and hence provide excellent soft tissue contrast within the images.

Most acquisitions are ECG-gated to minimize artefact due to cardiac motion. In addition and whenever possible, breath-holding is performed to prevent the degrading effect of respiratory motion on the images.

Gadolinium chelates

Gadolinium (Gd^{3+}) is a lanthanide element and highly paramagnetic, making it an excellent CMR contrast agent. Once injected intravenously, it distributes throughout the intravascular and interstitial space, enhancing signal intensity. Free Gd^{3+} is toxic, so for clinical use it must be complexed with one of a number of chelators, which can be linear or macrocyclic, ionic or non-ionic. At least nine products are commercially available. Gd^{3+} substantially shortens T1 relaxation time, hence its distribution can be imaged with appropriate T1-weighted imaging sequences.

The main applications of contrast CMR are:
- Tissue characterization, especially for assessment of cardiomyopathies
- Prediction of improvement of ischaemic LV dysfunction
- Contrast-enhanced angiography
- Stress CMR (see 📖 Stress cardiovascular magnetic resonance imaging, p. 494).

Advantages
- No ionizing radiation.
- Alternative to the radionuclide techniques in children, women of child-bearing age, and in those undergoing sequential studies who may otherwise receive a significant cumulative radiation dose.
- Avoids the use of iodinated contrast agents (although gadolinium chelates are not without risk, see below).
- Safe procedure; no adverse events related to exposure to a high-strength magnetic field (≤1.5T) have been described.

Limitations
- CMR should be avoided in patients with ferromagnetic implants.
- Allergic reactions may occur after injection of gadolinium chelates but they are usually mild and well-tolerated.
- Nephrogenic systemic fibrosis (NSF), a disorder characterized by fibrotic changes of the skin and other organs, has recently been ascribed to administration of gadolinium chelates.
- Patients with renal impairment are at ↑ risk of developing NSF and hence evaluation of renal function (i.e. serum creatinine levels, estimated glomerular filtration rate) before gadolinium injection is recommended in all patients undergoing contrast CMR.
- CMR machines feature a long tunnel with a narrow bore and may ∴ be unsuitable for patients with claustrophobia.
- Limited data on the prognostic power and impact of CMR on patient management.
- Constrained by high cost and limited availability.

Cardiovascular magnetic resonance in clinical practice

Indications

- Initial evaluation and follow-up of patients with complex congenital heart disease.
  - CMR is the gold standard for anatomical, morphological, and blood flow assessments in CHD. As the technique involves no ionizing radiation, it is suitable for serial assessments to evaluate progression and/or treatment response.
  - As for CTA, evaluation of anomalous coronary arteries is an indication for CMR. The lack of radiation exposure lends support to CMR, but the technique is not straightforward and visualization of the mid and distal coronary artery segments can be problematic. Currently, this condition remains within the domain of CTA unless the clinical question concerns only the origin and/or proximal course of the main coronary arteries.
- Quantification and monitoring of ventricular function in patients with heart failure or suspected ventricular dysfunction, especially in cases of limited echocardiographic access or inconclusive or unexpected results.
  - CMR, an examination that is free from geometric assumptions, is currently the reference standard for quantification of ventricular volumes, function, and mass. Because of its high interstudy reproducibility, CMR represents a reliable approach to sequential imaging in order to monitor changes in ventricular function and response to therapy.
- As part of the diagnostic workup of cardiomyopathy and myocarditis.
  - Comprehensive evaluation of patients with suspected cardiomyopathy involves the use of tissue characterization protocols and contrast enhancement.
  - This enables the detection of myocardial fibrosis and inflammation as well as infiltrative processes of the heart.
  - Given their characteristic appearances on CMR, several non-ischaemic causes of LV dysfunction and life-threatening dysrhythmias can be identified (Fig. 31.6), including:
    — Hypertrophic cardiomyopathy
    — Cardiac amyloidosis
    — Anderson–Fabry disease
    — Sarcoidosis
    — Arrythmogenic RV cardiomyopathy.

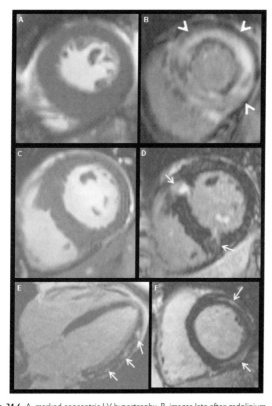

Fig. 31.6 A, marked concentric LV hypertrophy. B, images late after gadolinium injection show diffuse subendocardial enhancement (arrow heads). This pattern is characteristic of cardiac amyloidosis. C and D, mid-ventricular short-axis views before and after gadolinium injection in an asymptomatic subject with known mutation of myosin-binding protein C. They show asymmetrical septal hypertrophy with transmural fibrosis at the anteroseptal and inferoseptal walls (arrows). This appearance is most typical of hypertrophic cardiomyopathy. E and F, dilated left ventricle with widespread patchy subendocardial enhancement in the inferolateral, lateral, and anterolateral walls (arrows) consistent with myocarditis in a patient presenting with a history of acute viral illness and chest pain, ST-segment elevation on resting ECG, and troponin rise but normal X-ray coronary angiogram.

- Prediction of functional recovery after coronary revascularization in patients with coronary artery disease and left ventricular impairment.
  - In patients with known or suspected CAD, accurate characterization of myocardial infarction is possible with late contrast enhancement.
  - CMR is superior to other imaging techniques for the detection of small subendocardial infarcts because of its higher spatial resolution.
  - Stress CMR (see 📖 Stress cardiovascular magnetic resonance imaging, p. 494) allows evaluation of myocardial ischaemia.
  - CMR may help guide further management of patients early after an acute coronary syndrome by demonstrating the presence and extent of myocardial damage, areas of 'no-reflow', and jeopardized viable myocardium.
- Diagnosis and characterization of cardiac valve disease.
  - Although echocardiography is the technique of choice in the evaluation of cardiac valve disease, CMR can provide additional information and is especially indicated in cases of poor acoustic windows or discrepant findings.
  - CMR provides a reliable method of estimating the severity of valve stenosis and regurgitation, and compares favourably with conventional echocardiography.
  - More importantly, CMR may help identify the underlying mechanism of valve dysfunction as well as associated functional and morphological changes of prognostic importance (e.g. aortic dissection and myocardial fibrosis in aortic regurgitation).
- Diagnosis and characterization of cardiac masses.
- Assessment of vascular morphology with the acquisition of three-dimensional datasets during magnetic resonance angiography.

Stress cardiovascular magnetic resonance imaging

Stress CMR can be performed using stress agents suitable for the detection of either inducible wall motion abnormalities or heterogeneous myocardial perfusion.

Stress cardiac cardiovascular magnetic resonance imaging for wall motion

- Resting CMR study performed.
- Dobutamine stress within scanner.
- Cine loops obtained at each level: typically three short-axis and three long-axis views.
- Interpretation analogous to stress echo.

Stress cardiac cardiovascular magnetic resonance imaging for perfusion

- Resting CMR study performed.
- Dipyridamole or adenosine stress within scanner.
- Intravenous injection of gadolinium chelate paramagnetic contrast agent 0.05mmol/kg.
- First-pass perfusion imaging with strong T1 contrast, adequate coverage of the LV myocardium, and adequate spatial resolution: typically, three to four short-axis slices are acquired per R–R interval during the first pass and washout of contrast.
- Separate resting perfusion study at least 10min after stress study.
- Repeat imaging at least 5min after rest perfusion study to assess late gadolinium enhancement.
- Interpretation analogous to SPECT/PET, with inducible and fixed perfusion defects (Fig. 31.7), moreover:
  - Superior spatial resolution allows transmural extent of perfusion defects to be defined
  - Late gadolinium enhancement defines scar.

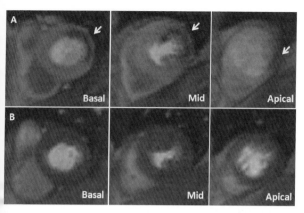

Fig. 31.7 Basal, mid, and apical ventricular short-axis views during perfusion CMR with intravenous adenosine. The stress (A) and resting (B) images show an extensive inducible perfusion abnormality involving the lateral wall (arrows) in a 58-year-old male with suspected angina.

Practical aspects of imaging techniques: infrastructure requirements

Imaging hardware

The scanners or cameras required for non-invasive imaging in CAD vary greatly in availability, the space required to accommodate them, and cost.

CT scanners
- Multidetector scanners now available in most radiology departments.
- Require significant space with appropriate shielding.
- Expensive.

Gamma cameras
- Available in any hospital with a nuclear medicine department.
- General purpose cameras similar in size to CT scanner, but dedicated cardiac cameras take up little more space than echo machine.
- General purpose cameras approximately 25% the cost of a CT scanner, dedicated cardiac cameras only 15%.

Positron emission tomography cameras
- Restricted availability.
- Require significant space with appropriate shielding.
- Expensive: perhaps 150% of the cost of a CT scanner.

Echo machines
- Available in almost every hospital.
- Small and highly mobile, making imaging extremely flexible.
- Inexpensive: approximately 10% of the cost of a CT scanner.

Cardiac magnetic resonance imaging scanners
- Restricted availability.
- Require significant space with appropriate shielding.
- Expensive: perhaps 150% of the cost of a CT scanner.

Staffing requirements

There is little to choose between the imaging modalities in terms of staffing levels and the level of expertise required, although the relative involvement of technical and medical staff varies widely between departments and countries. The training requirements for the safe provision of cardiac stress are identical for all of the functional techniques. Although CCT does not yet involve stress, there is still a need to administer high-dose β-blockade and sublingual GTN safely.

Cardiovascular CT
- Setting up and acquiring CCT is standardized and automated; expertise of staff manifested in the quality control of scans.
- At least two members of staff required to attend to the patient and run the scanner.
- Reporting is time-consuming and requires a high level of expertise.

Perfusion single photon emission CT

- Setting up and acquiring SPECT is standardized and straightforward; expertise of staff manifested in safe handling of radiopharmaceuticals and quality control of scans.
- Two members of staff for stress, one for image acquisition; roles separated in time with ^{99m}Tc-tracers, so overall staffing levels similar to other techniques.
- Reporting SPECT involves straightforward, qualitative assessment supported by quantitative software and skill required to recognize artefacts; images contain purely functional information, so reporting much quicker than CCT.

Perfusion positron emission tomography

- Staffing similar to SPECT, although imaging simultaneous with stress.

Stress echo

- Imaging straightforward in principle, but expertise required to obtain optimal images with reproducible positioning.
- At least two members of staff required, one to monitor stress and the other to image.
- Reporting subjective and requires experience, but quicker than CCT.

Cardiac magnetic resonance imaging

- Less standardized than other modalities, particularly with stress.
- Technical staffing requirements similar to other modalities, but need for expert medical decision-making during imaging.
- Reporting complete study is time-consuming and requires a high level of expertise.

Practical aspects of imaging techniques: patient-related issues

Patient convenience and comfort

Cardiovascular CT
- Patient in CT scanner for only ~20min.
- No stress required, but iodinated contrast causes flushing sensation.
- Short imaging time well-tolerated, breath-hold difficult for some patients.

Perfusion single photon emission CT
- Time-consuming: total time for test may be up to ~3h, although patient not required in imaging department for most of this time.
- Minor side-effects of stress.
- Prolonged acquisition time with arms above head can be uncomfortable.

Perfusion positron emission tomography
- Patient on PET camera for ~30min.
- Minor side-effects of stress.
- Short imaging time well-tolerated.

Stress echo
- Patient on echo couch for ~45min.
- Minor side-effects of stress.
- Semi-supine left-lateral position with left arm above head can be uncomfortable for prolonged period.

Cardiac magnetic resonance imaging
- Patient in MRI scanner for ~60min.
- Minor side-effects of stress
- Enclosed scanner impossibly claustrophobic for a proportion of patients, breath-hold difficult for some patients.

Patient safety

The risk of any of the imaging techniques for CAD is a composite of the short-term risk of the procedure and the long-term risk of exposure to any ionizing radiation. The ↑ lifetime risk of fatal cancer is ~5 × 10^{-5}/mSv. It should be remembered that the alternative in most cases is ICA, which carries a procedural risk of approximately 1 in 1000, and an effective dose equivalent (EDE) of ~5mSv.

Cardiovascular CT
- Risk of iodinated contrast: anaphylaxis, renal failure.
- EDE: scanner dependent. Retrospective gating 8–15mSv, prospective gating 1–5mSv.

Perfusion single photon emission CT
- Risk of stress: death 1 in 10,000, major complications <1 in 1000.
- No significant reactions to radiopharmaceuticals.
- EDE: ^{99m}Tc 6–10mSv, ^{201}Tl 14mSv.

Perfusion positron emission tomography

- Risk of stress: death 1 in 10,000, major complications <1 in 1000.
- No significant reactions to radiopharmaceuticals.
- EDE: ^{82}Rb 3–5mSv.

Stress echo

- Risk of stress: death 1 in 10,000, major complications <1 in 1000.
- Risk of anaphylaxis from echo contrast agent.
- No exposure to ionizing radiation.

Cardiac magnetic resonance imaging

- Risk of stress: death 1 in 10,000, major complications <1 in 1000.
- Risk of gadolinium chelate: anaphylaxis, nephrogenic systemic fibrosis in renal failure (incidence 3–5% with GFR <30mL/min).
- No exposure to ionizing radiation.

Index